E. Brähler (Ed.)

Body Experience

The Subjective Dimension of Psyche and Soma
Contributions to Psychosomatic Medicine

With Contributions by
H. Appelt H. Becker P. Bernhard D. Bongers C. Brähler
E. Brähler W. Dahlmann H. C. Deter P. Diederichs R. Ernst
H. Felder U. Gieler W. Hettich C. Heintze-Hook M. Jarka
P. Joraschky M. Lohs P. Möhring H. Müller-Braunschweig
A. Otten B. Strauss P. M. Wiedemann

With 13 Figures

Springer-Verlag Berlin Heidelberg New York
London Paris Tokyo

Professor Dr. rer. biol. hum. Elmar Brähler
Akademischer Oberrat
Zentrum für Psychosomatische Medizin
des Klinikums der Justus-Liebig-Universität Gießen
Abt. Medizinische Psychologie
Friedrichstraße 36, D-6300 Gießen
Federal Republic of Germany

Original title: E. Brähler (Ed.): *Körpererleben*

Front cover illustration: 'The Mad Girl' by Rik Wouters
Koninklijk Museum voor Schone Kunsten Antwerpen

ISBN-13: 978-3-642-73414-4 e-ISBN-13: 978-3-642-73412-0
DOI: 10.1007/978-3-642-73412-0

Library of Congress Cataloging-in-Publication Data
Körpererleben. English. Body experience : the subjective dimension of psyche and soma : contributions to psychosomatic medicine / E. Brähler, ed. ; with contributions by H. Appelt ... [et al.]. p. cm. Translation of: Körpererleben. Includes bibliographies and index.

1. Medicine, Psychosomatic. 2. Mind and body. 3. Mind and body therapies. I. Brähler, E. (Elmar), 1946- . II. Appelt, H. (Hertha) III. Title. RC49.K66313 1988 616.08-dc19
88-12341 CIP

Softcover reprint of the hardcover 1st edition 1988

2119/3145-543210 - Printed on acid-free paper

Preface

The past few years have seen a renaissance of the body. Having started off on its road to popularity in certain select therapy and encounter group circles, the return of the body is now a well-established phenomenon in art, literature, film and theatre, and even in the world of science a 'change of heart' is becoming apparent. The number of books and articles on the body has recently risen dramatically, the issues involved being many and varied. This renewed interest in the body, which can by now almost be said to have become a fashion, surely has its roots in social, political and scientific developments of recent years.

I would like to explain my motives in bringing out this book on body experience. They are based on my strong interest in a holistic approach to psychosomatic medicine, an approach that takes seriously the individual as subjective being, that is patient-oriented, and does away with all claims to omnipotence, including those clad in the guise of psychosocial concern. The individual's personal experience of his or her own body, which is always a subjective experience, is still not taken seriously enough. In modern iatrotechnics body experience plays only a marginal role; medicine nowadays is founded upon organic findings, it seeks to repair people like machines. In many cases this approach is indeed successful, but in many cases it also flies in the face of the individual's reality.

Psychology, too, has developed on a major scale along the lines of the causal, mechanical way of thinking characteristic of the physical sciences in past centuries. It, too, is in danger of losing sight of individuals as subjects and of reducing them to mere objects of study, to be investigated quantatively from a nomothetical viewpoint. Psychoanalysis, on the other hand, seems to have withdrawn from many areas of activity altogether, medical included, and in practice often appears to be a purely neurosis-oriented form of therapy. A psychosomatic approach to medicine that builds on psychoanalysis will not be able to avoid paying more attention in future to the issue of body experience.

As long as the question of people's body experience is ignored, every form of therapy will fail to grasp the central point in many diseases. An exaggerated emphasis on the body, however, such as has become fashionable in many of the therapeutic approaches that have developed as part of the current 'psycho-boom', can easily give rise to unrealistic expectations which soon turn to disillusionment and disappointment. Every form of therapy should be subjected to scientific testing. In our culture, magical and mystical beliefs and attitudes have long been succeeded by science, and it should not be our aim now to return to the Middle Ages. Instead, we should be attempting to integrate what we have learned since then.

The present volume contains 18 contributions, all written especially for this book. The first five chapters cover various aspects of the significance of body experience, the first being concerned with the importance of body experience for the patient (Brähler). The position of psychoanalysis with regard to the body is discussed next by Müller-Braunschweig, who traces the vicissitudes of the body through the history of psychoanalysis and pleads the cause for greater involvement of the body in the psychotherapeutic process.

Joraschky offers in his contribution an integrative review of the extensive research that has been done on the topics of body schema, body self, body perception and body experience; the meanings and usage of the various terms are clarified. Bernhard deals with the problem of pain sensation and perception, particularly stressing the subjective component. A specialized aspect - the skin as a visible organ of body experience - is discussed by Gieler.

Three chapters are about therapeutic approaches which lay particular emphasis on the body and body experience: Becker outlines the psychoanalytically oriented method of 'concentrative movement therapy'; Deter and Heintze-Hook describe a combination of 'functional relaxation' and analytical group therapy; and Dahlmann introduces his 'concentrative body-perception exercises' for helping patients with conditions causing chronic pain.

Sex-related aspects of body experience are the topic of six chapters. Diederichs underlines the significance of disturbed body experience for men with prostatopathy. Bongers reports on the results of narrative interviews on male body awareness, stressing the differences between this approach and the usual questionnaires. Taking the problem of fluor genitalis in women as an example, Lohs demonstrates how doctors and patients deal with a bodily symptom.

Jarka's contribution concerns the role of women's body experience in their desire for children and during pregnancy, birth and the postnatal period.

C. Brähler discusses fertility disorders in men and women, which she sees both as injury and challenge connected with a central disturbance in body experience.

The last chapter in this section (Möhring and Brähler) describes the body experience of people who have recovered from cancer and their partners, which is seen as an essential part of the way in which these couples cope with the illness in the context of their relationships.

Four chapters are concerned with empirical approaches to body experience and body complaints, Weideman reviews critical concepts, data and methods in the analysis of body experience, Strauss and Appelt report on their findings using a questionnaire developed by themselves on body experience. The last two chapters deal with the empirical quantification of body complaints, one reviewing the results achieved so far with the Giessen Subjective Complaints List (Brähler and Möhring), the other describing body complaints found in school children between 8 and 15 years of age (Brähler et al.).

I had hoped to be able to include one or two more contributions in the book, e.g. on sexual disorders as central disturbances in body experience, but unfortunately some papers which had been promised failed to come to fruition. This may be taken as an indication that the role of body experience in many disorders and their treatment is by now regarded by many authors as very relevant, but that not enough empirical material is available yet.

I would like to thank Professor H. E. Richter and Professor D. Beckmann for their openness and readiness to accept new fields of research. Special thanks are due to Professor H. Müller-Braunschweig and Dr. P. Möhring for the many useful discussions which helped me in planning the present volume. Mrs. H. Nöring-Wiechers and Ms. J. Schäbler assisted with technical aspects of the production.

My thanks are due, last but not least, to the contributing authors.

Giessen, May 1988 Elmar Brähler

Table of Contents

A. The Significance of Body Experience

Body Experience: A Neglected Dimension in Medicine
E. Brähler 3

Psychoanalysis and the Body
H. Müller-Braunschweig 19

Body Schema and Body Self
P. Joraschky 35

Sensation and Perception of Pain
P. Bernhard 51

Skin and Body Experience
U. Gieler 62

B. Body Experience in Therapy

Body Experience and Alienation: Psychoanalytically Oriented Concentrative Movement Therapy as an Introduction to Psychotherapy for Psychosomatic Patients
H. Becker 77

Body Therapeutic Techniques in Disease-Oriented Psychoanalytic Group Therapy with Asthma Patients
H. C. Deter and C. Heintze-Hook 91

Exercises in Concentrative Body Perception: A Psychophysiological Therapy Technique
W. Dahlmann 104

C. Sex-Specific Body Experience

Body Experience of Men with Prostatosis
P. Diederichs 119

Male Body Image
D. Bongers 131

Fluor Albus: How Doctors and Patients React to a Body Symptom
M. Lohs 140

The Role of Body Experience in Women's Desire for Children and During Pregnancy, Birth and the Time after Delivery
M. Jarka 153

Infertility: Injury and Challenge
C. Brähler 171

Body Complaints Among Recovered Genital Cancer Patients and Their Partners
P. Möhring and E. Brähler 177

D. Measuring Body Experience and Body Complaints

Psychological Research into Body Experience: Models and Methods
P. M. Wiedemann 189

Results Obtained with a Body Experience Questionnaire
B. Strauss and H. Appelt 200

The Body and Its Complaints: A Review of Findings Using the Giessen Subjective Complaints List
E. Brähler and P. Möhring 211

Body Complaints in Children from 8 to 15 Years of Age
E. Brähler, R. Ernst, W. Hettich, H. Felder and A. Otten 232

Subject Index 245

List of Contributors

Appelt, Hertha, Dr. phil.
Abteilung für Sexualforschung der Psychiatrischen und Nervenklinik der Universität Hamburg, Martinistr. 52
D-2000 Hamburg 20, Federal Republic of Germany

Becker, Hans, PD Dr. med.
Psychosomatische Klinik des Klinikums der Universität Heidelberg, Thibautstr. 2, D-6900 Heidelberg 1, Federal Republic of Germany

Bernhard, Paul, Dr. med
Psychosomatische Klinik, Dr. Schröder-Weg 12
D-7542 Schömberg, Federal Republic of Germany

Bongers, Dieter, Dr. Dipl.-Psych.
Gestalt-Psychotherapeut, Irmgardstr. 32, D-1000 Berlin (West) 37
Federal Republic of Germany

Brähler, Christa, Dr. rer. med. Dipl.-Psych.
Hautklinik des Klinikums der Justus-Liebig-Universität Giessen
Abteilung Andrologie und Venerologie, Gaffkystr. 14
D-6300 Giessen, Federal Republic of Germany

Brähler, Elmar, Prof. Dr. rer. biol. hum. Dipl.-Math.
Zentrum für Psychosomatische Medizin des Klinikums der Justus-Liebig-Universität Giessen, Abteilung Medizinische Psychologie, Friedrichstr. 36, D-6300 Giessen, Federal Republic of Germany

Dahlmann, Wolfgang, Dr. med.
Arzt für Neurologie und Psychiatrie, Psychotherapie
Leitender Arzt der Klinik am Hainberg, Psychosomatische Klinik in Bad Hersfeld, Klinik am Hainberg, Ludwig-Braun-Str. 32
D-6430 Bad Hersfeld, Federal Republic of Germany

Deter, H. C., PD Dr. med.
Psychosomatische Klinik Zentralinstitut für seelische Gesundheit
J 5, D-6800 Mannheim 1, Federal Republic of Germany

Diederichs, P., Prof. Dr. med Dipl.-Psych.
Regensburgerstr. 25, D-1000 Berlin (West) 30, Federal Republic of Germany

Ernst, Roman, Dipl.-Psych.
Zentrum für Psychosomatische Medizin des Klinikums der Justus-Liebig-Universität Giessen, Abteilung Medizinische Psychologie, Friedrichstr. 36, D-6300 Giessen, Federal Republic of Germany

Felder, Hildegard, Dipl.-Psych.
Zentrum für Psychosomatische Medizin des Klinikums der Justus-Liebig-Universität Giessen, Klinik für Psychosomatik und Psychotherapie, Friedrichstr. 33, D-6300 Giessen, Federal Republic of Germany

Gieler, Uwe, Dr. med.
Hautklinik der Philipps-Universität Marburg, Deutschhausstr. 9
D-3550 Marburg, Federal Republic of Germany

Hettich, Wolfgang, Dr. med.
Am Hofacker 7, D-5421 Frücht, Federal Republic of Germany

Heintze-Hook, Christiane, M.A.
Lehrbeauftragte für Funktionelle Entspannung (FE)
Mönchhofstr. 15 a, D-6900 Heidelberg, Federal Republic of Germany

Jarka, Marianne, Dipl.-Psych.
Zentrum für psychosomatische Medizin des Klinikums der Justus-Liebig-Universität Giessen, Klinik für Psychosomatik und Psychotherapie, Friedrichstr. 33, D-6300 Giessen, Federal Republic of Germany

Joraschky, Peter, Dr. med.
Psychiatrische Klinik mit Poliklinik der Universität Erlangen-Nürnberg, Schwabachanlage 6 und 10, D-8520 Erlangen Federal Republic of Germany

Lohs, Margit, Dipl.-Psych.
Geibelstr. 14, D-1000 Berlin (West) 45, Federal Republic of Germany

Möhring, Peter, PD Dr. med.
Zentrum für Psychosomatische Medizin des Klinikums der Justus-Liebig-Universität Giessen, Klinik für Psychosomatik und Psychotherapie, Friedrichstr. 35, D-6300 Giessen, Federal Republic of Germany

Müller-Braunschweig, Hans, Prof. Dr. phil. Dipl.-Psych.
Zentrum für Psychosomatische Medizin des Klinikums der Justus-Liebig-Universität Giessen, Klinik für Psychosomatik und Psychotherapie, Friedrichstr. 33, D-6300 Giessen, Federal Republic of Germany

Otten, Albert, PD Dr. med.
Zentrum für Kinderheilkunde des Klinikums der Justus-Liebig-Universität Giessen, Feulgenstr. 12, D-6300 Giessen Federal Republic of Germany

Strauss, Bernhard, Dr. phil., Dipl.-Psych.
Abteilung für Psychotherapie und Psychosomatik im Zentrum Nervenheilkunde der Universität Kiel, Niemannsweg 147 D-2300 Kiel 1, Federal Republic of Germany

Wiedemann, Peter M., Dr.
Technische Universität Berlin, Institut für Psychologie Dovestr. 1-5, D-1000 Berlin (West) 10, Federal Republic of Germany

A. The Significance of Body Experience

Body Experience: A Neglected Dimension in Medicine

E. Brähler

Introduction

Any consideration of the status of body experience in medicine, such as will be undertaken here, very soon finds itself caught up in the deep-rooted polarization between psyche and soma, between subjective experience and objective findings, which goes back to Descartes and his dualistic concept of man.

Since the last century medicine has regarded itself as a natural science. This has led to a very one-sided view of the human race as an object of scientific investigation, in which the subjective aspect of body experience has been relegated to a marginal role. This deficit inevitably gives rise to scientific attitudes which tend to exaggerate the importance of the body and which, where they are linked with more general reactionary leanings, all too easily end up by claiming to hold the key to man's salvation. Such oscillations between extreme views can be found in a similar form in the history of biology, where vitalistic and mechanistic concepts alternate in popularity (c.f. Wuketits 1985).

Von Uexküll (1961, 1985) regards the concept of the body as one of the major problems facing psychoanalysis and psychosomatic medicine:

> 'Medical science today possesses two paradigms which are mutually exclusive: the "machine definition", for the body, and Freuds paradigm of the psychic apparatus for the mind. The consequence is a dualistic medicine, the one being for bodies without minds and the other for minds without bodies. Modern medicine is in need of a new paradigm that can offer a solution to the hitherto insoluble psycho-physical problem,'

Von Uexküll claims that this paradigm has existed since the beginning of this century but has so far been ignored by both medicine and psychoanalysis: J. von Uexküll's *Funktionskreis* (functional circuit; von Uexküll 1920). Like von Weizsäcker's *Gestaltkreis* (gestalt circuit; von Weizsäcker 1947a), this may be seen as a precursor of the modern systems theory approaches, which are today attempting to step into the inheritance of subject philosophy (Habermas 1985c). In place of the 'subject-object' relationship we now have the 'system-environment' relationship, and the mind-body question becomes irrelevant (Habermas 1985c). Whether this paradigm is really capable of replacing the old one is impossible to tell - as impossible as it is to predict what new problems it may bring with it.

Independently of current theories, however, human body experience as everyone's own reflection of their living reality is still of major importance, quite apart from philosophical constructs such as the mind-matter problem or the system-environment approach. Paying more attention to body experience is a vital part of any patient-centred medicine (Balint 1957) and serves to introduce the concept of the subject into medical science (von Weizsäcker 1951).

Since any consideration of body experience is incomplete without first reflecting on its context, we shall begin on the following pages by taking a look at the renaissance of the body. After that, it will be shown how far the dimension of body experience is lacking in modern iatrotechnical medicine and how, to all intents and purposes, it has even been neglected by psychosomatic medicine - in spite of its theoretical claims to the contrary. Finally, the necessity of a far greater involvement of body experience in a patient-centred medicine will be demonstrated.

The Renaissance of the Body

In recent years we have experienced a renaissance of the body in the media. After the body's achievement of considerable status in the therapeutic and encounter group movements of the 1970s - consider the teachings of the Bagwhan or Gestalt therapy, for example, and also bio-energetics, which has built particularly upon the ideas of Wilhelm Reich - we now observe a return of the body in art, literature, film and theatre. The 'rediscovery of the body' has reached the world of science as well and an avalanche of books on the subject has appeared on the market.

The various facets of this phenomenon are reflected in the numerous characteristics attributed to the body in the titles of these publications. In German, we find works on the dismembered body (Kamper 1982), the spoken body (Wimmer 1982), the other body (Kamper and Wulf 1984; Pfleiderer 1984), the infamous body (Dressen 1984), the ceremonial and cloned body (Baudrillard 1982), the staged body (Peitmann 1984), the organic and psychoanalytical body (Dieckmann 1984), the female body (Shorter 1984), the transfigurative body (Tibon-Cornillot 1982), the incapable and absent body (Virilio 1982), one's own body (Paulus 1982; Paulus and Otte 1979), the human body (Bernhard 1978, Bleker 1983; Winau 1983; Roloff 1983), the fearless body (Duhm 1980), the endangered body (Bleker 1983) and the communicative body (Ochmann 1981).

The body is considered in connection with death (Wulf 1982), work and social class (Waldhubel 1983), identity (Poppe 1982), movement and mind, and names and senses (Lipowatz 1984); with being possessed (Schott-Billmann 1979), with resistance (Mindell 1981), emotion (Nitzschke 1983) and speaking (Anzieu et al. 1982); with the murder of reality (Chasseguet-Smirgel 1981), birth and rebirth (Le Camus 1983), dreams (Matisson 1982) and with immobility and gestures (Werner 1984).

The body is seen as partner (Eicke 1973), tool (Gensch 1983), statue (Küchenhoff 1983), medium (Lermer 1981) and 'signifier' (Warsitz 1983). We are offered descriptions of the expansion (Tibon-Cornillot 1982), the techniques (Mauss 1975), the proportions (Hufschmidt 1977) and the dynamics of the body (Reindell 1981); of its disappearance (Halfmann and Zillich 1982), its reappearance (Kamper and Wulf 1982), its resurrection (Hart-Nibbrig 1985), its history (Kamper and Rittner 1976), its libidinal re-cathexis (Dieckmann 1981), its trail (Anzieu 1982), its significance (Giegerich 1983), its sexualization (Haug 1983), its messages (Kurtz and Prestera 1976), its symbolic function (Gebauer 1982), its socialization (Orban 1981), its proper use (Barlow 1973), its diagnosis (Rumpf and Schomann 1983), its signals (Seittner 1982), its social perception (Rittner 1982) and its languages (Heinrichs 1985).

These works reflect, on the one hand, how the body is seen as an object, to be studied or ignored. On the other hand, it is given the status of an autonomous living being which has certain characteristics and attributes and is capable of acting, interacting, experiencing and suffering, quite independently of that which is not body. This is reminiscent of the cynic method of Sloterdijk (1983) which is described by Habermas (1985a) as working

> through its strategy of denying argumentation, its subversive intent and the manner in which it submerges contradictions in the expressiveness of the body, through a principle of embodiment that aims at securing the existential unity of theory and life, through the materialist way in which it musters the lower organs against the higher, in the subjectivist revolt of the private against the public and the nominalism of its situationally determined manner of thinking, which in its very approach is a protest against generalizing thought.

In the field of medicine and psychotherapy numerous subjective aspects of human beings are investigated via the body, such as body image (Freyberger 1983; Grunert 1977; Kiener 1973, 1974; Pankow 1982; Rechenberger 1983; Siblik 1973), body schema (Baumann 1976; Bay 1983; Conrad 1933; Joraschky 1983; Meermann and Fichter 1983; Schilder 1923; Schulte-Herbrüggen 1983), body self (Joraschky 1983), body self-image (Bongers 1984; Martin 1982), body concept (Mrazek 1984), body ego (Battenberg 1978; Hoffer 1978), body perception (Meermann 1983), body position (Fischler et al. 1977), bodily symptoms (Schmidt-Atzert 1984), body complaints (Brähler and Scheer 1983), body experience (Strauss and Appelt 1983), body disorders (Meyer 1963), body picture and body co-ordination (Schneider 1979). These studies will be reviewed more closely in the chapters by Joraschky and Wiedemann in this volume.

Body structure and its relationship to personality has long been an object of research (Buse and Pawlik 1984; Kretschmer 1977).

The communicative aspect of the body is emphasized in studies on body contact (Montagu 1971; Winau 1982), body posture (Lermer 1977), body shape (Jürgens 1978), body expression (Lowen 1973), body language (Argyle 1975; Gniech 1984; Hauschild 1983; Heinrichs 1985; Kummer 1984) and body orientations (Seittner 1984).

In the field of psychotherapy, publications have appeared on body work (Besuden 1983; Fuchs 1949; Lowen 1975; Painter 1984; Seidel 1981), body co-ordination (Brambring and Dawidowski 1980), body control (Dreitzel 1981), and body therapy (Petzold 1977). These will be discussed by Becker, Dahlmann, and Deter and Heintze-Hook in their contributions below.

In reviewing the German literature one is struck by the way in which the word *Körper* (for body) has overtaken the old term *Leib*, which appears less and less frequently. It is very difficult to reach differential definitions for these terms, even though every German can name individual associative differences, because the range of connotations for each has changed so much in the course of history. Whereas *Leib* was once understood as referring to the animated body, nowadays both terms are generally used synonymously. Not so very long ago, physical education and sports in West German schools were still called '*Leibes*übungen' and '*Leibes*erziehung', whilst the East Germans consistently referred to '*Körper*erziehung' and '*Körper*kultur' (Brockhaus 1973).

Whilst a few decades ago *Körper* still carried rather the implication of something material or dead - similar to our use of the word 'body' in medicine and physics (e.g. 'solid body', 'antibody' or 'corpuscle'), or even in mathematics - nowadays its meaning has shifted towards the concept of a body as the bearer or epitome of life and living matter. Meanswhile the term *Leib* has come to be seen as something old-fashioned or reactionary, best left to theologians or philosophers, who still go on arguing about the *'Leib/Seele'* (literally: 'body/soul or mind', or 'psyche/soma') problem.

The modern use of the word *'Körper'* may also be seen in terms of an effort to overcome the *'Leib/Seele'* dualism and, via language, to move towards a unified view of mankind.

Habermas (1985b) sees the pragmatic attempts of linguistics and anthropology at countering the Cartesian dualism of psyche and soma by elevating third categories such as action, language or *Leib* to the rank of philosophical concepts, as a preliminary to overcoming the paradigms of a philosophy of awareness. However, the category *Leib* has by now been replaced quite clearly by the term *Körper.*

The renewed interest in the body which is to be found in many branches of science today surely has its roots in social, scientific and political developments over the past few years. As Heinrichs (1985) observes, 'Many people nowadays, believing it is high time they tried to save their own souls at least, all else apparently being lost, are turning more and more resolutely to their bodies - massaging, feeding or dieting them with special care. In their bodies they seek salvation, life, nature, refuge'.

The omnipresent threat to our fundamental biological base, whether through the progressive destruction of our environment or the atomic threat, the split between the highly technical and functional aspects of our modern world and the menacing, archaic elements dormant in manking - all this frequently leads to an individual's withdrawal into private life, first back to nature in the garden and then, by logical progression, into the privacy of one's own body. Many people feel that if the ideal of wholeness cannot be realized in the world at large, they can at least endeavour to fulfil it in their personal lives.

Besides its many achievements in overcoming magic, mysticism and superstition, which had kept people in a state of immaturity for centuries, modern thought has also had inhuman and self-destructive consequences. The European concept of progress was rendered possible by the typically Western separation of body and mind (Kamper and Wulf 1982), but at the price of a culture permanently removed from - or even living in hostile antagonism to - the body. Religious, military, educational and economic forces have between them brought about a 'large-scale abuse of the body' (c.f. Becker, this volume).

Many people hope to find solutions to these problems - to find themselves - in body-oriented therapies and other forms of body experience. They dream of the good, untamed, archaic body deep down inside themselves, which has become buried and only has to be released to achieve a meaningful, harmonious and happy existence. Parallel to this we can observe a revival of interest in other cultures which is based on the assumption that the populations of other societies lead innocent, happy and uncomplicated lives. There is a tendency to glorify and romanticize nature, which is raised up as the new banner of hope (Bergfleth 1984). The fathers of enlightenment are assumed to have failed; refuge is sought in a mysticized version of Mother Nature. Beckmann (1984) describes how among the Indians of North America mystical movements only arose in periods of crisis, whereas their usual relationship to nature was based on a sound knowledge of natural processes.

Habermas (1985 c) talks about a tendency in many people nowadays to believe that they can enter 'the anarchistic free space of post-modernism', whereby the implied criticism of subject philosophy is linked with a total rejection of Reason. The modern dismissal of Descartes includes rejection of 'his virtues: all methodical thinking, all scientific responsibility ... The crusade against a scientific instrumental Reason that has become inflated to a totality, itself begins to take on a totalitarian character.'

It remains to be seen whether the present interest in the body will turn out to be a passing phenomenon, a serious reversal in scientific thinking or even the first sign of a rejection of science itself.

Iatrotechnical Medicine and the Body

In most countries, medical students generally make their first acquaintance with the human body as a corpse, once they have learnt the scientific basics at the beginning of their course. During the early part of their studies they usually have no contact with patients at all. Instead, they have to study for examinations, mainly consisting of multiple-choice items, in which the question of the validity of this kind of testing is forced almost completely into the background by claims to objectivity. The students are taught to think and work in the manner of iatrotechnical medicine, even if they are offered a few cosmetic improvements such as medical sociology, medical psychology or psychosomatics on the way. Rothschuh (1978) sees the following principles as basic to the concept of iatrotechnical medicine:

1. The organism is not controlled by particular vital forces; there is no life force.
2. Vital processes are basically physical and chemical processes, although specially organized in relatively complex structures.
3. Relations between these functional units are strictly determined by laws of nature; in principle living organisms are organized no differently from inanimate nature. Natural laws are causal laws. The aim is to find the causes or conditions underlying all physiological and pathological processes and explain them in minute detail.
4. To this end the organism must be divided up into its component parts and elements. The investigation must proceed along causal, analytical lines.
5. The means employed to find out how the parts function is the experiment, as in

physics and chemistry. But here the experiment must be carried out on a living organism or on isolated, living parts. Thus, experimental medicine using live animals is the standard method upon which iatrotechnical medicine is based.
6. This way of abstracting from the whole organism results in a very reduced view of mankind, but guarantees reliability in the choice of methods when diagnosing and treating disorders.
7. The analysis of the laws governing relationships in the healthy and diseased body may not be considered complete until every detail needed for repairing these causal relationships has been elucidated. The body is viewed as a technically functioning object, to be dissected and manipulated as required.

Iatrotechnical medicine set out in the last century to lead mankind towards a happier future. The medical world was convinced that the human race could create its own salvation here on earth (Schipperges 1968). Richter (1979) refers in this context to a 'God complex'. After the many successes achieved by iatrotechnical medicine, the belief arose that disease and even death could be conquered if only one researched intensively enough. This has long since been proved a utopian idea (Schipperges 1968). Nevertheless, the optimism of medical science remains unbroken, even though its consistent objective of conquering all disease and gaining control over other vital processes, such as ageing, seems to be slipping further and further out of reach. The enthusiasm of iatrotechnical medicine for the technically possible has resulted in two lines of medical development receiving special attention and being followed with particular zeal at the moment: one is gene technology and reproduction techniques, and the other is the extension of human life through organ transplants or machine replacements. The special danger inherent in gene technology is that it may unknowingly find itself carrying on a most unfortunate line of tradition.

As early as 1903, the German scientist Schallmayer published the results of his much-acclaimed study on racial degeneration and genetics, entitled *Vererbung und Auslese in ihrer soziologischen und politischen Bedeutung* ('Heredity and Selection: Their Sociological and Political Significance', quoted by Schipperges, 1968). This work promulgated the organic perfection of mankind and especially the physical and mental purification of the Germanic race. Schipperges (1968) remarks, 'These are the consequences, the realization of which we have partly experienced. There is no reason why the attempt should not be repeated, with a more precise understanding of nature and more extensive powers - even at the price of still greater sacrifice. The idea of higher revelations resulting from the united forces of true science is too fascinating to fail to move the hearts of men, to fire their minds and to force their hands to take action now and make the dream come true.'

Modern gene technology promises to eradicate all hereditary disease. Hobom (1985) writes, 'The logical consequence of prenatal diagnostics, where genetic defects are found, is abortion ... One consequence of prenatal diagnostics in any form is, however, a gradual change in the attitude of society to the birth of a handicapped child - towards both the child and its parents.' What this can mean was clearly expressed by Glass in 1971, in his inaugural speech as President of the American Society for the Advancement of Science (quoted by Kayser 1985): 'No parents in the future will have the right to burden society with deformed or idiot children'.

Nordhoff and Hohlfeld (1985) describe our present situation in the following way: 'Either we stick to the maxim of progress ... in which case we must alter our concept of man and our moral standards, or we keep hold of the latter - then the traditional idea of progress will have to go.'

This judgement applies equally well to modern developments towards the technical perfection of the human organism, which is most strikingly represented by the project Cyborg (cybernetic organ) by Kline and Clynes (1961).

The first artificial hearts have been implanted, and the following experimental objectives are on the way to becoming reality (Tibon-Cornillot 1984):

- Sharper human eyes through optical cells
- Liver stimulators and adrenal stimulators
- Several areas of the head can be replaced by artificial elements (a magnetically fixed artificial eye can be better co-ordinated with the healthy eye; jawbones made of Lecithin; nylon dentures with plastic teeth); arteries made of polyethylene to maintain a constant temperature; aortas of nylon; totally artificial (plastic) limbs; a pelvis artificially supported or replaced
- An exoskeleton is envisaged and already partially realized, a modern 'suit of armour' which would increase the strength and resistance of the human body through a framework whose parts are directly connected and perfectly co-ordinated with human movements by means of electromotors.

Underlying all such developments is still the unreflected assumption that the history of science, albeit with occasional detours and temporary setbacks, is still a one-way street to progress, as von Uexküll (1985) put it in his criticism of his generation's socialization. Other traditions have certainly survived in medicine as well, but these are in danger of being forced almost totally into the background by the current trend. The successes of medicine in healing have been consistently overestimated (Göckenjan 1985). The increase in chronic diseases in particular confronts modern medicine with enormous tasks for the future, which should not be neglected in favour or a few spectacular successes in individual fields. Preventive medicine and after-care are under-represented. That is not to say that the doctors have failed to offer a great deal of advice. We are at present caught up in a constant stream of new health trends, which promote sport, jogging, keep-fit, aerobics and more. All of these, however, never had the intention of helping people towards a more positive kind of body experience; their real objective is the achievement of greater control over the body, by keeping it fit through activity. Instructions on how to do this are given in such a way that one cannot help feeling that what is being talked about is how best to extend the lives of machines. Diet regimes are being produced on an inflationary scale, partly contradicting each other, depending on which single aspect of the mechanically-viewed human metabolism is being over-emphasized. Every field of medicine has its own precise views on what it considers to be healthy behaviour, offering a mass of recommendations on prevention that are partly contradictory and often impossible to follow. This all results from the mechanistic approach which fails to take into account the full complexity of the living body.

It would not be proper to attack medicine on the ground that its basic approach is that of a natural science, but a science must also recognize facts which do not fit in with past or present theories and must constantly be in search of better models. The problem of not perceiving unwelcome facts has been admirably demonstrated by Devereux (1967, 1972) in other branches of science. Body experience is the indicator reflecting one's state of physical wellbeing; discomfort and bodily complaints are feelings which make us aware that there is something wrong. When a certain level of discomfort has been reached, one feels ill. The doctor in iatrotechnical medicine, however, makes his diagnosis according to functional disorders and organic findings - he is symptom-oriented. The patient's body experience is of interest only insofar as it offers information about symptoms.

If medicine really exists to benefit mankind and not just for the scientific gratification of the medical experts, then it must pay due attention to its patients' experience of their bodies, taking it just as seriously as the organic findings - otherwise it will go on passing by the patients' reality, which is made up of subjective experiences. Von Uexküll and Wesiack (1981) stress that this is a language problem and that statements can be understood and interpreted on various levels of meaning (Wesiack 1984).

Since it is the lives and feelings of patients that lie at the centre of the practice of medicine, it is not too much to demand that a doctor should try to understand these aspects as well and see them as the true reality with which he or she is dealing. It is wrong to take the opposite approach and expect the patients to fit their experience to the organic findings. No amount of goodwill on the part of patient or doctor will make such attempts at reconstituting the patient's reality work.

Psychosomatics and the Body

Psychosomatic medicine is in many ways the exact opposite of iatrotechnical medicine. It is not tied to the mechanistic way of thinking of traditional medicine but stresses the importance of psychological causes in the development of physical disease; thus it provides quite a different approach to illness, which it sees in terms of disturbances in the relationship between body and mind (von Weizsäcker 1951). Psychoanalytical psychosomatics in particular follows Freud in countering the machine paradigm for the body with the idea of a 'psychic apparatus' for the mind (von Uexküll 1985).

Although this way of contrasting iatrotechnical medicine (body-without-mind) with psychoanalytical psychsomatics (mind-without-body) may be rather an exaggeration (von Uexküll 1985), there is still an undeniable tendency in psychoanalytical theory and practice to neglect the role of the body. But this applies equally much to psychosomatics in general, whose historical development was dominated for a long time by arguments between the psychic and the somatic camps about its name (Bräutigam and Christian 1983). This polarization continues today, making it very difficult to arrive at a generally acceptable theoretical model in psychosomatics.

In practice, advocates of the psychosomatic approach often talk about the psychological origins of physical illnesses. Psychosomatics is understood as a one-way street from mental conflict to physical suffering (cf. Overbeck and Overbeck 1978), even though von Weizsäcker stated as early as 1949 that 'the mind expresses itself in the language of the body and the body in that of the mind; there is no causality, and if one talks about psychogenesis, then one should only mean a historical development, in which bodily changes occurred in place of mental processes and vice versa' (quoted in von Weizsäcker and Wyss 1957).

Much effort has been put into attempting to trace the route taken by mental conflicts during their conversion into physical suffering - which has repeatedly been perceived and understood by the patients themselves as a meaningful process - in order to describe it scientifically in an objective, mechanistic way. This one-sided, psychogenetic approach had its historical function in the past but is now out of date (Bräutigam and Christian 1983).

The search for an explanatory model in psychosomatics has produced many theoretical concepts: dualism, parallelism, complementarism, epiphenomenalism, the doctrine of identity, interactionism (cf. Fahrenberg 1981, 1983; Wuketits 1985), none of which has really managed to assert itself. Neither have the high hopes of the psychophysiologists that they would be able to find objective, organically or psychophysiologically measurable correlates to body experience and subjective feelings been fulfilled so far (Fahrenberg 1983). Even the orgasm, which was long assumed to be a fairly homogeneous experience, has turned out to be a psychophysiological process accompanied by many different qualities of feeling.

Now that the euphoria about bio-feedback and its claims to achieving conscious control over the body has ebbed, recent hopes have been pinned on the idea of psycho-immunological links, which are meant to elucidate the way in which body and mind act in harmony.

Much as it is to be welcomed that psychosomatics no longer views itself as a branch of medicine specializing in certain specified 'psychosomatic diseases', but rather as a general manner of approach, here, too, we find inexcusable simplifications. For every disease certain personality profiles, family constellations or psychosocial variables, expressed in mathematical models, are pinpointed as the supposed causes of the illness. The psychosomatics specialists are no more proof against fantasies of omnipotence than those in iatrotechnical medicine - as, for example, when they try to prove that cancer is purely psychogenic and so argue that it can be cured more effectively by psychotherapy than by iatrotechnical medicine. Neither iatrotechnical medicine nor psychosomatics, nor any form of alternative medicine will ever be able to protect people from suffering, pain, illness and death, which are just as inseparably a part of life as birth, pleasure, joy and health, all of which are also experienced with the body.

Medicine must commit itself to the concept of a 'life-circuit', to trying to arrive at a humane position which lies between the extremes of omnipotence and impotence (Richter 1979). From the psychosomatic quarter there is evidence of a move in this direction, as, for example, where illness is understood in the context of social adjustment (Overbeck 1984) or as self-cure (Beck 1981); or where the social background to health and disease is taken into account (Totman 1979) and multiple perspectives or multi-factor approaches to health and illness are put forward (Wesiack 1983; Weiner 1983).

There is a danger at present that with a new systems theory paradigm the human individual as subject will be neglected in favour of the systems approach. In this connection, body experience takes on a special significance in that, quite apart from any theoretical models, it is the elementary expression of human life and as such may not be taken merely as an indication of organic or psychic malfunctioning.

The Role of Body Experience in a Patient-Oriented Medicine

Health, ill-health and disease can be approached on two different planes: the objective plane of organic, medically observable symptoms and the subjective plane of complaints and feelings of discomfort as reflected in body experience (cf. Brähler and Scheer 1983, 1984). Underlying these are two different systems of reference and two different languages, which begin to become irreconcilable particularly when a patient either feels ill without an organic finding or feels well in spite of a pathological one. This can have far-reaching consequences for the patient, since the asymmetry in the power relations between doctor and patient means that the doctor's view usually wins. At the same time, the doctor is often in danger of losing sight of his or her ideal of helping the patient in the best possible way. In more patient-oriented medicine, stronger emphasis on the patients body experience is indispensable.

Somatopsychic influences have so far received too little attention in both organic and psychosomatic medicine - from the former because it is only interested in organic processes, and from the latter because it is an unattractive area to work in. Meanwhile, many patients suffer from complaints and disturbances in their body experience which do not seem to stand in any causal relation to the illness in question. These patients in particular are in danger of being no longer perceived as whole people but being defined purely through their illness. The result is that their subjective feelings, inasmuch as they are not related to the disease, slip right out of the focus of the doctor's interest. In many chronic diseases, for example, the subjective state does not correspond with the organic condition. Here, help for the patient in the form of tertiary prevention is required, i.e. trying to avoid unnecessary further suffering resulting from an existing illness. Instead, 'rehabilitation', although seldom achieved, is a popular concept nowadays.

Both in administering actual medical treatment, such as operations or courses of drug therapy, and in carrying out subsequent examinations in after-care, the doctors attention is always focused on symptoms and organic findings and not on the patient's subjective state or body experience. After operations on the stomach or heart, for instance, it is not infrequent that in spite of organic improvement the patient's subjective complaints remain unchanged or even exceed the pre-operative level (Möhlen and Brähler 1984; Brähler and Möhring, this volume).

It is in the interest of a patient-oriented medicine to pay more attention to subjective states, which inevitably leads one away from a purely individual-oriented point of view towards an approach which includes the social and family environment, in which the patient's subjective feelings are always embedded. Bodily complaints are very closely related to partner-relationships, for example (cf. Brähler and Möhring, this volume).

In some areas of medicine there is evidence of improvement, giving grounds for hope that the polarization between the physical and mental compartments of human beings within medical thinking may sometime be dissolved. In obstetrics, for example, a change is taking place whereby the one-sided approach that can boast such achievements as the totally programmed delivery is being corrected in favour of a far greater consideration for the subjective feelings of the pregnant mother. In children's departments, too, efforts are under way to improve the special situation of children in hospital by involving parents in their treatment.

There are many diseases with physical manifestations which have no apparent organic basis. Here, traditional medicine is often itself at a loss and is ready to acknowledge 'psychogenic' disorders in such cases. This diagnosis is usually reached by a process of elimination and has led to a distinction being drawn between organic and psychogenic forms of a whole series of illnesses, e.g. impotence, sterility, prostatitis; retention of urine, bed-wetting and bed-soiling by children; anorexia, bulimia, paralysis, heart disease, fluor and many forms of skin disease. This distinction is very dubious, partly because it is very probable that refined methods of investigation in the future may well discover an organic basis for the cases hitherto diagnosed as psychogenic, and partly because even those cases diagnosed as organic often have a psychogenic element in them too. For the patients, it is initially unimportant whether their complaints are diagnosed as organic or psychogenic, as such categories are not applicable to what they themselves feel.

The doctor's diagnosis can, however, have enormous consequences for an individual's future 'career' as a patient. In particular, the distinction between psychogenic and organic makes the limitations of the mechanistic and psychoanalytical approaches clear, there being no evidence of such a dichotomy in the patient's subjective experience (cf. the chapters by Diederichs and Lohs in this book). It is time that psychosomatics, especially psychoanalytical psychosomatics, overcame its abstinence and anxiety about contact with the body, otherwise it will find itself becoming increasingly irrelevant to many diseases. Although the potential dangers inherent in many body-oriented forms of psychotherapy cannot be dismissed (cf. Kind 1985), there are numerous cases where it is impossible to get through to patients without involving their own experience of their bodies, especially when disturbances in this very body experience are the main symptom (cf. Müller-Braunschweig, Deter and Heintze-Hook, Becker, Dahlmann in this volume). Further aspects of body experience will not be discussed here as they will be considered in detail in the other chapters in this book.

References

Anzieu D (1982) Die Spuren des Körpers im Geschriebenen. Eine psychoanalytische Untersuchung des Erzählstils. In: Anzieu D, Gibello B, Gori R, Bion WR (eds) Psychoanalyse und Sprache. Vom Körper zum Sprechen. Innovative Psychotherapie und Humanwissenschaften, vol 19. Jungfermann, Paderborn

Anzieu D, Gibello B, Gori R, Bion WR (1982) Psychoanalyse und Sprache. Vom Körper zum Sprechen. Innovative Psychotherapie und Humanwissenschaften, vol 19. Jungfermann, Paderborn

Argyle M (1975) Bodily communication. Methuen, Ltd London

Balint M (1957) Der Arzt, sein Patient und die Krankheit. Klett, Stuttgart

Barlow W (1973) The Alexander technique. Knopf, New York
Battenberg F (1978) Das Körper-Ich und seine nachholende Entwicklung im Rahmen der Milieutherapie. Dynam. Psychiatr 11: 510-527
Baudrillard J (1982) Vom zeremoniellen zum geklonten Körper. Der Einbruch des Obszönen. In: Kamper D, Wulf C (eds) Die Wiederkehr des Körpers, vol 132. Suhrkamp, Frankfurt, p 350
Baumann S (1976) Der Einfluß des Körperschemas auf die Qualität der sportmotorischen Gewandtheit. Thesis, Department of Philosophy, University of Salzburg
Bay E (1983) Organisch-neurologische Aspekte zum Körperschema. Mater Psychoanal Anal Orient Psychother 9: 14-18
Beck D (1981) Krankheit als Selbstheilung. Insel, Frankfurt
Beckmann D (1984) Grundlagen der Medizinischen Psychologie. Vandenhoeck & Ruprecht, Göttingen
Bergfleth G (ed) (1984) Zur Kritik der palavernden Aufklärung. Matthes & Seitz, Munich
Bernhard M (1978) Der menschliche Körper und seine gesellschaftliche Bedeutung. Limpert, Bad Homburg
Besuden F (1983) Körperarbeit in einer psychosomatischen Klinik. Mater Psychoanal Anal Orient Psychother 9: 18-21
Bleker J (1983) Der gefährdete Körper und die Gesellschaft - Ansätze zu einer sozialen Medizin zur Zeit der bürgerlichen Revolution in Deutschland. In: Imhof AE (ed) Der Mensch und sein Körper. Beck, Munich
Bongers D (1984) Körperselbstbildnis. Eine explorative Studie mit offenen Interviews. Research report no 4. Institute of Psychology, Technical University, Berlin
Brähler E, Scheer JW (1983) Der Giessener Beschwerdebogen (GBB) - Handbuch. Huber, Bern
Brähler E, Scheer JW (1984) Subjektive Beschwerden und objektiver Befund. In: Scheer JW, Brähler E (eds) Ärztliche Maßnahmen aus psychologischer Sicht - Beiträge zur medizinischen Psychologie. Springer, Berlin Heidelberg New York
Bräutigam W, Christian P (1983) Psychosomatische Medizin. 3rd edn. Thieme, Stuttgart
Brambring M, Dawidowski B (1980) Training der Körperkoordination bei blinden Kindern. Heilpädag Forsch 8: 278-289
Brockhaus FA (1973) Der Sportbrockhaus. Brockhaus, Wiesbaden
Buse L, Pawlik K (1984) Kretschmers Konstitutionstypologie als implizite Persönlichkeitstheorie: Selbst-Attributions-Effekte in Abhängigkeit vom Körperbau-Persönlichkeits-Stereotyp. Z Different Diagn Psychol 5: 111-129
Chasseguet-Smirgel J (1981) De Sade: Der Körper und der Mord an der Realität. Psyche (Stuttg) 35: 237-252
Conrad K (1933) Das Körperschema. Eine kritische Studie und der Versuch einer Revision. Z Ges Neurol Psychiatr 147: 346-369
Devereux G (1967) From anxiety to method in the behavioral sciences. Mouton, The Hague
Devereux G (1972) Ethnopsychanalyse complémentariste. Flammarion, Paris
Dieckmann B (1984) Der psychoanalytische und der organische Körper. In: Kamper D, Wulf C (eds) Der andere Körper. Mensch und Leben, Berlin
Dieckmann H (1981) Die libidinöse Wiederbesetzung des Körpers in der Psychosomatik. Anal Psychol 12: 269-285
Dreitzel HP (1981) Körperkontrolle und Affektverdrängung. Zum gesellschaftlichen Hintergrund körper- und gefühlsbetonter Therapieformen. Integr Ther 7: 179-196
Dressen W (1984) Infame Körper. Widerstand im Erziehungsprozeß. In: Kamper D, Wulf C (eds) Der andere Körper. Mensch und Leben, Berlin
Duhm D (1980) „Schön ist die erotische Bewegung eines angstlosen Körpers". Psychol Heute 7: 60-63
Eicke D (1973) Der Körper als Partner. Kindler, Munich
Fahrenberg J (1981) Zum Verständnis des Komplementaritätsprinzips. Z Klin Psychol Psychother 29: 205-208
Fahrenberg J (1983) Psychophysiologische Methodik. In: Groffmann KJ, Michel L (eds) Verhaltensdiagnostik, Psychologische Diagnostik, Enzyklopädie der Psychologie. Hogrefe, Göttingen
Fischler M, Kongehl G, Kornhuber HH (1977) Informationstheoretische Untersuchungen zur menschlichen Wahrnehmung der Körperlage im Raum bei seitlicher Kippung. Arch Psychiatr Nervenkr 224: 141-149

Freyberger H (1983) Klinisch-psychosomatischer Beitrag zum Thema „Körperbild“. Mater Psychoanal Anal Orient Psychother 9: 21-26
Fuchs M (1949) Über Atemtherapie und entspannte Körperarbeit. Psyche (Stuttg) 3: 538-548
Gebauer G (1982) Ausdruck und Einbildung. Zur symbolischen Funktion des Körpers. In: Kamper D, Wulf C (eds) Die Wiederkehr des Körpers. Suhrkamp, Frankfurt
Gensch R (1983) Der Körper als Werkzeug - der Körper als Werkstück: Die Professionalisierung der Beziehung von Körper und Arbeit. In: Imhof AE (ed) Der Mensch und sein Körper von der Antike bis heute. Beck, Munich
Giegerich W (1983) Die Bedeutung des Körpers in Psychologie und Psychotherapie. Anal Psychol 14: 264-284
Gniech G (1984) Die Körpersprache des Menschen als Hilfsmittel für das Erkennen und die Beurteilung. Bremer Beiträge zur Psychologie, Series A: Psychological Research Report no 25. Psychology course, Bremen University
Göckenjan G (1985) Kurieren und Staat machen. Gesundheit und Medizin in der bürgerlichen Welt. Suhrkamp, Frankfurt
Grunert J (ed) (1977) Körperbild und Selbstverständnis. Psychoanalytische Beiträge zur Leib-Seele-Einheit. Kindler, Munich
Habermas J (1985a) Zwischen Heine und Heidegger. Ein Renegat der Subjektphilosophie. In: Habermas J (ed) Die neue Unübersichtlichkeit. Suhrkamp, Frankfurt
Habermas J (1985b) Untiefen der Rationalitätskritik. In: Habermas J (ed) Die neue Unübersichtlichkeit. Suhrkamp, Frankfurt
Habermas J (1985c) Der philosophische Diskurs der Moderne. Suhrkamp, Frankfurt
Halfmann J, Zillich C (1982) Das Verschwinden des Körpers (Bildessey). In: Kamper D, Wulf C (ed) Die Wiederkehr des Körpers. Suhrkamp, Frankfurt
Hart-Nibbrig CL (1985) Die Auferstehung des Körpers im Text. Suhrkamp, Frankfurt
Haug F (ed) (1983) Sexualisierung der Körper. Special issue 90. Frauenforum 2. Argument, Berlin
Hauschild T (1983) Körpersprache, Magie und medizinische Heilerwartung. In: Imhof AE (ed) Der Mensch und sein Körper von der Antike bis heute. Beck, Munich
Heinrichs HJ (1985) Der Körper und seine Sprachen. Qumran, Frankfurt
Hobom G (1985) Gentechnologie - Herausforderung und Verantwortung. JLU-Forum. Z Justus-Liebig-Univ (Giessen) 15: 5-9
Hoffer W (1978) Die Entwicklung des Körper-Ichs. In: Overbeck G, Overbeck A (eds) Seelischer Konflikt, körperliches Leiden. Rowohlt, Reinbek
Hufschmidt HJ (1977) Körperproportionen in Plastik und Malerei. Ein anthropometrischer und kulturhistorischer Versuch. Arch Psychiatr Nervenkr 224: 187-202
Imhof AE (ed) (1983) Der Mensch und sein Körper von der Antike bis heute. Beck, Munich
Joraschky P (1983) Das Körperschema und das Körper-Selbst als Regulationsprinzipien der organischen Umwelt-Interaktion. Minerva, Munich
Jürgens HW (1978) Der Mensch und seine Umwelt. Die menschliche Körperform im sozialen Umfeld. Ärztl Kosmetol 8: 61-75
Kamper D (1982) Das Phantasma vom ganzen und zerstückelten Körper. In: Kamper D, Wulf C (eds) Die Wiederkehr des Körpers. Suhrkamp, Frankfurt
Kamper D, Rittner V (eds) (1976) Zur Geschichte des Körpers. Hanser, Munich
Kamper D, Wulf C (eds) (1982) Die Wiederkehr des Körpers. Suhrkamp, Frankfurt
Kamper D, Wulf C (eds) (1984) Der andere Körper. Edition Corpus. vol 1. Mensch und Leben, Berlin
Kayser G (1985) Industrialisierung der Menschenproduktion - Zum faschistischen Charakter der Entwicklung neuer Technologien der Geburtenkontrolle. Beitr Femin Theor Praxis 1 (14): 55-67
Kiener F (1973) Untersuchungen zum Körperbild, Teil 1. Z Klin Psychol Psychother 21: 335-351
Kiener F (1974) Untersuchungen zum Körperbild, Teil 2. Z Klin Psychol Psychother 22: 45-66
Kind H (1985) Kritisches zu körperbezogenen Therapieformen. Psychother Psychosom Med Psychol 35: 167-170
Kline M, Clynes M (1961) Drugs, space and cybernetics: Evolution to Cyborg. Columbia University Press
Kretschmer E (1977) Körperbau und Charakter. Untersuchungen zum Konstitutionsproblem und zur Lehre von Temperamenten. Springer, Berlin Heidelberg New York

Küchenhoff J (1983) Body Building: Der Körper als Statue. Fragmente 9: 6-32
Kummer I (1984) Körpersprache als Ausdruck des Lebensstils. Z Individualpsychol 9: 142-152
Kurtz R, Prestera H (1976) Botschaften des Körpers. Kösel, Munich
Le Camus J (1983) Praxis der Psychomotorik in Frankreich: Geburt, Wiedergeburt und differenzierte Auseinandersetzung mit dem Körper. Motorik 6: 1-10
Lermer SP (1977) Entwicklung und Überprüfung einer Methode zur Beobachtung von Körperhaltungen in der analytischen Gruppenpsychotherapie. Faculty of theoretical medicine, Ulm university
Lermer SP (1981) Die Visualisierung von Einstellungen und Emotionen durch das Medium „Körper". Eine ausgewählte Literaturübersicht zur Bedeutung der Körperhaltung (posture) in der Psychotherapie. Gruppenpsychother Gruppendyn 17: 219-233
Lipowatz T (1984) Der Körper, der Name und die Sinne. In: Kamper D, Wulf C (eds) Der andere Körper. Mensch und Leben, Berlin
Lowen A (1976) Bioenergetics. Penguin, New York
Lowen A (1973) Depression and the body: The biological basis of faith and reality. Penguin, New York
Martin M (1982) Körperselbstbild und Neurotizismus bei Kindern und Jugendlichen. Prax Kinderpsychol Kinderpsychiatr 31: 213-218
Matisson MD (1982) Der Traum und der Körper im analytischen Psychodrama. In: Petzold H (ed) Dramatische Therapie. Neue Wege der Behandlung durch Psychodrama, Rollenspiel, Therapeutisches Theater. Hippokrates, Stuttgart
Mauss M (1975) Körpertechniken. In: Mauss M (ed) Soziologie und Anthropologie. Hanser, Munich
Meermann R (1983) Verzerrungen und Körperwahrnehmung bei Anorexia nervosa: Einige diagnostische und therapeutische Implikationen. In: Minsel WR, Herff W (eds) Studien zur pädagogischen und psychologischen Intervention, vol 4. Lang, Frankfurt
Meermann R, Fichter M (1983) Störungen des Körperschemas bei Pubertätsmagersucht. Psychother Psychosom Med Psychol 132: 161-169
Meyer AE (1963) Körperstörungen und Sexualität, dargestellt am Beispiel des gemeinen Hirsutismus. Prax Psychother 8: 1-7
Mindell A (1981) Widerstand und Körper. Überlegungen aus Jungianischer Sicht. Integr Ther 7: 197-203
Möhlen K, Brähler E (1984) Beschwerdebild und Selbstkonzept von Patienten mit Ulcus duodeni vor und 4 Jahre nach einer Operation. Z Psychosom Med Psychoanal 30: 150-163
Montagu A (1971) Touching: The human significance of the skin. Columbia University Press, New York
Mrazek J (1984) Selbstkonzept und Körperkonzept. Psychologie. Schweiz Z Psychol 43: 1-23
Nitzschke B (1983) Körper und Emotion in der Philosophie Schopenhauers. Eine perspektivische Betrachtung der Psychoanalyse aus dem Blickwinkel des 19. Jahrhunderts. Anal Psychol 14: 285-304
Nordhoff HB, Hohlfeld R (1985) Humane Grenzen des technisch Machbaren. Mabuse Z Gesundheitswesen 10 (37): 36-42
Ochmann HJ (1981) Nichtverbale Kommunikation und Adoleszenz. Ein Beitrag zur Sozialisation des kommunikativen Körpers unter besonderer Berücksichtigung der mikrosozialen Interaktionswelten von Jugendlichen. Campus Forschung, vol 211. Campus, Frankfurt
Orban P (1981) Psyche und Soma. Über die Sozialisation des Körpers. Akademische Verlagsgesellschaft, Wiesbaden
Overbeck G (1984) Krankheit als Anpassung. Suhrkamp, Frankfurt
Overbeck G, Overbeck A (1978) Seelischer Konflikt - körperliches Leiden. Rowohlt, Reinbek
Painter J (1984) Körperarbeit und persönliche Entwicklung. Wie wir durch Tiefenentspannung zur Harmonie von Leib, Seele und Geist gelangen. Kösel, Munich
Pankow G (1982) Körperbild, Übergangsobjekt und Narzissmus. Ein Beitrag zu vor-konfliktuellen Strukturen. In: Beland H, Eickhoff FW, Loch W, Meistermann-Seeger E, Richter HE, Scheunert G (eds) Jahrbuch der Psychoanalyse. Beiträge zur Theorie und Praxis, vol 14. Frommann-Holzboog, Stuttgart
Paulus P (1982) Zur Erfahrung des eigenen Körpers. Theoretische Ansätze, therapeutische und erziehungswissenschaftliche Aspekte sowie ein empirischer Bericht. Beltz, Weinheim

Paulus R, Otte R (1979) Zur Erfassung der Zufriedenheit mit dem Aussehen des eigenen Körpers. Psychother Psychosom Med Psychol 29: 128-141
Peitmann H (1984) Der inszenierte Körper. In: Kamper D, Wulf C (eds) Der andere Körper. Mensch und Leben, Berlin
Petzold H (ed) (1977) Die neue Körpertherapie. Jungfermann, Paderborn
Pfleiderer B (1984) Das Spiel mit dem anderen Körper. In: Kamper D, Wulf C (eds) Der andere Körper. Mensch und Leben, Berlin
Poppe U (1982) Zum Verhältnis von Körper und Identität. Einige sozialisationstheoretische Zusammenhänge. Sportunterricht 31: 165-172
Rechenberger I (1983) Haut und Körperbild. Werkstattgespräche zum Thema Körperbild. Mater Psychoanal Anal Orient Psychother 9 (1): 31-34
Reindell A (1981) Körperdynamik der Angst. Prax Psychother Psychosom 26: 265-273
Richter HE (1979) Der Gotteskomplex. Rowohlt, Reinbek
Rittner V (1982) Krankheit und Gesundheit. Veränderungen in der sozialen Wahrnehmung des Körpers. In: Kamper D, Wulf C (eds) Die Wiederkehr des Körpers. Suhrkamp, Frankfurt
Roloff HG (1983) Der menschliche Körper in der älteren deutschen Literatur. In: Imhof AE (ed) Der Mensch und sein Körper von der Antike bis heute. Beck, München
Rothschuh K (ed) (1978) Konzepte der Medizin in Vergangenheit und Gegenwart. Hippokrates, Stuttgart
Rumpf D, Schomann H (1983) Die Möglichkeiten der Körperdiagnostik in der Therapie. Gruppendynamik 14: 25-33
Schilder P (1923) Das Körperschema. Ein Beitrag zur Lehre vom Bewußtsein des eigenen Körpers. Springer, Berlin
Schipperges H (1968) Utopien der Medizin. Müller, Salzburg
Schmidt-Atzert L (1984) Die Auswirkung wahrgenommener Körpersymptome auf die Emotionen. Arch Psychol 136: 35-47
Schneider FJ (1979) Eine Untersuchung über den Einfluß einer Sportunterrichtseinheit: „Schöpferische Bewegung und Pantomime" auf das Körperbildnis, das Selbstbildnis und die Körperkoordination. Sportunterricht 28: 133-138
Schott-Billmann F (1979) Körper und Besessenheit als Medien der Psychotherapie in primitiven Gesellschaften. Integr Ther 5: 277-296
Schulte-Herbrüggen UW (1983) Die Bedeutung des Körperschemas für die Technik psychoanalytischer Behandlung von psychosomatisch Erkrankten. Mater Psychoanal 9: 27-31
Seidel U (1981) Psychodrama und Körperarbeit. Prax Kinderpsychol Kinderpsychiatr 30: 154-159
Seittner W (1982) Das Wappen als Zweitkörper und Körperzeichen. In: Kamper D, Wulf C (eds) Die Wiederkehr des Körpers. Suhrkamp, Frankfurt
Seittner W (1984) Körperrichtungen. In: Kamper D, Wulf C (eds) Der andere Körper. Mensch und Leben, Berlin
Shorter E (1984) A history of womens bodies. Penguin, Harmondsworth
Siblik E (1973) Körperbild und motorische Geschicklichkeit. Faculty of philosophy, Vienna University
Sloterdijk P (1983) Kritik der zynischen Vernunft, 2 vols. Suhrkamp, Frankfurt
Strauss B, Appelt H (1983) Ein Fragebogen zur Beurteilung des eigenen Körpers. Diagnostica 24: 145-164
Tibon-Cornillot M (1982) Die transfigurativen Körper. Zur Verflechtung von Techniken und Mythen. In: Kamper D, Wulf C (eds) Die Wiederkehr des Körpers. Suhrkamp, Frankfurt
Tibon-Cornillot M (1984) Die Expansion des Körpers. In: Kamper D, Wulf C (eds) Der andere Körper. Mensch und Leben, Berlin
Totmann R (1979) The social causes of illness. Souvenir, London
Uexküll J von (1920) Theoretische Biologie. Springer, Berlin
Uexküll T von (1961) Der Körper als Problem der psychosomatischen Medizin. Psyche (Stuttg) 15: 76-87
Uexküll T von (1981) Lehrbuch der psychosomatischen Medizin, 2nd edn. Urban & Schwarzenberg, Munich
Uexküll T von (1985) Der Körperbegriff als Problem der Psychoanalyse und der somatischen Medizin. Prax Psychother Psychosom 30: 95-103

Uexküll T von, Wesiack W (1981), Das Leib-Seele-Problem in psychosomatischer Sicht. In: Uexküll T von (ed) Lehrbuch der Psychosomatischen Medizin, 2nd edn. Urban & Schwarzenberg, Munich

Virilio P (1982) Transpolitik. Vom unfähigen zum abwesenden Körper. In: Kamper D, Wulf C (eds) Die Wiederkehr des Körpers. Suhrkamp, Frankfurt

Waldhubel T (1983) Arbeit, Körper und Klasse. Zur Kritik des Belastungsbegriffes. Forum Krit Psychol 12: 146-158

Warsitz P (1983) Der Körper als Signifikant. Zum Zweifel an der Einheitserfahrung des Körpers im Anschluß an D Wyss und J Lacan. Fragmente 9: 35-58

Weiner H (1983) Gesundheit, Krankheitsgefühl und Krankheits-Ansätze zu einem integrativen Verständnis. Psychother Psychosom Med Psychol 33: 15-34

Weizsäcker V von (1947a) Der Gestaltkreis, 2nd edn. Thieme, Stuttgart

Weizsäcker V von (1947b) Körpergeschehen und Neurose. Klett, Stuttgart

Weizsäcker V von (1951) Der kranke Mensch. Eine Einführung in die medizinische Anthropologie. Köhler, Stuttgart

Weizsäcker V von, Wyss D (1957) Zwischen Medizin und Philosophie. Vandenhoeck & Ruprecht, Göttingen

Werner R (1984) Stehen - Sitzen - Liegen. Versuch über den Körper zwischen Stillstand und Gebärde. In: Kamper D, Wulf C (eds) Der andere Körper. Mensch und Leben, Berlin

Wesiack W (1983) Einführung in die psychosomatische Medizin. In: Loch W (ed) Die Krankheitslehre der Psychoanalyse. Hirzel, Stuttgart

Wesiack W (1984) Grundzüge der psychosomatischen Medizin, 2nd edn. Springer, Berlin Heidelberg New York

Wimmer M (1982) Der gesprochene Körper. Zur Authentizität von Körpererfahrungen in Körpertherapien. In: Kamper D, Wulf C (eds) Die Wiederkehr des Körpers. Suhrkamp, Frankfurt

Winau R (1982) Krankheitskonzept und Körperkontakt. In: Kamper D, Wulf C (eds) Die Wiederkehr des Körpers. Suhrkamp, Frankfurt

Winau R (1983) Die Entdeckung des menschlichen Körpers in der neuzeitlichen Medizin. In: Imhof AE (ed) Der Mensch und sein Körper von der Antike bis heute. Beck, Munich

Wuketits F (1985) Zustand und Bewußtsein. Hoffmann & Campe, Hamburg

Wulf C (1982) Körper und Tod. In: Kamper D, Wulf C (eds) Die Wiederkehr des Körpers. Suhrkamp, Frankfurt

Psychoanalysis and the Body

H. Müller-Braunschweig

The discovery that bodily symptoms can arise with no apparent somatic cause was one of the major stimuli behind the development of the theory and therapy of psychoanalysis. Starting from his clinical experience of patients with such symptoms, Freud evolved his ideas on unconscious psychic dynamics. One of the many afflictions of the patient he describes in *Studies on Hysteria* as Cäcilie M., for example, was a violent pain in her right heel. This pain started the moment she wanted to present herself in the company of strangers and was afraid that she might not 'find herself on a right footing' with them. As soon as this connection was cleared up, the symptom disappeared (Freud 1895).

Continued investigations into such phenomena led Freud further and further back into his patients childhoods. Surprisingly often they came up with reports about traumatic sexual seductions in their early years, which had originally been repressed. Through reliving such repressed experiences, first in hypnosis and later in a wakeful state by means of associations coupled with the analyst's interpretations, the patients' pathological symptoms could often be cured. Subsequently Freud gave up the 'seduction theory' (for the most recent discussion on this theory see Schmidtbauer 1985). The reported seductions often turned out to be fantasies. These fantasies he now assumed to be based on instinctual wishes of a sexual nature which, because of a predetermined process of psychosexual development, had become attached to certain parts of the body - the oral, anal and genital zones. An instinct arising from a somatic source thus led to pleasurable sensations in certain areas of the body (erotogenic zones), which Freud assumed to exercise a decisive influence on future psychic development, especially in the period between the 1st and 5th-6th years of life (Freud 1905). If special events in adult life caused the individual to regress to the level of these 'component instincts' and thus also to revert to corresponding wishes and fantasies, feelings of anxiety and guilt were aroused. The wishes were repressed and finally reappeared in symbolic form, as (frequently somatic) symptoms.

The psychoanalytical theory of the origins of neurosis that has just been outlined so very briefly here contributed largely to the body-relatedness of the theory of psychoanalysis but also to a form of therapy in which the fantasies, ideas and actions of the adult patient were often related to basic physical needs and processes such as touching, incorporating, repelling, eliminating, demarcating, penetrating, etc. To this extent the therapy was also body-related. At the same time, however, psychoanalysts sometimes show a peculiar reserve towards their patients body language, which can go as far as plain ignorance[1]. One explanation for this attitude - apart from the analyst's own personal defences - is probably to be found in Freuds early discovery that behind the neurotic, frequently physical symptom there lay concealed a neurotic conflict. If the patient C. mentioned at the beginning was suffering from a conversion symptom - the pain in her heel - then this pain could be removed by discovering its unconscious mental causes, i.e. the bodily aspect had to give way, so to speak, to the psychological explanation. For this reason, a tendency to 'desomatization' [to use the term later coined by Max Schur (1955)] has continued in psychoanalytical theory and practice to this day. The concept of 'desomatization' also applied to a therapeutic line which, starting from a relatively undifferentiated, unconscious, body-oriented and preverbal mental state, moved in the direction of a more differentiated, conscious, body-unrelated and verbalizing psychic condition, so also following the line of phylogenesis. This tendency to desomatization arose out of the efforts of psychoanalysts to effect a reversal of the regressive psychic states mentioned above. In the process of developing his therapeutic technique further, Freud then came upon the phenomena of transference and resistance, which were soon to take their place alongside the basic postulates about unconscious psychic processes as part of the essential equipment of every psychoanalyst. Because the patient's transference was meant to be allowed develop with as little outside influence as possible, the concept of 'therapeutic abstinence' was introduced for psychoanalysts, which applied to physical contact as well (cf. Cremerius 1984). In the discussion on body therapies later on I shall be coming back to this issue.

The beginnings of psychoanalysis thus led from physical symptoms to their psychic origins, from somatic treatment to verbal interpretations, from the search for physiological changes to an understanding of underlying mental dynamics. This new line of approach was subject to vehement attacks, which soon forced Freud and his associates to overemphasize the differences between their ideas and the strongly natural scientific leanings of their contemporaries, in order to be able to follow their own line consistently. Even in 1932, in a letter to Viktor von Weizsäcker, Freud still stressed that the 'study of innervations, vasodilatation and nervous tracts ... (would be) dangerous temptations' for the analysts. All the same, he himself was partially committed to the natural scientist's approach, as is born out in his metapsychological models, in which he 'aligns mental manifestations (such as instinct, stimulation, unpleasure, pleasure, wish) with physical processes (like quantum of energy, energetic tension and discharge ...)' (Habermas 1968, cited in Mertens 1981b). In developing his metaphors Freud drew upon the terminology of three different scientific disciplines: neurophysiology, hydrodynamics and mechanics (König 1981). In spite of his psychological approach he always hoped one day to be able to trace mental processes back to physical (neurophysiological) causes.

The problematical relationship between the causal scientific approach, working according to the precepts of physics and chemistry, and the psychodynamic

[1] Cf. also the introduction by Grunert (1977) to a collection of psychoanalytical contributions on this subject that includes further important aspects and works by psychoanalytical authors that could not be discussed here.

understanding of psychic and psychosomatic phenomena has continued to this day. Especially in the past decade, however, it has also brought forth new insights into the way in which mental and biological processes work together, as demonstrated by the new psychobiological approaches to psychosomatics (cf. Deutsch 1980; Lipowski 1975; Weiner 1979). Putting aside all momentary polemicism, both lines of research can supplement one another.

With respect to the body, the emphasis of psychoanalysis has nevertheless always been upon reverting to the earliest stages of somatic development, when soma and psyche were still relatively undifferentiated, and so also to mental phenomena (especially needs) which were strongly influenced by the nature and import of the physical functions with which they were so closely bound up. This applies both to the early assumptions about erotogenic zones mentioned above and to a more modern view in which the role of body zones is seen as being largely determined by the early mother-infant interaction (see below). This aspect has been dominant throughout the history of psychoanalysis, regardless of the various changes that have taken place in its theory and practice.

The conversion symptoms brought up the question of the precipitant experiences that had triggered off symptom formation, but above all they stressed the issue of their underlying psychic dynamics. The assumptions about erotogenic zones proved to be fruitful here for both the theory and therapy of psychoanalysis. When, for example, a female patient began suffering from nausea and vomiting shortly after her fathers death, the analytical therapy, by means of associative bridges, was able to bring to light her unconscious fantasy that she could (orally) incorporate her father and in this manner keep hold of him, thereby alleviating the 'work' of mourning. But this incorporation contained the aspect of sexual union as well (Fenichel 1945). The early body modus of ingestion and incorporation was in these cases also associated with pleasurable sensations ('cathected with libido') and, furthermore, placed in the service of the psychic economy.

The theoretical conception of libido has been the subject of much critical discussion in recent years (see Klein 1976; Holt 1976; Mertens 1981b). Nowadays it is assumed that innate sensorimotor patterns are stimulated by similarly innate instinctive stimuli ('nuclei') as well as by external stimuli. Maturational and learning processes accumulate on this basis, forming a close network of motives (see König 1981).

The biologically important body functions, which in the early stages of development represent the starting point and model for differentiated mental processes, still retain their significance in later life. An image attributed to Viktor von Weizsäcker compares the human being with a tube that is open at the top and bottom. Without intake, absorption und elimination processes (whether in the area of the body or the mind) the human organism cannot survive. This was also the reason for the central significance of the so-called erotogenic zones, which could then later serve to symbolize unconscious thoughts and fantasies. 'Incorporative tendencies are better expressed through the mouth, the respiratory organs and the skin, eliminative tendencies through the intestinal tract and likewise through the respiratory organs' (Fenichel 1945). Fenichel goes on to point out that 'convex organs like the hand, nose, foot and breasts' can assume phallic significance, whilst 'concave organs like the mouth, anus and nostrils . . . represent feminine wishes'.

These early ideas on the erotogenic zones have since been expanded through the addition of other vitally important areas of experience. The range of early body experiences now considered relevant includes skin and balance sensations as well as visual and auditory perception; the manifold sensori-motor impressions gathered whilst learning to walk have also been added. All these areas of experience are only conceivable in the context of the interaction with the mother, the earliest nurturing object. The notion that mental development was determined largely by instincts following genetically predetermined laws therefore gave way to the idea of a development determined from the start by the interaction between mother and child. 'Thus one can show how the vocalization of affects, mimetic interactions and body rhythms that go on between mother and child have a quasi-dialogue structure right from the start, representing precursors to spoken language. Only very slight deviations in chronological sequence structure are apparently responsible for the breakdown of the dialogue ... The child can ... open the interaction with visual behaviour and the mother continue it with a tactile response; the child answers vocally and the mother with a mimetic reaction. The quality of the dialogue depends upon the chronological synchronization' (Krause 1983). Body phenomena thus play a vital role in early communication behaviour. Such sequences have also been termed 'tonic dialogue' (Mertens 1981 a). Also relevant in this connection is Spitz's observation that the early communication between mother and child is carried on by means of 'balance, tension (of muscles and other organs), body posture, temperature, vibrations, skin and body contact, rhythm, tempo' (Spitz 1960).

These insights, along with experiences gathered whilst treating deeply disturbed patients, have resulted in the emergence of object relations theory to take its place alongside the instinct-defence aspect upon which the the neurosis model briefly described above was based.

Let us now return to the question which arose earlier of the significance of the erotogenic zones in normal development. Building upon the ideas of Stolorow (1979), Mertens (1981 b) describes their role as follows: 'Experiences and fantasies in the oral-incorporative mode (cf. Erikson 1964) not only signal the achievement of rudimentary self-object boundaries but also further the process of differentiation between self and object representatives, in that they help the child to learn the difference between inner and outer, between the self as a container and the non-self that can be taken into the body (mouth). These incorporation fantasies also enable the young child to ascribe valued and admired characteristics of its key object to itself, which has a further structurizing influence on its self-image'.

Thus it is clear that basic experiences associated with body functions also play a vital role in the genesis of the ego functions. Following its emphasis on 'driving' forces leading to unconscious wishes and fantasies, the psychoanalytical construct of the ego as a cognitive and controlling element now comes into the picture. Ego development is likewise influenced by early body experience. Freud had already pointed this out in his description of the sensations arising when one touches one's own body. *Two* sensations actually occur here: one in the touching finger and one in the part of the body that is touched. The latter sensation can amount to an 'inner perception". This double form of perception which arises upon touching one's own body, as opposed to touching objects in the outside world, constitutes an important foundation for the perception of one's own body and, furthermore, for distinguishing between it and the outside world. 'The ego is first and foremost a body ego' (Freud 1923). From here one can trace a line to the present-day concept of body self. Whereas the ego is nowadays regarded rather as an accumulation of controlling structures (Sandler and Joffe 1969), the concepts of self and body self lay greater emphasis on the area of experience. In the definition by Lichtenberg (1978), the latter term 'refers to the individual's full range of experiences that center on his body - its surface, its interior, and all the images ... that comprise it.' Besuden (1983) suggests that deficits in ego structure could be connected with deficits in the area of body image. Similarly, early efforts to integrate body image into a structured psychosomatic whole and the transient experience of 'unity' could be models for later creative processes, which also produce greater, inherently structured units (cf. Niederland 1967; Müller-Braunschweig 1977).

I have already mentioned how the form and function of biologically important organs can become bound up with unconscious wishes and verbal expressions. The significance acquired early on is then retained in later development, whereby the earlier psychic phenomena may be overlaid by the later, but do not lose their potential effectivity (Rapaport and Gill 1959; see also Mertens 1981b). Thus, the incorporative tendencies referred to above can also appear in more differentiated interpersonal relationships and may, for example, play an important part in emotionally working through a loss, as in the case described above of the patient who lost her father (Freud 1916).

In spite of the critical influence that early infantile development indubitably has on later life and of the overlaying process mentioned above, psychosomatic experience cannot be evaluated entirely in terms of 'earlier-later' or 'undifferentiated-differentiated'. Mental incorporation, for instance, is not only a symbol 'for' the 'real' act of physical incorporation. Ingestion or incorporation, like penetration or elemination, are processes which can occur mentally or physically, spatially or not. The following quotation from *Studies in Hysteria* appears two pages after the report on the pain in the heel of patient C.:

> I have not found such an extensive use of symbolization in any other patient. It is true that Frau Căcilie M. was a woman who possessed quite unusual gifts, particularly artistic ones, and whose highly developed sense of form was revealed in some poems of great perfection. It is my opinion, however, that when a hysteric creates a somatic expression for an emotionally-coloured idea by symbolization, this depends less than one would imagine on personal or voluntary factors. In taking a verbal expression literally and in feeling the 'stab in the heart' or the 'slap in the face' after some slighting remark as a real event, the hysteric is not taking liberties with words, but is simply reviving once more the sensations to which the verbal expression owes its justification. How has it come about that we speak of someone who has been slighted as being 'stabbed to the heart' unless the slight had in fact been accompanied by a precordial sensation which could suitably be described in that phrase ...? What could be more probable than that the figure of speech 'swallowing something', which we use in talking of an insult to which no rejoinder has been made, did in fact originate from the innervatory sensations which arise in the pharynx when we refrain from speaking and prevent ourselves from reacting to the insult? [And finally,] it may be that [hysteria] does not take linguistic usage as its model at all, but that both hysteria and linguistic usage draw their material from a common source. (Freud 1895)

The expression 'common source' was to my knowledge not eplained further by Freud, but one is reminded first of all of Fenichel's description of the 'appropriateness' of certain organs for symbolizing conscious and unconscious feeling (see above). The 'precordial sensation' mentioned by Freud is a reference to the physical 'affect correlates' that were to become so central in psychosomatic medicine later on. But the expression 'common source' must surely also mean not just that one symbolizes the other (the psychic the somatic) but rather that, for example, the concepts of 'penetration' or 'incorporation' represent processes which can find expression on the psychic or the somatic level, as suggested above. Thus, a partner in love or indeed in a conversation can, in such an interaction, be almost as thoroughly 'incorporated' as a steak (cf. also Fenichel 1945, p 65 and Hoffmann 1979, p. 161).

This brings us to the term 'attitude' which has both psychic and somatic connotations (Grace and Graham 1952; Bräutigam & Christian 1981, p 52). The German world *Haltung* is in fact used to apply equally to body posture and to attitude in the mental sense. In the same way, the reference made by Freud in his example above to 'finding oneself on the right footing' (in German: *das rechte Auftreten*) has the twofold meaning of 'setting one's foot on the ground' (and so standing firmly) and simultaneously 'presenting oneself before other people'. This 'putting ones best foot forward' will only have the desired effect, however, if one 'treads firmly', if one is 'steadfast', able to 'stand on one's own two feet', and so 'passes' the test of an audience. The state of 'steadfastness' can thus express itself physically or psychically. If in the above quotation Freud refers to his patient's feeling for form, the way he uses this term also implies the possibility of expressing psychic events in the form of body posture or movement.

In another (philosophical) context, it has been pointed out whilst considering these processes that psyche and soma can 'only signify two different perspectives on the same phenomenon'. (Mertens 1981b, p 41; see also von Uexküll 1963)

The capacity for self-reliance just referred to in connection with being able to 'stand on one's own two feet' can, however, be critically disturbed early in a child's development. If a child's first attempts at walking, which are normally undertaken with excited enjoyment, are obstructed by an anxious mother or if the mother cannot tolerate the spatial separation which begins in this 'practice phase' (Mahler et al. 1975), then a development will be started off in which every subsequent 'step' towards independence, every 'pro-gression' is coupled with anxiety, guilt and insecurity.

Now, these lines of thought have their practical consequences for therapy. The fact that mental and physical processes become associated with one another at a very early stage provides a starting point for the body-oriented treatments that are practiced in many centres for psychosomatics nowadays (cf. Chap 6, this volume). However, even in the 1920s, analysts were already concerned with the question of body phenomena occurring during analytical treatment. Their observations have only recently been taken up on a larger scale. In 1928 Fenichel pointed out that 'in every neurosis, even the commonest minor inhibitions, full control over mobility ... suffers to a certain extent' and that this could be observed in psychoanalytical treatments as well.

If, for instance, a patient can no longer escape a correct interpretation, but still makes the attempt, it often happens that he convulsively innervates all his skeletal muscles as if he were striving for muscular protection to prevent repressed impulses that are hidden deep down inside him from coming to the surface, as if he wanted to counteract the pressure of the repression from within with a muscular pressure from without. ... Since thoughts are rehearsed actions, inhibited thoughts must manifest themselves, like inhibited actions, in movement and changes in tonus - in a short paper on 'Thinking and Muscle Innervation' Ferenczi has shown that this is in fact the case. (Fenichel 1928, cited in J. Grunert 1977)

In the light of these suppositions, a number of clinical observations become easier to understand. Ferenczi (1921) writes, 'It is the neurotics who are distinguished by their excessively cautious, calculated, weighty manner of walking and moving,' and elsewhere he comments, 'occasionally one feels it is necessary to draw the patients attention to his posture (muscular tensions in his body) and so to "mobilize" him a little. Subsequently, it is often possible to talk about many things which had hitherto been hidden or unconscious'. (Ferenczi 1925, cited in Grunert 1977, p 37).

Fenichel claims that where unconscious thoughts and fantasies manifest themselves in the equally unconscious image of an organ, the struggle between an impulse (for instance, a sexual one) and its repression can give rise to spasmodic cramps in the muscles of the pelvis, the pelvic floor or the hip joint. The obsessional neurotic's anal pleasure in retention shows itself, for example, in sphincterismus, i.e. in muscle innervations which are perpetuated beyond the physiologically functional degree. This hypertonus can be displaced 'onto the entire skeletal muscular system'. 'Such people unconsciously live in constant fear of incontinence ...' (Fenichel, cited in Grunert 1977, p. 39).

However, a high degree of 'counter-cathexis' can ultimately also lead to a blockage of inner perceptions and so to feelings of depersonalization in those areas of the body which are conflictingly cathected. In the early years of his work Fenichel had already stated that 'the struggle for repression between a cathected instinct and the ego's counter-cathexis ... [could] only be physiologically reflected in constant changes in the skeletal muscular system. ... "And now we hear that individuals with certain, especially hysterical, tendencies, whilst attempting to relax their tensely contracted muscles, sometimes get into affective states comparable only to the behaviour shown by patients in whom a "significant trauma" has been touched upon in a psychocathartic therapy' (Fenichel 1928, cited in Grunert 1977, p. 36).

In 1933, in his *Character Analysis,* Wilhelm Reich also stressed the parallels between psychic structure and body posture, as demonstrated in the stimultaneous occurrennce of 'characterological armour' and 'body armour'. Here he regards the chronic tension in the body as being also responsible for the emotional blockage. These ideas led A. Lowen (1976) in the USA to develop his technique of bio-energetics, which among other things aims, by loosening chronic muscular tension, to achieve a more relaxed overall attitude. Representatives of this and other directions also point out the significance of individual body zones such as the regions of the mouth and jaw, or of the neck. Tension in the neck is interpreted as inhibited vocal expression and the repression of an impulse to cry, shout and scream (cf. Kurtz and Prestera 1976).

A patient who in a psychoanalytical group therapy had successfully maintained the position of the superior 'co-therapist' - the others called him 'boss' - for 2 years and who himself showed hardly any emotions, went on to partake in a 'psychoanalytical primal therapy' which also involved elements of body therapy. Here he commented on the tenseness in his jaw. During one session the therapist tapped his on the jaw, encouraging him to 'relax there', whereupon the participant broke out in a loud laugh, described by the others as 'horrific'. This laugh really did 'break' out of him, coming in bursts and finally turning into loud crying. After this, he was able for the first time to talk about very painful experiences he had had with his mother as a child[1].

Here we find a vivid example of a 'stiff upper lip' and how a brief touch by the therapist in the 'holding' environment of the group sufficed to release the doggedly restrained emotions.

Psychosomatic imbalances of tension such as this, if continued for a long time in the areas either of the voluntary motor system or of the autonomic nervous system, can lead to illness. Particularly in such cases, depth-oriented body therapies - perhaps combined with other somatic and verbal psychotherapeutic methods - can prove astoundingly successful. This also applies to the area of subjective pain.

The statements quoted above by Fenichel and Ferenczi (on the latter see also Cremerius 1983) had little influence on the future development of psychoanalysis. Ruitenbeek (1970) attributes this to the stronger taboo on physical contact prevalent in the USA which, after all, became the major centre of psychoanalysis after 1933. Furthermore, the early patients had not been deprived of affection and warmth to the extent that became the norm later on. The reasons for the withdrawal of the body from the focus of interest are surely more complex. In recent years, however, new approaches to the treatment of narcissistic and borderline disorders and the discovery of the special psychic characteristics typical of psychosomatic patients, as well as direct observations of the mother-child interaction, have all contributed to a broadening out of psychoanalytically oriented forms of treatment and with it to a renewed interest in the body.

This brings us back to the more recent psychoanalytical theories in the field of psychosomatics. It is well-known that the emphasis these days is less on the conversion symptoms with their clear symbolism, as described above, than on a 'physiological reaction of the vegetative organs to continued or periodically recurring emotional states' (Alexander 1950) - even though the boundaries between this and symbolization may not always be clear. The developments in this field, like those discussed so far, can again only be presented here through a few examples (see also Kapfhammer 1983; von Rad 1983; Wesiak 1977).

The importance of the form and function of the various organs as a basis for the development of content and meaning in later mental processes was indicated above. I have already described how early psychic phenomena, although overlaid by the later, still retain their potential effectivity so that there always remains an archaic psychic level that is closely linked with physical phenomena; the incorporation tendencies discussed above were an example of this. An important aspect to note here is that the physiological accompaniments of emotions and affects do not undergo such extensive modifications as is usually the case in mental development, so that, even in adult life, the whole breadth and depth of the physiological and sensori-motor body reactions are still potentially there, as indeed is the entire spectrum of psychic reactions, from the more primitive to the more differentiated.

---

[1] This example is taken from an intensive workshop on psychoanalytical primal therapy led by the late Dr. H.-J. Manthey, who died in 1984 (see also Damm 1978).

The inhibitory mechanisms and the capacity for symbolization acquired in later life have removed us from these underlying archaic forms of experience and their accompanying somatic affects. Under great pressure, however, we can still be overwhelmed by such early response forms. This happens particularly where the early nucleus of the psychosomatic self, including the body self, was strongly influenced in childhood by traumatic, overwhelming experiences and correspondingly violent physiological processes.

An example of such a development in early life is given by R. Krause (1983). He describes how a baby's apparently unaccountable gastric colics could finally be understood on discovering that the mother always carried on telephone conversations with her friends whilst breast-feeding. Another 6-month-old baby developed a cough, accompanied by vomiting, with no known somatic cause. Close observation revealed that the mother 'responded to every negative expression of affects in her infant by pushing her nipple into its mouth in a manner which, though clearly intended to appear as a sort of routine action, was in fact so aggressive that the baby could not get enough air. The child's screams only reinforced her response' (Krause 1983). Such children become overwhelmed by unpleasurable affects to a degree that can only be called traumatic. Here we are no longer dealing primarily with an early sexual trauma, as described by the early psychoanalysts, but of repeatedly unempathic actions by the person caring for the baby. Krystal (1978) defined infantile trauma as a state in which the infant's still rudimentary controlling functions are powerless in the face of unpleasurable affects. These early experiences amount to a 'hell' from which there is no escape, a timeless horror, since the child, of course, cannot visualize this state ever coming to an end. (It is easy to imagine that later anxiety about emotional or physical closeness to a partner can have its roots in just such experiences.) A first after-effect of such treatment, according to psychoanalytical psychosomatics (see McDougall 1974) is that a tendency develops to split off affects, since not feeling anything offers the only chance of escaping the infinite torment. Such an autoplastic change is the only means available to the infant of countering early unempathic treatment, if the appropriate expressions of affect (crying) have proved useless. However, the splitting off of affects and emotions brings with it the further consequence that a state of inner emptiness becomes established, which is reinforced still further by the fact that the infant's initially diffuse affect forerunners have no chance of becoming more fully differentiated in the course of supportive interactions. Around or over an early nucleus of the self that has been damaged in this way, a personality structure develops which, because of the damage done to its own subjective experience (insensitivity to its own impulses and needs) is often forced into an extreme overadjustment to the outside world. One's own needs can no longer serve as a compass with which to orientate oneself in the world. Along with the damaged nucleus described here, the self also acquires a 'psychosomatic sector' (Stephanos 1973) or a 'psychosomatic fixation point' (Fain 1966), in which archaic, undifferentiated affects (Kutter 1980) and physiological processes become closely interwoven, forming a 'psychosomatic subsystem' (Müller-Braunschweig 1980). With appropriate stimulation, psychosomatic illness can be the result.

In connection with the splitting-off processes mentioned above, McDougall (1974) has also referred to the 'robot-like' way of experiencing and functioning which is typical of psychosomatic patients. This also includes a mechanized attitude to one's own body and its functions (cf. Schöttler 1981).

Apart from the aspect of the 'primitive sector', there is another developmental line which should be mentioned in connection with the undifferentiated body self. Margret Mahler (Mahler et al. 1975) describes how a (normally developed) child, at the beginning of the differentiation phase, frequently seeks to push itself away from its mother's body in order to explore its surroundings with its own perceptions. This is also a symbolic expression of the child's first move towards self-reliance and 'setting itself apart' from its mother. The child thus creates for itself a 'potential space' (Winnicott 1971) in which to develop its mental and emotional abilities. Many authors hold the view that the creation of this potential space is only possible with the help of a 'transitional object' - a cushion, or piece of cloth, that is invested with the mother's attributes and so symbolizes her presence (cf. Winnicott 1953; Mitscherlich 1978). The transitional object can be kept by the child in situations when it is alone (e.g. going to sleep) and so represent a step towards independence from the mother. Out of the outward symbol there gradually develops an inner symbol, its mother's internal representative, which makes the child less dependent on her immediate presence. Kestenberg (1971) sees forerunners of this development in what she calls 'intermediate objects' - such as milk, later on excrement or secreta and, later still, even sexual fantasies in the early oedipal phase - which she assumes to form 'bridges' between mother and child.

Successful differentiation in the individuation phase would appear to be of central significance to the body image as well. Kestenberg (1971) has also introduced the concept of the 'organ-object image'. She assumes that in the early stages of infancy representatives develop in which, for example, the mother's breast is joined to the child's own lips and mouth cavity (and, may I add, perhaps also the upper digestive tracts) in one unified ideational representative. A successful dialogue in infancy allows this image to develop to the full without disturbance. During the continuing process of differentiation and ego formation, the infant will integrate the whole ideational complex (including the maternal element) into its image of its organs - it becomes internalized. The good or bad feelings arising during the interaction will become localized in the corresponding organs. An irritation during feeding, as in the example quoted above, will then lead to a distorted body image and a corresponding susceptibility to future disturbances in the organ concerned (bearing in mind how, under hypnosis, vegetative processes can be strongly influenced by thoughts and images).

The early body representatives described before may similarly be expected to have a disturbing influence on the functioning of the affected organ (in this case the upper digestive tract) in the child's later life. The psychosomatic patient's strong dependency on an object, which likewise becomes established in the early mother-infant interaction, is well known. If a part of the body, an organ, is strongly bound up with a maternal image - i.e. later also with a partner with whom the subject has formed a close symbiotic relationship - this naturally also has its consequences for future physiological responses, whether to object-loss or to damage or illness affecting one's own body, this being experienced as a form of object-loss as well. The idea of being 'whole' or 'complete' or 'viable' has remained bound to the image of a caring object. This puts me in mind of expressions used by cardiac neurotic patients and recorded by Richter and Beckmann (1973): 'My heart is unreliable' or 'I am afraid my heart could leave me.' The analogy between mother and heart is clear. In an unpublished manuscript, Cecil Mushatt (1980) stresses the importance of the gradual dissolution of the early symbiosis, which is so central in the therapy of these disorders. He points out that 'the more severe physical and psychic reactions are to be seen in those patients who show marked impairment of the individuation process.' He describes among others a patient with ulcerative colitis who, whilst sitting at the bedside of his mother, who is fatally ill, suddenly had the, for him, shocking fantasy of pulling off his mother's breasts and other parts of her body and pushing them under his skin. 'Then I would have my mother with me.' In this phase of treatment (after years of psychotherapy and psychoanalysis), which was accompanied by violent emotional outbursts, he experienced the wish to be united with his mother simultaneously with sadistic, murderous impulses towards her. Earlier intimations of such fantasies had in the past always led to a worsening of his colitis.

In many cases the mother - or, to be more precise, the 'bad' interactions with her - thus remains literally embodied in an organ. Those parts of the body and organs which are experienced as being the seat of the bad affects therefore frequently remain split off from conscious experience. The affected body zones are later often described by the patient in psychotherapy or analysis as strangely 'lifeless', 'separate' or 'shadowy'. Such patients are not permitted to perceive themselves to the full, either mentally or physically. They must live restrictedly, cut off from vital sources of mental or physical energy. This splitting will be perpetuated all the more strongly the more the early mechanism of discharge through somatic symptoms has, so to speak, become set in. Giving up this somatic discharge would lead to a repetition of the early traumatic anxiety which, as described above, was probably experienced as completely destroying. It would also reinstate the condition of total dependence against which the adult patient often seeks to defend himself through an almost desperate show of self-reliance.

The impairment of the 'nucleus of the self' - i.e. a disturbance in the subjective aspect of the first interaction which has resulted in the splitting-off of archaic, body-related affects or whole body zones - often leads to a feeling of 'vacuity' or being 'anuclear'. 'Who am I anyway?' or 'Do I have a base?', 'What can I hold onto?' Such expressions bring us back to the new dimensions in psychoanalytically oriented therapy which have been introduced in many clinics for psychosomatics nowadays. One such dimension involves the inclusion of the patient's subjective body experience as an integral part of therapy, loosening the taboo on physical contact upheld by classical analysts (and not to be confused with the exclusively cathartic gratification offered by some of the so-called encounter groups). An example of this approach which has become very widespread in the Federal Republic of Germany is a type of movement therapy called *Konzentrative Bewegungstherapie* (KBT). It is closely related to the technique of 'sensory awareness' developed by Charlotte Selver in the United States (cf. Brooks 1974), both methods sharing common roots in the early pioneering work of Elsa Gindler. Therapeutic emphasis is placed on sensory awareness of oneself and one's movements within a group (see Chap 6 this volume). The somatic element (the subjectively experienced body) is the 'foundation and field of reference for ... physical, psychosomatic and psychic processes' (Stolze 1984). It is often possible subsequently to understand these experiences analytically in verbal phases of therapy inserted between movement sessions. The leader of a KBT group may himself be sparing with physical contact (although with some patients it can be necessary). Physical contact takes place rather among the group members themselves. Experience has shown that intensive transference processes develop, which can then be taken up for therapeutic purposes. However, the extreme reaction to a touch on the jaw described above shows especially clearly how affects which are hardly or not at all accessible by verbal means can be reached by working more directly on the body. There are a great many such instances. The therapeutic potential here can be decisive in treating rigid character-neurotic or alexithymic patients.

But this does not only apply to such patients. The issue is a more general one these days. Krystal (1977) has made the observation that nowadays, in contrast to the period around the turn of the century, one can by no means always expect that when patients are confronted with interpretations, alongside the intellectual insight, they will really experience the corresponding affects as well. It is more likely that the therapist's interventions will be 'considered with some interest', but that the affect will be more or less isolated. By twisting them into (unemotional) clichés, many patients manage to render the best interpretations ineffective. However, this defensive use of cliché formation as described by Krystal often fails in the face of body experiences and the affects associated with them.

A further example of a well-tried, body-oriented form of therapy is the method known in Germany as *funktionelle Entspannung* (literally: functional relaxation), or FE, which was developed by Marianne Fuchs in the course of her work with psychosomatic patients in Heidelberg, in the days of von Weizsäcker (Fuchs 1949, 1974; Rosa and Rosa-Wolff 1976). In contrast to KBT, this technique lays heavier emphasis on working with the individual. In a state of relaxation (but without suggestive directions) the patient learns to experience areas and zones of the body intensively and so bring about vegetative changes.

Combinations of KBT and FE with analytical psychotherapy have been tried out extensively with in-patients in many West German centres (see, e.g. Arfsten and Hoffmann 1978; Bräutigam 1978; Becker and Lüdecke 1978; Bepperling and Klotz 1978; Janssen 1978; Müller-Braunschweig and Möhlen 1980; Müller-Braunschweig et al. 1981). The success of this sort of combination of body-related methods with (verbal) out-patient analytical therapy has to my knowledge hardly been studied systematically as yet, but clinical experience has shown that occasional supplementary body therapy during psychoanalysis or an analytically oriented psychotherapy can achieve important therapeutic results of the type described above. The transference processes which would arise if analytical and body-oriented therapies were to proceed permanently side-by-side would have to be traced in detail before one could recommend this approach to be practised on a large scale. [It was only after writing this article that I heard about the work of H. Dieckmann (1981). There are many parallels between his approach and mine.]

A combination of verbal dialogue and attention to bodily sensations (including breathing and muscles) is also the objective behind George Downing's 'body-oriented psychotherapy'. 'Affectless association' in the sense described above is prevented through constant reflection on one's own physical sensations (especially breathing), whereby here again the individual is in the foreground. By involvement of the body and, where necessary, of 'holding' contact with the therapist, a way through to the emotions is found. This applies most particularly to those emotions associated with very early experiences. Cathartic discharge of affects is involved, but is not the main objective of the psychotherapeutic work. In the attention it pays to transference, counter-transference, defences and the significance of childhood, this approach has much in common with psychoanalysis.

Thus it seems that the future development of psychoanalysis, as well as providing more and more differentiated descriptions of mental phenomena, could lead to a rediscovery of body experience. An integration of these new insights into theory and therapy is clearly on its way. In the area of therapy this also means a more flexible approach to the whole spectrum of experience, ranging from the vegetative and sensori-motor physical processes with their attendant 'basic' emotions, to the more differentiated mental processes that are relatively removed from the body. The term 'desomatization' applies in this connection to only one, if an important, developmental sequence in the emergence of the psychosomatic personality (see also Becker 1981) - a sequence which, among other things, includes the acquisition of the important ability to symbolize. The progressive differentiation between body and mind must repeatedly be supplemented by integrative steps in the direction of psychosomatic unity. Such an integration is nowadays especially threatened from without by modern developments in science and technology, with their constantly fluctuating demands, their overemphasis on rationality and their dangerous destruction of our biological basis. These threats may have contributed to the renewed interest in the body discernible today. The ever-present reality of the atomic threat is yet another factor promoting narcissistic withdrawal (Wangh 1983; Richter 1984), perhaps also withdrawal into 'mute' psychosomatic symptoms. A further consequence of this situation is that a dangerous split develops between a highly technologized functional approach, on the one hand, and often seemingly archaic mental processes, on the other. In therapeutic work with the individual, combined methods, including combinations of verbal and body therapies, can facilitate access to the various sides of the psychosomatic personality and so reduce the tendency to (individual) splitting processes. The experience gained through working with body-related therapies against a background of psychoanalytical understanding could also help to keep alive the creativity of psychoanalysis in theory and therapy.

References

Alexander F (1950) Psychosomatic medicine: its principles and applications. Allen and Unwin, London

Arfsten AJ, Hoffmann SO (1978) Stationäre psychoanalytische Psychotherapie als eigenständige Behandlungsform. Prax Psychother 23: 233-245

Becker H (1981) Konzentrative Bewegungstherapie. Thieme, Stuttgart

Becker H, Lüdecke H (1978) Erfahrungen mit der stationären Anwendung psychoanalytischer Therapie. Psyche (Stuttg) 31: 1-20

Bepperling W, Klotz M (1978) Analytische Psychotherapie und funktionelle Entspannung als kombinierte Behandlungsmethode. Hippokrates, Stuttgart

Besuden F (1983) Das Körperbild als Matrix des Körpererlebens. Vortrag vor der DKPM in der Psychosomatischen Klinik, Bad Neustadt/Saale

Bräutigam W (1978) Verbale und präverbale Methoden in der stationären Therapie. (Neue therapeutische Zugänge zum psychosomatisch Kranken.) Z Psychosom Med Psychoanal 2: 146-155

Bräutigam W, Christian P (1981) Psychosomatische Medizin. Thieme, Stuttgart

Brooks CVW (1974) Sensory awareness. Viking, New York

Cremerius J (1983) Sandor Ferenczis Bedeutung für Theorie und Therapie der Psychoanalyse. Psyche (Stuttg) 37: 988-1015

Cremerius J (1984) Die psychoanalytische Abstinenzregel. Psyche (Stuttg) 38: 769-800

Damm S (1978) Primärtherapie aus psychoanalytischer Sicht. Mater Psychoanal Analyt Orient Psychother 2: 126-148

Deutsch F (1926) Der gesunde und kranke Körper in psychoanalytischer Betrachtung. In: Grunert J (ed) Körperbild und Selbstverständnis. Kindler, Munich

Deutsch L (1980) Psychosomatic medicine from a psychoanalytic viewpoint. J Am Psychoanal Assoc 1: 653-701

Dieckmann H (1981) Die libidinöse Widerbesetzung des Körpers in der Psychosomatik. Anal Psychol 12: 269-285

Erikson EH (1964) Childhood and society. Norton, New York

Fain M (1966) Regression et Psychosomatique. Rev Fr Psychoanal 30: 451-456

Fenichel O (1928) Über organlibidinöse Begleiterscheinungen der Triebabwehr. In: Grundert J (1977) Körperbild und Selbstverständnis, Kindler, Munich

Fenichel O (1945) Psychoanalytische Neurosenlehre, vol 2. Walter, Freiburg

Ferenczi S (1921) Psychoanalytische Betrachtungen über den Tic. Int Z Psychoanal 7: 33-62

Ferenczi S (1925) Zur Psychoanalyse von Sexualgewohnheiten. Int Z Psychoanal 11: 6-39

Ferenczi S (1926) Kontraindikationen der aktiven Therapie. Int Z Psychoanal 12: 3-14

Freud S (1895) Studien über Hysterie. Frl Elisabetth v R Gesammelte Werke, vol 1. Fischer, Frankfurt

Freud S (1905) Drei Abhandlungen zur Sexualtheorie. Gesammelte Werke, vol 5. Fischer, Frankfurt. Standard edn, vol 7

Freud S (1916) Trauer und Melancholie. Gesammelte Werke, vol 10. Fischer, Frankfurt. Standard edn, vol 14

Freud S (1923) Das Ich und das Es. Gesammelte Werke, vol 13. Fischer, Frankfurt. Standard edn, vol 19

Freud S, Breuer J (1974) Studies on hysteria. Penguin, Harmondsworth

Fuchs M (1949) Über Atemtherapie und entspannende Körperarbeit. Psyche (Stuttg) 3: 538-548

Fuchs M (1974) Funktionelle Entspannung. Hippokrates, Stuttgart

Grace WJ, Graham DT (1952) Relationship of specific attitudes and emotions to certain bodily diseases. Psychosom Med 14: 243-251

Grunert J (ed) (1977) Körperbild und Selbstverständnis. Psychoanalytische Beiträge zur Leib-Seele Einheit. Kindler, München

Hoffmann O (1979) Charakter und Neurose. Suhrkamp, Frankfurt

Holt RR (1976) Drive or wish? A reconsideration of the psychoanalytic theory of motivation. Psychol Issues Monogr 36

Janssen PL (1978) Zu einigen psychotherapeutischen Aspekten der Beschäftigungstherapie in einer psychiatrischen Klinik. Psychother Med Psychol 28: 183-193

Kapfhammer HP (1983) Psychoanalytische Psychosomatik. In: Mertens W (ed) Psychoanalyse. Ein Handbuch in Schlüsselbegriffen. Urban and Schwarzenberg, Munich

Kestenberg JS (1971) From organ-object imagery to self and object representations. In: McDevit JB, Settlage CF (eds) Separation-Individuation. Essays in honor of Margaret S. Mahler. Int Univ Press, New York

Klein GS (1976) Freuds two theories of sexuality: Perspectives to change in psychoanalytic theory. In: Berger L (ed) Clinical-cognition psychology models and integration. New York

König WH (1981) Zur Neuformulierung der psychoanalytischen Metapsychologie: Vom Energie-Modell zum Informationskonzept. In: Mertens W (ed) Neue Perspektiven der Psychoanalyse. Kohlhammer, Stuttgart

Krause R (1983) Zur Onto- und Phylogenese des Affektsystems und ihrer Beziehung zu psychischen Störungen. Psyche (Stuttg) 11: 1016-1043
Krystal H (1977) Aspects of affect theory. Bull Menninger Clin 41: 1-26
Krystal H (1978) Trauma and affects. Psychoanal Study Child 33: 81-116
Kurtz R, Prestera H (1976) Botschaften des Körpers. Kösel, Munich
Kutter P (1980) Emotionalität und Körperlichkeit. Anmerkungen zu einer Emotiogenese psychosomatischer Störungen. Psychother Psychosom 25: 131-145
Lichtenberg J (1978) The testing of reality from the standpoint of the body self. J Am Psychoanal Assoc 26: 357-383
Lipowski ZJ (1975) Physical illness, the patient and his environment: Psychosocial foundations of medicine. In: Reiser MF (ed) American handbook of psychiatry, vol 4. Basic Books, New York, pp 3-42
Lowen A (1975) Bioenergetics. Penguin, New York
Mahler M, Pine F, Bergmann A (1975) Die psychische Geburt des Menschen. Fischer, Frankfurt
McDougall J (1974) The psychosoma and the psychoanalytic process. Int Rev Psychoanal 1: 437-459
Mertens W (1981 a) Psychoanalyse. Kohlhammer, Stuttgart
Mertens W (1981 b) Krise der psychoanalytischen Theorie? In: Mertens W (ed) Neue Perspektiven der Psychoanalyse. Kohlhammer, Stuttgart
Mitscherlich M (1978) Die Bedeutung des Übergangsobjektes für die psychosomatische Theorie. In: Overbeck G, Overbeck A (eds) Seelischer Konflikt - körperliches Leiden. Rowohlt, Reinbek
Müller-Braunschweig H (1975) Die Wirkung der frühen Erfahrung. Klett, Stuttgart
Müller-Braunschweig H (1977) Aspekte einer psychoanalytischen Kreativitätstheorie. In: Kraft H (ed) Psychoanalyse, Kunst und Kreativität heute. Die Entwicklung der analytischen Kunstpsychologie seit Freud. DuMont, Cologne
Müller-Braunschweig H (1980) Gedanken zum Einfluß der frühen Mutter-Kind-Beziehung auf die Disposition zur psychosomatischen Erkrankung. Psychother Med Psychol 30: 84-59
Müller-Braunschweig H, Möhlen K (1980) Bericht über die stationäre Behandlung eines Patienten mit einem psychogenen Anfallsleiden unter besonderer Berücksichtigung der averbalen Therapieformen. Psyche (Stuttg) 12: 1073-1091
Müller-Braunschweig H, Müller-Braunschweig H, Korn H (1981) Zur therapeutischen Funktion der Mal- und Bewegungstherapie. Musik und Medizin 17: 51-62
Niederland WG (1967) Klinische Aspekte der Kreativität. Psyche (Stuttg) 26: 900-928
Rad M von (1983) Alexithymie. Springer, Berlin Heidelberg New York
Rapaport D, Gill MM (1959) The points of view and assumptions of metapsychology. Int J Psychoanal 40: 153-162
Reich W (1933) Charakteranalyse, Technik der Grundlagen. Selbstverlag, Berlin
Richter HE (1984) Sterbeangst und Destruktivität. Psyche (Stuttg) 38: 1105-1123
Richter HE, Beckmann D (1973) Herzneurose. Thieme, Stuttgart
Rosa KR, Rosa-Wolff LR (1976) Psychosomatische Selbstregulation. Hippokrates, Stuttgart
Ruitenbeek HM (1970) Die neuen Gruppentherapien. Klett, Stuttgart
Sandler J, Joffe WG (1969) Auf dem Wege zu einem Grundmodell der Psychoanalyse. Psyche (Stuttg) 23: 461
Schmidtbauer W (1985) Unter der Couch. (Review of JM Masson: Was hat man dir, du armes Kind, getan?) Psychol heute 1: 69-70
Schöttler C (1981) Zur Behandlungstechnik bei psychosomatisch schwer gestörten Patienten. Psyche (Stuttg) 2: 111-141
Schur M (1955) Zur Metapsychologie der Somatisierung. In: Overbeck G, Overbeck A (eds) Seelischer Konflikt - körperliche Leiden. Rowohlt, Reinbek
Spitz R (1960) Die Entstehung der ersten Objektbeziehungen, 2nd edn. Klett, Stuttgart
Stephanos S (1973) Analytisch-psychosomatische Therapie. Jb Psychoanal [Suppl 1]
Stolorow RD (1979) Psychosexuality and the representional world. Int J Psychoanal 60: 39-45
Stolze H (ed) Die konzentrative Bewegungstherapie. Mensch und Leben, Berlin
Uexküll T von (1963) Grundfragen der psychosomatischen Medizin. Rowohlt, Reinbek

Wangh M (1983) Narzissmus in unserer Zeit. Psyche (Stuttg) 37: 16–40
Weiner H (1979) Psychobiology and human disease. Elsevier, New York
Wesiak W (1977) Einführung in die Psychosomatische Medizin. In: Loch W (ed) Die Krankheitslehre der Psychoanalyse, 3rd edn. Hirzel, Stuttgart
Winnicott PW (1953) Transitional objects and transitional phenomena. Int J Psychoanal 34: 89–97
Winnicott DW (1971) Playing and reality. Tavistock, London

Body Schema and Body Self

P. Joraschky

Terminology

I cannot exactly say that I have a body, but the mysterious link which unites me with my body is the root of my whole potential. The more I am my body, the more of reality is available to me. Things only exist inasmuch as they are in contact with my body and are perceived by it.
Gabriel Marcel (1953)

The controversy about the interaction between 'being a body' and 'having a body' has lost none of its relevance today. The success of the natural-scientific approach in medicine has meant that especially the aspect of 'having a body' has been pushed into the foreground and the body has become increasingly isolated as an object of investigation, so that it has become necessary, in the words of Viktor von Weizsäcker (1947), to 'introduce the subject into medicine'. This began to be important when the removed, objectivist approach that had been productive in the scientific investigation of organic functions began to dominate the doctor's encounter with his patients and increasingly to alienate him from them. In the 1950s, the exponents of anthropological medicine and phenomenology felt the time had come to call attention back to the most natural phenomenon of all, the wholeness of our bodies and our corporality. In recent years, interest in the body as the subject of all experience has markedly increased. More attention is being paid to the body as 'partner' (Eicke 1973). Listening to our body, being more aware of it, sensing it more fully, asking whether it is ready to go along with psychosocial changes or not - all these things have become the concern of many therapeutic techniques nowadays.

The ambiguous position of the body as both subject and object of experience has given rise not only to the age-old philosophical issue of 'being a body' vs. 'having a body', but also to a state of conceptual and terminological confusion. In the German language one comes across expressions such as *'Körperschema'*, *'Körperbewußtsein'*, *'Körperbild'*, *'Körperfühlbild'*, *'Körper-Ich'* or *'Körper-Selbst'*. In English the terminology is even more confused; it is not uncommon to encounter several terms being used interchangeably in the same article. Here we find the concepts 'body image', 'body schema', 'postural model', 'corporeal awareness', 'body percept', 'body concept', 'somatopsyche', 'somatognosy', 'body experience', 'body ego'.

The attempt will be made below to take various different concepts which may be seen as separate facets of the general conception of 'corporality', considering each with regard to its own conceptual plane, and so to arrive at a series of definitions. This will be supplemented by brief reference to some empirical approaches to research on the aspects in question (for a more detailed review, see Joraschky 1983).

The Phenomenology of Corporality

The human being is the subject and object of every anthropology. This unique paradox has its parallel in the concept of corporality as an integral part of the self, as opposed to the body as an object among other objects. For the phenomenologist, the body is *my* body in the sense that it is simultaneously the body which I possess and the body which I am. My body as an object is set apart from all other objects through the special relationship it has with myself, as is demonstrated, for example, in the concept of 'the perceiving-perceived body' (Ricoeur 1965). Merleau-Ponty (1945) has attempted to conceptualize this double aspect in the term 'ambiguité'. Taking up the line of the French phenomenologists Marcel (1953), Sartre 1943) and Merleau-Ponty (1945), who first made us aware of the relevance of our bodies for the way in which we experience the world and come to terms with it, Buytendijk (1967) has also stressed the significance of corporality for our experience of our environment. Blankenburg (1983) draws together the threads which were identified and elaborated by the phenomenologists when he describes the body as: centre of orientation in our perception of our environment, focus of subjective experience, field of reference for subjective feelings, organ of expression and articulatory node between the self and the environment.

The special contribution of the phenomenologists lies in their emphasis on wholeness; they exercise a necessary integrative function, since an approach involving the investigation of parts is in constant danger of losing sight of the whole. On the other hand, many of their statements remain very general. However much we may strive to seek and live out the immediacy of our environmental experience, which was the concern of the phenomenologists, it can never be the same for the adult (for example) as it once was for the child. For the adult, abstract thinking has become second nature, so to speak: we live and think primarily in the subject-object dichotomy. We are more likely to come closer to the ambiguity of 'being a body' and 'having a body' if we review the different functional ranges covered by each of these two aspects.

Body Schema

Historical Review of the Concept of Body Schema

As early as the end of the last century neurologists observed bizarre body percepts in patients with brain lesions. In keeping with the clinical approach, they attempted to group these into a systematic symptomatology under one main heading. The main research in this field goes back to Head and Holmes (1911), Pick (1908, 1915) and the Vienna School (Hoff and Schilder 1927; Engerth; Gerstmann 1924; Schilder 1923, 1935; Pötzl).

The use of the term 'schema' in connection with the investigation of physical disorders was introduced by Bonnier (1905). He uses the term 'coenesthaesia' to describe the body percept which arises out of the integration of various sensory impressions from the muscles, joints and skin. He draws particular attention to the spatial quality of corporality, which had been the concern especially of Munk (1890) before him.

The basic neurophysiological studies and experiments were carried out by Head, who worked his findings into a theory which is still of interest today. In cooperation with Holmes he developed the concept of *postural schema* (Head and Holmes 1911). Head not only described the marked disturbances in body perception occurring as a result of some cerebral lesions, but also developed a model and frame of reference for normal body perception which particularly stressed the importance of the postural schema for body posture and spatial orientation. On the basis of their investigations the authors postulated a central representation that served as a 'standard' for the integration of sensory stimuli. The patterns formed by sensory and kinaesthetic representations they called 'schemata', which they conceptualized as a series of dynamic functional principles. These are constantly reorganizing themselves according to the continually changing afferences, and yet are also predetermined. For Head and Holmes they were a priori existent in the form of a potential sensitivity to touch before the first touch, a capacity for movement before the first move.

The term *body schema* was introduced by Pick (1908), who stressed that there are 'several body schemata for every sensory quality of the body'. Pick speaks of the body as having 'spatial images' that develop in the course of one's life on the basis of sensory information and uses this concept to explain certain clinical observations, especially phantom limbs and body-schema disorders. In the 1920s there followed a wave of descriptions of such disturbances, which were so varied that the first priority was their classification. It was Schilder (1923) who first recognized that in connection with the issue of disturbed body perception the experiential aspect of corporality should not to be excluded - with the result that neurophysiological aspects, i.e. problems of central localization, became confused with the issue of body experience. The final consequence was that the term *body image* - which had been introduced by Schilder (1935) and soon became popular especially in the American literature - came to be used in a far broader sense than its original definition as the content of Heads schema, so that by now it embraces all subjective body experience as well as the whole issue of the role of corporality in our experience of the outside world. The concept of 'image' has not so much the meaning of a 'picture', but was intended by Schilder rather to come closer to the Freudian concept of 'imago', i.e. it was expressly intended also to include the unconscious contents of body experience. One consequence of this was that a whole series of very different and still unclarified functions all came to be subsumed under one collective term, which is especially noticeable in the investigation of the so-called body schema disorders, earlier known as 'aschematia'.

Body Schema Disorders

A great variety of disturbances in body perception occur in connection with lesions, particularly in the parietal cortex. These perception defects are unsystematic and frequently transient: e.g. the wrong name is given for a part of the body or the wrong word for a position on the body.

Under the influence of the clinical approach the early authors did their best to order and describe various syndromes, inventing such terms as 'autotopagnosia' (coined in 1908 by Pick to describe some patients inability to localize and name parts of their own body), 'finger agnosia' and 'prosopagnosia', which was Gerstmans term (1924) for an inability to perceive faces correctly. Further disturbances included right-left disorientation with respect to ones own body, and 'anosognosia', which refers to the phenomenon of a patient disregarding or refusing to accept the impairment or disappearance of a bodily function or performance, especially common in hemiplegia.

Following these initial descriptions, clinical neurologists concentrated on discovering further body-related disorders. In the process, the name 'body schema' soon came to be seen as a collective term for a whole variety of clinical symptoms, so that it ultimately amounted to nothing more than a common denominator which indicated that they all in some way had to do with the human body and body perception. Thus there were soon subsumed under the general heading 'aschematia' such varied phenomena as phantom limbs, anosognosia, pain asymbolia and autoscopy (the illusion of seeing ones own double), as well as psychiatric disorders (see the review by Frederiks 1969), making the construct still more heterogeneous.

Closer neuropsychological investigations revealed that such disturbances in perception are linked up with particular methods of investigation or situations and that most of them are in fact specific manifestations of more general neuropsychological insufficiencies. Any hopes that the study of severe perceptional disorders would lead to conclusions as to the normal functioning of the body schema have not been fulfilled. Nevertheless, recent studies have brought to light interesting connections between disturbances in perceiving ones own body and environmental perception; thus, right-left disorientation is manifested both in poor body orientation and in defective perception of the environment. The more generalized cognitive defects that have been discovered include such things as problems with localization in general or difficulties in identifying the parts out of a whole and perceiving complex structures, as is required for facial perception, for example.

The complexity of interacting factors that is to be found on different levels of organization can best be illustrated through the example of the *phantom limb*. The phantom limb, i.e. the continued perception of a nonexistent or deafferentated extremity, is generally regarded as the most conspicuous evidence of the existence and functioning of a body schema. As a natural consequence of having an extremity amputated, patients always perceive a phantom limb for a longer or shorter period of time. This perceptual phenomenon may be seen as a classic example by which to demonstrate the various planes which are important to the concept of body schema (cf. Joraschky 1983):

a) The amputation involves a complete severance of all the normal afferences, i.e. not just the tactile but also the postural and above all kinesthetic impulses. The effect of the subsequent sensory deprivation is particularly stressed by the 'peripheral theories' of the phenomenon, the evidence for which is based above all on electrophysiological processes at the cut surface and on the additional influence that neuroma formation, wound infection, etc., can have on the phantom and its development.
b) Neurophysiological hypotheses suggest that the absence of normal afferences brings about spontaneous cortical activity, causing the body percept to persist in consciousness. The abnormal peripheral stimuli can alter the experience of the phantom, which is why it is initially sensed more acutely than the remaining extremity; 'sensory attention' (Frederiks 1969) has been affected. Body perception is, however, an integrative achievement of the central nervous system and linked to cortical structures.
c) The individual nature, above all, of the phantom sensation, the phantom pain and its involution or persistence reveals the significance of individual psychological factors. Investigations involving patients with phantom pain and persisting phantoms, in particular, bring out the importance of the manner in which the patient responds to the loss of the limb on a psychic level. Here we find parallels to working through a loss after bereavement and the wish to reinstate the body's integrity. This process, however, must be considered separately from the actual perception of the phantom limb, which is related to the body schema on the level of the central nervous system.

In summary, we may say that the phantom limb is a product of perceptual processes that regularly occurs after the amputation of an extremity, due to the tendency of the neurophysiological body schema not to adjust to the change immediately but rather to persist in its old form for a certain time. The close link between subjective body experience and the central processing of information coming from the body, with the resulting perception of a phantom limb, comes out clearly in the variability between patients with regard to their manner of working through the phantom.

The various facets of the spatial regulation of body posture, of orientation and of body perception can be considered on different levels, discussed in the sections which now follow.

Principles Underlying the Neurophysiological Regulation of Body Schema

Information concerning our own body - the location of its limbs, the balance of tension between its muscles, its spatial position - comes to us from organs which do not belong to the classical 'five senses' and whose functional homogeneity is expressed through no single composite term: the postural receptors in and on the joints and vertebrae, the tonicity receptors in the tendons, the muscle spindles and the vestibular apparatus. In the terminology of sensory physiology one can speak of the senses of posture and position, of kinaesthesia and of the 'somaesthetic sense' as a collective term for deep and superficial sensibility (Nafe and Kenshalo 1966).

The multisensory coordination which results in unified perception comes about through the central integration of sensory messages. Even a simple tactile sensation involves a complex multisensory integration of pressure, temperature and positional afferences with sensori-motor muscular coordination, the final result being the sensation of touching as an experiential unit. For central integration, the thalamus and parietal cortex (Critchley 1953) play a central role. Hypotheses as to how this body schema is able to function in the central nervous system as a regulatory principle for achieving spatial posture and orientation have already been put forward by Hoff and Schilder (1927). This is best imagined as a system of spatial co-ordinates which first of all establishes the position of the main axis of the limbs taken as a whole; from this the spatial locations of individual postures or attitudes are derived as secondary processes.

Starting from the problem of body orientation, the feedback mechanism theory was developed, which has since become a basic paradigm in cybernetics. In connection with the historical background of the concept of body schema it is worth noting the particular part played by the principle of the *'Funktionskreis'* (literally: functional circuit) postulated by J. von Uexküll (1920) and the *'Gestaltkreis'* (Gestalt circuit; V. von Weizsäcker 1947) as well as Holst and Mittelstaedt's 'reafference principle' (1950).

Control-system models have since proved useful especially in explaining simple movement patterns. Such schemata include, for example, walking movements, which involve the organization of the simplest reflex in the spinal cord, via preconditioned behaviour schemata with instinctive regulation in the brain stem, right up to the co-ordination of finely regulated voluntary movements in the motor cortex, where higher-order movement schemata are adjusted to the environmental conditions and hierarchically ordered. So far, only lower-order motor patterns can be represented in control-system block diagrams. The simultaneous and automatic heterosensory co-ordination of body perception brings about 'recognition and memory, with the arousal of feelings and their comparison with earlier experiences' (Jung 1972 - all higher psychic accomplishments which take us into the field of the psychological theories.

Body Schema and Spatial Orientation

In the psychology of perception the problem of spatial orientation is considered from an 'egocentric' and an 'exocentric' viewpoint (Bischof 1966), which can be well related to the functions of 'being a body' and 'having a body'. In conceptualizing perceptual space one can distinguish between an evidential and a functional structure: in the evidential (phenomenal-spatial) system of reference, the naive observer's access to perceptual space is based upon the structure of his experiential reality (subjective, egocentric), whilst the functional system is concerned with the psychological laws determining the mental content of 'space'.

a) In the *phenomenal-evidential system of reference* we relate our environment to ourselves and experience it as being pervaded by our own corporality. This perceptual space is not a neutral stage for our actions and movements but rather a subjective one. It presents itself differently to every individual at every stage of their life. The phenomenologists (Dürckheim 1932; Bollnow 1963) have described the evidential structure of perceptual space as the *gelebte Welt* (the world as we live it).

b) The term *functional orientation in space* refers to the way in which we can localize and move our bodies according to spatial laws. Spatial orientation is achieved with astounding precision. The organism responds not only to afferences but is simultaneously receiving reafferences from its own actions. The working diagram of a feedback control system characterizes such processes. This self-regulated feedback mechanism abolishes all notions of the perceptive and motor aspects of orientation working independently. The organization of perceptual space is founded upon the motor systems involved in spatial orientation and cannot possibly be understood without these: positional and postural sensations, superficial sensibility and visual impressions form a spatial model of our body. In building up its perceptual world the organism can 'rely' on certain 'expected' regularities (redundancies) in the physical world (Köhler 1961).

Important contributions to describing the active communication between a perceiving subject and its perceived world in terms of a dynamic process have been made by the tonus theories (Goldstein 1934; Werner and Wappner 1949). According to Gibson (1973) the alternation between active and passive readjustment, between changed and changing situations, constitutes the basic process in orientation. Orientating motion enables the sense organs to pick out existent environmental stimuli, whereby the human organism is capable, in Gibsons view, of identifying invariant elements in a stimulus situation by using higher-order parameters such as relative intensities and stimulus proportions, which are unchanging. This enables us to achieve a perceptive performance that is relatively independent of environmental factors.

Spatial orientation can be described from the level of simple movement schemata right up to complex co-ordination and control of spatial and environmental schemata by the subject. In the process, the schemata can be called up unconsciously and automatically compared and co-ordinated with one another. This capacity for exocentric positioning allows us to orientate ourselves as an object among objects in our environment.

Perception of the Body as Object

Research in the psychology of perception is concerned with processes - how the body is perceived in comparison with other objects in the environment - and with structures - to what extent conscious information about bodily dimensions corresponds with the physical facts. The main focus of interest is on the issue of *perceptual constancy:* how far do we perceive our bodies as being invariant in comparison with objects in the environment? In evaluating the results of psychological studies on body perception it is important to take into account the method applied in each case, as the results are influenced to varying degrees by situational, motivational, affective and other factors. For the formalist question of how far body perception corresponds to the objective physical-spatial facts, the *linear method* is most suitable. With this method, the subject is asked to estimate the distance, in a straight line, between two points on the body as defined by a suitable stimulus instrument; the stimulus distance is estimated on a measuring scale projected onto a screen. Using this method, a great many studies (reviewed in Shontz 1969) found constant differences between body perception and object perception: a regular finding is that subjects overestimate the breadth of their head and the length of their forearm and underestimate the length of their hands and feet. In interpreting the so-called body perception disorders, as in anorexia nervosa, it is important to ascertain whether the method applied has also included subjective body experience or whether a maximally objective, impersonal perception of body dimensions has been measured. Under redundant stimulus conditions one finds - even among schizophrenics with the most bizarre disturbances in body experience - a constancy of body perception as long as it is viewed as an object (Weckowicz and Sommer 1960). This particularly striking discrepancy between body experience and the precision of body perception is in principle not so surprising when one considers that in schizophrenia the cognitive functions are not as a rule subject to specific disturbances. This is just an illustration to show that it is useful to distinguish between studies in the psychology of perception and methods which aim specifically at investigating body experience. Thus the body schema, which is interpreted by perception psychologists as a cognitive structure, operates under natural stimulus conditions (i.e. with redundant information) on the whole very precisely when compared with object perception, in spite of the discrepancies mentioned above.

Relationship Between Body Experience and Body Perception

The constancy of body perception, the body schema as a cognitive structure, enables us to rely on our body as an object among objects. The body's spatial orientation goes on 'automatically'; our awareness of our bodies is only 'peripheral' (Frederiks 1969), i.e. self-experience and body experience are inseparably interrelated, they are regulated unconsciously and they only enter our consciousness under special circumstances (pain, joy, external influences etc.). The relationship between body experience and body perception is regarded by the phenomenologists as immediate, whereas perception psychologists assume the two to be dissociated. This discrepancy can best be explained when one views the relationship in question against the background of psychogenetic maturation.

Association and Separation Between Body Experience and Body Perception as a Developmental Process

The detailed studies on the development of motor activity and the construction of environmental schemata by Piaget (1969, 1979) were an important contribution to clarifying the role played by the body schema in the construction of reality. Piaget showed how the simplest movement and perception patterns develop progressively via primitive schemata with which the handling and manipulation of objects is practised, until they finally lead to whole action sequences. As he describes it, the gradual transition from subjective, body-centred activity to a logic of action occurs in the following manner.

To begin with, the child's point of reference, the centre of its field of action, is its own body. As it learns to orientate itself by means of its body, its ability to perceive its environment also becomes organized. As long as its perception is centred on its own bodily activity, the infant's subjective space, which is parcelled up according to sensory qualities, predominates - until finally, at the end of the 1st year of life, its oral, tactile, visual, auditory and postural perceptual fields become coordinated. Piaget shows how the various body-centred perceptual fields finally become joined up into larger groups and how, from the age of about 4 onwards, following the principles of the topological distribution of space with its categories of closure and association, the development of spatial-geometric relationships becomes possible, bringing with it the ability to distingusih clearly between self and object. Egocentric, body-oriented perception draws to a close around the age of 6 or 7 years, as the dimensions front-back, up-down and right-left become stabilized. But only at the age of 12 or 13 years is it possible for the child to leave the egocentric standpoint forever, to give up its body as the point of reference and to see itself in space from another's point of view as well.

Simultaneously included in this process of integrating the child's body-centred perceptual fields and 'body zones' is the development of mental distance. Taking the development of the child's animistic view of the world as an example, we can clearly see how the 'living space' with its permeable boundaries becomes little by little, and within the framework of increasingly stabilized body boundaries, a more removed, impersonal field for action.

Piaget describes structures and the continuity of structures where researchers before him had at best seen a sequential accumulation of elements of knowledge. He demonstrates how schemata are formed and organized in a series of stages and shows how, through redundant information, the object acquires substantiality in the eyes of the child and finally, through the child's own active repetition, attains 'practical permanence'. In connection with the formation of the permanent object, the child learns to distinguish between the recognized thing and the recognizing subject. This subject-object distinction is of vital importance for both cognitive and affective development (which in psychoanalytical theory is related to the development of the body self).

We cannot concern ourselves here with details of the developmental process and comparisons between affective and cognitive development, but it is important to take note of how, in individual stages, first of all processes related to the child's body experience develop in direct association with its experience of its surroundings and secondly, in a parallel process, the cognitive development of its body as an object progresses as well. Both developmental processes are equally relevant, both for the child's experience of itself as subject and for its perception of objects. A mature, successful development is defined through the capacity to assess objects in a clear and removed manner and the ability to centre on one's own experience when necessary. This is demonstrated by empirical studies on field dependence and independence.

Psychological Experiments on the Relationship Between Body Experience and Body Perception

The influence of personality variables on perceptual constancy has been investigated using methods which try to eliminate cognitive controls. Such methods include drawing tests, such as the Draw-a-person test (Goodenough 1962), investigations with distorting lens systems or tachistoscopic presentations of parts of the body, presentations of parts of the body on photographs (Secord and Jourard 1953), construction tasks using parts of photographs (Gellert 1975) etc. Most well-known of all are the studies by Wapner (1965), Witkin (1973) and Witkin et al. (1962).

In their famous perception studies on field dependence, Witkin et al. (1962) and Witkin (1973) are concerned with developmental aspects of the capacity for psychic distance. They describe how the infant's initially diffuse body boundaries become stabilized in accordance with the 'successive articulation of the body schema', whereby 'field independence' is defined as the achievement of sufficiently stable body boundaries. In analogy to this 'articulation' of the body boundaries, Bain (1973) speaks of 'decreasing participation' until mature 'body flexibility' is finally established. This latter term refers to the oscillation between subjective and objective perception, the freedom to 'open oneself' at the same time as possessing a stable capacity for maintaining mental distance. 'Body flexibility' has been the subject of various experiments by perception psychologists.

With adults it is possible to study the influence of personality variables on perceptual constancy by eliminating redundant information. In his most famous series of experiments Witkin placed his subjects in a dark room on a tilting chair in order to find out, when they were asked to set a rod on the vertical plane, how far they orientated themselves according to signals from their own bodies, i.e. bodily sensations of position, and to what extent they were influenced by stimuli from their surroundings. Subjects who are strongly influenced by their surroundings are assumed to be field-dependent whilst those who are more able to orientate on the basis of their body experience are considered to be field-independent.

Witkin attaches great importance to the role of body experience in the development of body boundaries and the articulation of environmental perception. As evidence to support his ideas on the central significance of body experience for the development of psychic distance as a cognitive style, Witkin draws upon the fact that influences on body experience, the stimulation of body boundaries and the concentration on external or internal body signals all have their effect on the individual's capacity for demarcation from the environment.

In summary, it may be said that the integration of the sensori-motor system and of spatial orientation can be seen as a function of the body schema. The body as an object of perception has a stable perceptual structure which makes possible its use as a 'tool' in action sequences and as an object in spatial perception. The emotionally coloured processes related to dependence and independence can be seen within the framework of self-object differentiation, whereby the formation of a coherent body self and the stability of body boundaries are critical parameters in the individual's interaction with the environment. The integration of processes based on body experience into a coherent structure with clearly developed boundaries has been followed most closely by psychoanalysis, which has set it, under the rubric of 'body self', in a metapsychological context.

The Body Self

In connection with the concept of 'being a body', the phenomenologists have drawn attention above all to the body's role as the focus of self experience and as articulatory node between the individual and environment (Blankenburg 1983). In psychoanalytical terms, the issue is that of the relationship between body experience and self-awareness or, viewed metapsychologically, of the structure of the body self and the demarcation between body and environment, defined as the separation of the representation of self from object representations.

Structure of the Body Self

Classical instinct theory in psychoanalysis represented the first attempt ever made to develop a dynamic theory of human behaviour based upon bodily needs. Particularly Freud's concept of the erotogenic zones and the role of the id in his structural model (1923), both of which are closely bound up with his instinct model, are relevant in this connection. Even in his repeatedly revised versions, Freud's own descriptions of the id remain imprecise and contradictory. At one point he talks of it as a sort of energy reservoir, understanding it in this sense as unchangeable, whilst at another he sees it, in connection with the psychosexual phases, as being subject to a process of maturation. Ego psychology offers no solution to these contradictions either; on the contrary, A. Freud (1968) stresses the constancy of the id and regards the chances of changing the individual's instinct structure as slight.

The model of the phases of the libido describes how the different erotogenic zones successively take their place as the focus of experience and how they are gradually integrated into a structure. In contrast to Piaget's permanent object (1969), this structure is more readily reversed and moulded, which constitutes the basis for the functional principles of fixation and regression. For this structure Freud invented no special term, but it is seen above all as being relevant for the development of self-constancy.

Within the framework of his structural model Freud (1923) assumed the 'body ego' to exercise an important function, particularly during the early stages of development: 'The ego is first and foremost a body ego.' However, Freud did not pursue this idea further and never drew a clear distinction between the body ego and the ego and ego functions.

Spiegel (1959) points out that the concept of 'self' in the theoretical terminology of psychoanalysis only became popular relatively late because for Freud the German word *Selbst* was, in meaning or at least as a name, synonymous with the everyday use of the word he chose for ego, *Ich* (literally; 'I'). In Freud's writings on the structural aspects of his theory, the ego appears in a contradictory light, applying both to individual functions and to the experiencing 'I', so that in many places the term 'ego' should really be replaced by 'self'. In contrast to the elements of Freud's structural theory the concept of self, like the concepts of personality and identity, has its origins in a system which has more to do with the observation of interpersonal interactions and the description of self-experience (cf. Thomä 1980).

A vital contribution to our understanding of the structure of the body self was made by the object-relations psychologists, who describe how the individual body, self- and object representations are formed against the background of specific interaction patterns within the mother-infant relationship. This manner of approach enables one to leave the frequently abstract models of ego psychology and come closer to directly observable phenomena. Concentration on the progressive development of those psychic functions which contribute to the development of psychic distance and autonomy easily makes one forget that even after the first 3 years of life, the body self (though no longer so much in the foreground) is still continually involved in the interaction of the self with its surroundings.

Unlike the id, the body self does not exist a priori but rather takes shape gradually as a developmental process in the course of the individual's interactions with the environment. The conceptualization of body self as a way of describing the organization of body zone representations goes back to the ideas of Glover (1956) and Erikson (1968) on the fundamental processes that take place in the interaction between self and object. In his model of the 'ego nuclei' Glover was the first to combine traditional aspects of instinct theory with the newer theses on ego development. According to this model, a system of 'multi-nuclear', discrete ego nuclei gradually fuses to form a coherent structure. Erikson in particular provided the framework for the theory on how 'nuclear cores for the development of identity' (Greenacre 1958), through the 'co-ordination of individual islands of the body', finally become formed into a 'coherent body image' (Linn 1955). This integration of ego nuclei happens during the interplay between self and object representations as part of a 'simultaneous bio-psycho-social event' (Loch 1971). The process whereby the body representations become integrated finally leads to a body self with an 'individual structure' corresponding to the self-representations, in which varying body zones dominate.

As to clinical relevance, it is only possible here to point to the importance of the structure of the body self in connection with disturbances in self-awareness. The partial body representations which are integrated into the sense of the self manifest themselves above all in severe regressive and disintegrative processes, as in psychoses, where a *fragmentation* on the unified sense of self and of body experience can occur.

Role of Body Experience in the Separation and Discrimination between Self and Environment

The model of the body-self boundaries provides a link with newer developmental lines in psychoanalytical theory. The body self as a model for the integration of the partial body representations proved to be closer to observable reality than the structural model. The same applies to the boundary concept in relation to the self concept. In its conception of self, psychoanalysis refers more closely to the models of psychological personality theory, in which the importance of demarcation processes is similarly stressed. In her developmental studies on the growth of body experience, beginning with the 'symbiotic membrane' and continuing via the 'inner-outer separation', Mahler, together with her colleagues (1978), elaborates the concept of body boundaries further.

Federn (1956) had already recognized the importance of flexible body boundaries in connection with the sense, and the regulation of the sense, of one's own value, but his conception is still closely linked to instinct theory. Nevertheless, his clinical approach and his analysis of severe boundary disorders in depersonalization states, in regressive phenomena and in psychoses made Federn an important influence on further research on disturbances in boundary regulation.

Work on the metapsychology of the body-self boundaries goes back to Jacobsen (1954) and Mahler (1968). Starting from the 'undifferentiated' stage, via the stage of 'nuclear identity' with its still diffuse body and object boundaries, the individual 'body-self nuclei' (Hoffer 1950) become fused and finally form the structure of the body self. However, such metapsychological constructs have yet to prove their worth for explaining clinical phenomena.

On the subject of clinical relevance, Schilder's (1935) and Federn's (1956) clinical and self-observations in particular led to important contributions on the flexibility of self boundaries, the fluctuation of self-awareness and boundary dynamics. They describe at length the variations in body-boundary experience which can accompany regressive phenomena like going to sleep, orgasm or mental illness, as well as the different patterns which are formed as individual body zones come to prominence in varying degrees in the course of self-experience. Boundary disorders manifest themselves in depersonalization experiences which simultaneously affect one's relations with one's own person, with one's body and with the environment. Here it is only possible to mention in passing modern research on the stability and flexibility of the body self and body boundaries in connection with psychoses, borderline syndromes and psychosomatic disorders (Scharfetter 1976; Joraschky 1983). This also includes studies on how pacemakers, organ substitutes and similar encroachments on bodily integrity (such as the introduction of an artificial anus, prostheses etc.) are integrated into the body self.

Psychometric Studies on Body Self and Body Boundaries

Since the 1950s, Fisher and Cleveland (1968; Fisher 1970, 1973) stand out among those who have worked hard on finding measures for the stability of body boundaries and the structure of the body self. After trying out all sorts of test procedures in a large number of studies on different boundary dimensions (drawing tests, various creative performance tests, thematic apperception tests, interviews), Fisher and Cleveland (1968) found that above all the dimensions relating to boundary and contour descriptions in the Rorschach test are capable of reflecting unconscious boundary articulations. They quantified boundary stability and permeability by means of barrier and penetration scores, which later became standard criteria in the Holtzman test (1961).

By investigating the direct effects of physical stimuli on Rorschach responses, Fisher demonstrated how outer or inner body stimulation could affect the barrier score. In this way he revealed the close link between body experience and the cognitive style of psychic distance. Patients with a high barrier score have a better capacity for adjustment and a higher stress tolerance. Fisher depicts firm body boundaries as 'buffers' against external stimuli, allowing the individual greater freedom for action. In a series of studies Fisher goes on to show that the location of diseases in the body reflect an outer-inner distribution; patients with high barrier scores often suffered from disorders affecting the outer regions of the body whilst those with a low barrier score tended to have more internal illnesses (e.g. breast cancer as compared with stomach and colonic cancer). Measures of physiological responsiveness also have their equivalents in such an inner-outer pattern (heart rate as opposed to skin resistance etc.).

Landis (1970) also used Rorschach cards to investigate the 'permeability' and 'impermeability' of body boundaries. Landis, however, sees the stability of body boundaries less in terms of polar dimensions than as various degrees of intensity within a continuum. This interpretation comes closer to the psychoanalytical theories on boundary dynamics than the rather more static interpretation by Fisher.

For investigating body-self structure Fisher has tried out various psychometric methods in recent years (1970, 1973). Using the 'Body Focus Questionnaire' he has attempted to pursue the question of how far it is possible, using empirical methods, to differentiate between individual body zones with respect to their varying prominence within the body self, with the ultimate aim of developing a 'body map' specific to each individual. The subjects are asked to give one response each time to alternative regions of the body, indicating which areas stand in the foreground of their own self-experience. The answers are subsequently categorized (front/back of body, heart, eyes, mouth, head and arms). By this means Fisher was able to demonstrate, for example, the close link between prominence of the back of the body and an anal character. Prominence of the back of the body in the test was associated with themes like anxiety about loss of control, avoidance of ridicule, defiance, negativism and expressions of hostility, as well as homosexuality. Direct stimulation of the back of the body led to a significant increase in memories of anal terms.

With a 'Body Prominence Index' Fisher measures 'global body experience' and with the 'Body Distortion Questionnaire' the nature and intensity of distorted body experience (principally for use with schizophrenics).

The results of psychometric studies so far support the approach which distinguishes between the structure of the body self and the dynamics of body boundaries. They offer promising beginnings to objectifying unconscious aspects of body experience with respect to the structure of the body self and to the quantitative assessment of the stability of the body-self boundaries.

In summary, one can say that this chapter has attempted to present on an abstract level the terms relating to body orientation, body perception and body experience and to clarify the concepts behind them. The concepts of 'body schema' and 'body self' were chosen as general headings, these being the most commonly used in the literature, and their very different scientific applications were discussed. Thus, 'body schema' refers to the neurophysiological aspects of body perception: its heterosensory processing, regulation by the central nervous system and cognitive structure (which is also known as 'body concept'). The term 'body self' applies to the regulation of body experience and our mental image of our bodies; the terms 'body image' and 'body ego' also belong here.

References

Bain BC (1973) Toward at theory of perception: Participation as a function of body-flexibility. J Gen Psychol 89: 157-296
Bischof N (1966) Psychophysik der Raumwahrnehmung. In: Metzger W (ed) Handbuch der Psychologie, vol 1. Hogrefe, Göttingen, pp 307-408
Blankenburg W (1983) Der Leib als Partner. Psychother Med Psychol 33: 206-212
Bollnow OF (1963) Mensch und Raum. Kohlhammer, Stuttgart
Bonnier B (1905) L'aschématie. Rev Neurol 13: 604-609
Buytendijk FJH (1967) Prolegomena einer anthropologischen Physiologie. Müller, Salzburg
Critchley M (1953) The parietal lobes. Arnold, London
Dürckheim Graf K (1932) Untersuchungen zum gelebten Raum. Neue Psychol Stud 6: 4
Eicke D (1973) Der Körper als Partner. Kindler, Munich
Erikson EH (1966) Identität und Lebenszyklus. Suhrkamp, Frankfurt
Federn P (1956) Ichpsychologie und die Psychosen. Klett, Stuttgart
Fisher S (1970) Body experience in fantasy and behavior. Appleton-Century-Crofts, New York
Fisher S (1973) The female orgasm. Allen Lane, London
Fisher S, Cleveland SE (1968) Body image and personality. (New revised edition). Dover, New York
Frederiks JAM (1969) Disorders of the body schema. In: Vinken PJ, Bruyn GW (eds) Handbook of clinical neurology, vol 4. North-Holland, Amsterdam
Freud A (1968) Wege und Irrwege in der Kinderentwicklung. Huber, Berne, and Klett, Stuttgart
Freud S (1923) Das Ich und das Es. Gesammelte Werke, vol 13. Fischer, Frankfurt
Gellert E (1975) Children's constructions of their self-images. Percept Mot Skills 40: 307-324
Gerstmann J (1924) Fingeragnosie: Eine umschriebene Störung der Orientierung am eigenen Körper. Wien Klin Wochenschr 37: 1010-1012
Gibson JJ (1973) Die Sinne und der Prozeß der Wahrnehmung. Huber, Berne
Glover E (1956) Grades of ego-differentationen. In Glover E (ed) On the early development of mind. Imago, New York
Goldstein K (1934) Der Aufbau des Organismus. Einführung in die Biologie. Unter besonderer Berücksichtigung der Erfahrung am kranken Menschen. Den Haag
Goodennough FL (1962) Measurement of intelligence by drawings. Harcourt, Brace & World, New York
Greenacre (1958) Early physical determinants in the development of the sense of identity. J Am Psychoanal Assoc 6: 612-627
Haynal A (1975) Freud and Piaget. Psyche (Stuttg) 29: 242-272
Head H, Holmes G (1911) Sensory disturbances from cerebral lesions. Brain 34: 102-254
Hoff H, Schilder P (1927) Die Lagerreflexe des Menschen. Springer, Vienna
Hoffer W (1950) Development of the body ego. Psychoanal Study Child 5: 18-23
Holst EV, Mittelstaedt H (1950) Das Reafferenzprinzip. Naturwissenschaften 464-476
Holt RR (1967) Beyond vitalism and mechanism: Freud's concept of psychic energy. In: Massermann HH (ed) The ego: Scientific proceedings of the American Academy of Psychoanalysis. Grune & Stratton, New York (Science and psychoanalysis, vol 11)
Holtzman WH, Thorpe JS, Swartz JD, Herron EW (1961) Inkblot perception and personality. University of Texas Press, Austin
Jacobson E (1954) The self and the object world. Psychoanal Study Child 9: 75-127
Joraschky P (1983) Das Körperschema und das Körper-Selbst als Regulationsprinzipien der Organismus-Umwelt-Interaktion. Minerva, Munich
Jung R (1972) Einführung in die Sinnesphysiologie. In: Jung R (ed): Somatische Sensibilität, Geruch und Geschmack, vol 11. Urban and Schwarzenberg, Munich
Kohler I (1961) Interne und externe Organisation in der Wahrnehmung. Psychol Beitr 6: 426
Kolb LC (1959) Disturbance of the body-image. In: Arieti S (ed) American handbook of psychiatry. Basic Books, New York, pp 749-769
Landis B (1970) Ego boundaries. Psychol Issues Monogr 24
Linn L (1955) Some developmental aspects of the body image. Int J Psychoanal 36: 36-42
Loch W (1971) Grundriß der Psychoanalytischen Theorie (Metapsychologie). In: Loch W (ed) Die Krankheitslehre der Psychoanalyse. Hirzel, Stuttgart

Mahler MS (1968) Symbiose und Individuation, vol 1. Psychosen im frühen Kindesalter. Klett, Stuttgart
Mahler MS, Pine F, Bergmann A (1978) Die psychische Geburt des Menschen. Fischer, Frankfurt
Marcel G (1953) Etre et avoir. Aubier, Paris
Merleau-Ponty M (1945) Phenomenologie de la perception. Gallinnard, Paris
Munk H (1890) Über die Funktionen der Großhirnrinde. Hirschwald, Berlin
Nafe JP, Kenshalo DR (1966) Somästhesie. In: Metzger W (ed) Handbuch der Psychologie, vol 1. Hogrefe, Göttingen, pp 221-249
Pankow G (1968) Gesprengte Fesseln der Psychose. Reinhardt, Munich
Piaget J (1969) Das Erwachen der Intelligenz beim Kinde. Klett, Stuttgart
Piaget J (1979) Der Aufbau der Wirklichkeit beim Kinde. Klett, Stuttgart
Pick A (1908) Über Störungen der Orientierung am eigenen Körper. Arb Dtsch Psychiatr Univ Klin Prag 1-19
Pick A (1915) Zur Pathologie des Bewußtseins vom eigenen Körper. Ein Beitrag aus der Kriegsmedizin. Neurol Centralbl 34: 257-265
Plügge H (1967) Der Mensch und sein Leib. Niemeyer, Tübingen
Poeck K, Orgass B (1971) The concept of the body schema: A critical review and some experimental results. Cortex 7: 254-277
Ricoeur P (1965) De l'interprétation. Essai sur Freud. Massan, Paris
Sartre J-P (1943) L'être et le néant. Gallinnard, Paris
Scharfetter C (1976) Allgemeine Psychopathologie. Thieme, Stuttgart
Schilder P (1923) Das Körperschema. Ein Beitrag zur Lehre vom Bewußtsein des eigenen Körpers. Springer, Berlin
Schilder P (1935) The image and appearance of the human body. Kegan Paul Trench Trubner, London
Secord PF, Jourard SL (1953) The appraisal of body cathexis: Body cathexis and the self. J Consult Psychol 17: 343-347
Shontz FC (1969) Perceptual and cognitive aspects of body experience. Academic, New York
Spiegel LA (1959) The self and perception. Psychoanal Study Child 14: 81-109
Thomä H (1980) Auf dem Weg zum Selbst. Bemerkungen zur psychoanalytischen Theorieentwicklung in den letzten Jahrzehnten. Psyche (Stuttg) 34: 221-245
Uexküll J von (1920) Theoretische Biologie. Paetel, Berlin
Wapner S (ed) (1965) The body percept. Random, New York
Weckowicz TE, Sommer R (1960) Body image and self-concept in schizophrenia. J Ment Sci 106: 17-39
Weizsäcker V von (1947) Der Gestaltkreis. Theorie der Einheit von Wahrnehmen und Bewegen, 3rd edn. Thieme, Stuttgart
Werner H, Wapner S (1949) Sensory-tonic field theory of perception. J Pers 18: 88-107
Witkin HA (1973) Psychologische Differenzierung und Formen der Pathologie. Psyche (Stuttg) 27: 555-593
Witkin HA, Zyk RB, Faterson HF, Goodenough DR, Karp SA (1962) Psychological differentation. Wiley, New York

Sensation and Perception of Pain

P. Bernhard

Pain is still widely viewed as being a somatic phenomenon (Cohn 1983), even though the subjectivity of pain perception is generally well known, as in, for example, the placebo effect, alleviation of pain by hypnotic suggestion or the discrepancy between pain complained of and observable body lesions (Reischauer 1957). In fact, it is still not clear whether pain is a symptom or an illness (Baar 1982).

'Feeling pain is often equated with "being sick" and pain is the main symptom that sends people to the doctor' (Adler 1975). Although research into somatic pain has greatly increased during the past few years, with interdisciplinary co-operation led by anaesthesiologists, there remains a conspicuous lack of research into psychosomatic interrelationships, even though it is precisely in the realm of pain perception that the body-mind unity is most apparent. An attempt to find an explanation for this leads to the hypothesis that even Freud hardly dealt with the topic of pain, although - or more likely because - he himself constantly suffered pain: from functional cardialgia, migraines and, after 1923, also from the effects of his jaw carcinoma. Consequently, research on pain perception also seems to have been unattractive or even taboo to subsequent generations of psychoanalysts (Berning 1980).

Pathophysiology of Pain

Pain perception is a complex psychophysiological event consisting of afferences with peripheral reception extending to central conception, localization and emotional colouring, and of efferences with central control mechanisms at the spinal level (Melzack 1970). Pain occurs as surface pain resulting from a trauma to the body surface, as deep pain largely from chemosensitive perivascular receptors, as conduction pain resulting from irritation in a region of sensitive nerve fibres, and as transmission pain resulting from the viscerocutaneous afferent connection with the corresponding Heads zones (Struppler 1975).

Afferent pain perception occurs at three synaptic junctions (Melzack 1970). At the first spinobulbar junction in the posterior horn of the spinal cord, diffuse pain can be felt as the result of the summation of a spatial and temporal convergence effect. Pain is first perceived in the second junction, in the brain stem with the thalamus. The local reaction becomes a total reaction, for example, podalgia results in escape behaviour. The cortex, the third junction, is where the pain is consciously perceived. The subjective evaluation of the pain as danger, for example, or as punishment, occurs via pain engrams from previous experience in an individuals life history and from sociocultural influences. Comparative measurements made among different ethnic groups have shown that, in spite of a constant objective pain sensation threshold, as far as subjective pain perception is concerned, there is definitely a lower threshold of pain tolerance among Italian and Jewish housewives than among American and Irish housewives (Sternbach and Tursky 1965). Sociocultural differences were also found in anthropological observations of women who perceive no pain when giving birth, but whose husbands lie in bed at the same time and moan with pain (Kröber 1948, quoted in Larbig 1982). Whereas 'pain sensation' with localization in time and space is attributed to the neospinothalamic tract of the subcortical pain path, the paleospinothalamic tract - because of its connection to the limbic system and the hypothalamus - is responsible for the 'feeling of pain' with its emotional colouring and torturous component of suffering (Hassler 1960).

By modulating the afferent pain impulses at the level of the spinal cord, the efferences of the brain cortex make possible the internal regulation of pain intensity by means of the gate control system described by Melzack (1970). An in vivo pain analysis of Greek firewalkers and Indian fakirs was made by Larbig (1982), who was able to show that a subcortical dissociation of the central nervous system from the motor activity brought about a trancelike state in which 'the brain is asleep and the body is awake.' As a result, the central process of becoming conscious of pain is inhibited and quantitative pain perception thus becomes a 'phenomenon of attentiveness' (Melzack 1970). These processes are suspected of playing a role in hypnosis, religious ecstasy and orgasm. It was said of Napoleons personal physician Larrey that he was able, during by amputations, to distract his patients to such an extent by constantly talking to them that they hardly complained of any pain.

In recent research Popp (1983) describes deoxyribonucleic acid photons from ultraweak electromagnetic waves with a control function in the cell nucleus. He proposes that the DNS photons use the pain system as a generalized psychosomatic alarm system to control and maintain all of the body functions.

Psychoanalytical Foundations

Psychoanalysis has dealt mainly with psychogenic pain. In this context pain is seen mainly as a somatic conversion product of repressed psychological conflicts. A pain symptom appears when the old repressed childhood conflicts are revived in a releasing conflict situation, resulting in the collapse of the fragile balance that has so far existed between drive impulse and defence (Freud 1915a, 1920, 1926).

Among the numerous models of the psychophysiological conversion of emotional pain into physical pain, a few of the major hypotheses will be considered in more detail. In his conversion theory, Freud (1894) describes the symbolic representation of repressed conflicts in the form of motor symptoms such as paralysis and also in terms of sensory symptoms such as pain. When pain arises in this manner, whole complexes of ideas are repressed from the consciousness and the affects associated with these thoughts are converted into pain. Symbolization and linguistic usage both draw upon this common source, giving rise to expressions like 'stabbed to the heart', 'a slap in the face'; here the notion of pain corresponds to an associative as well as a symbolic impairment of function (Berning 1980).

Fenichel (1964) differentiates between two types of conversion: if a painful functional disturbance in the experience of a child is associated with an emotional conflict that had to be repressed, then the conflict repeated later on as an adult can once again mobilize the painful functional disturbance; it is the childhood emotional conflicts, which remain repressed, that provide the drive energy for the conversion. On the other hand, if another person, by means of pain, receives the affection and attention that the patient also desires, then this pain is due to a 'hysterical identification' with the other person. Fenichel gives this example: 'Do you want to be just as happy as Mrs. X? All right, in order to achieve that, here is the punishment that she received.'

Engel (1959) describes states of psychogenic pain especially in 'pain-prone' patients. Having been raised strictly, these patients, whenever they feel intense aggressive or sexual impulses, tend to remember the pain - perceptibly and physically, as it were - that was once inflicted upon them in harsh punishment for having had such impulses (Kallinke 1981). Here, too, the forbidden impulse is expressed symbolically and associatively, and hence prevented. Schur (1974), Freuds personal physician, proposed that conflict resolution comes from a deep psychophysilogical reversion to an infantile level of body experience. He described the mechanism of a regression with simultaneous resomatization and desublimation of instinctive energy, which could lead in particular to extensive organ lesions.

In a later metapsychology of pain, Freud (1917, 1926) sees pain perception more as a pathological mourning reaction following object loss or separation. 'The transition from physical pain to emotional pain corresponds to the shift from narcissistic cathexis to object cathexis.' In psychogenic pain the necessarily highly cathected object image plays the role of that part of the body narcissistically cathected due to somatic pain. In both cases the same psychological helplessness is experienced (Berning 1980). This helplessness is taken a step further by Engel and Schmale (1967) and defined as a system: 'given up - giving up', helplessness and hopelessness. This generally psychosomatic theory is probably significant for pain perception as well.

'Normal' Pain Perception and its Significance

While pathopsychological pain processes delimit the biological scope for pain perception, psychoanalytical theories link the origin and development of pain with an unconscious emotional conflict. As far as the experience of pain as a whole is concerned, 'normal' pain perception with its manifold somatic and psychic meanings is informative.

According to Engel (1969), pain is 'a fundamentally unpleasant sensation that is attributed to the body and that corresponds to the suffering caused by the psychic perception of a real, impending or imagined injury'. Pain is an essential control and alarm system for somatic and psychic dangers that upset the emotional and physical balance, thereby endangering normal psychophysiological functioning. In contrast to the sensory organs, pain perception is nonspecific (Janzen 1966).

In the somatic realm, the syndrome of syringomyelia illustrates the danger of painlessness. When pain and temperature sensation are absent due to dissociated sensory immobilization, in spite of the presence of touch and deep sensibility, the patient will frequently suffer injuries and hot or cold burns.

The significance of pain to the individual is not innate, but must be learned so that he can form an engram (Carrière 1983). If these pain experiences are absent, for example, as in deprivation, the results are self-destructive behaviours. Work with dogs has shown that, after sensory deprivation, there is a delay before they withdraw their muzzles from a flame (Melzack and Scott 1957). Similarly, children of rejecting and punishing mothers can be observed to have an undifferentiated and reduced pain reaction (Witkin et al. 1962). In *Die psychische Geburt de Menschen,* Mahler et al. (1978) ascribe great intrapsychic and interactional significance to pain perception. Those first pain experiences are necessary for the body surface and organs of perception to be cathected (Freud 1923). During the stage of primary narcissism, the infant learns through negative sensations to differentiate between inside and outside and to perceive its body. The separation of subject and object is important for the establishment of a body schema and a body ego (Kernberg 1979). Heidegger (1953) saw pain as 'access to the ground-plan of existence' and, according to Gebsattel (1938, quoted by Janzen 1966), being helplessly delivered up to pain led 'to the division of ego and body.' Mahler et al. (1978) describe in the 'third subphase' a reconciliation crisis of the infant with the 'struggle for detachment and individuation ... Oral, anal, early genital compulsions and conflicts coincide and accumulate at this important crossroads of personality development ... The body schema and physical discomfort are perceived more intensely.' The fear of losing the love of the object leads to increased psychic and somatic vulnerability; physical sensations and discomforts are perceived more consciously Mahler et al. (1972). Conversely, Mahler et al. (1978) observed that children who are poorly individualized and fixed in a symbiotic relationship with their mothers are less sensitive to pain. Aside from the cathexis of the body, the intensity of pain depends on the individual and the sociocultural significance attached to pain. A great deal of attention increases the pain; distraction reduces it. Depending on the body image, more conscious, more visible and more superficial pain is felt to be easier to bear than invisible, unknown and deep pain (Carrière 1983). Pain makes it possible to turn an insoluble intrapsychic conflict into an interactional appeal for help, to turn distress beyond hope into an actual illness (Hallen 1956), with the possibility of medical help and human sympathy.

Due to our largely somatic-oriented health care system, physical pain acquires psychosocial significance. As quoted earlier, 'Feeling pain is often equated with "being sick"' (Adler 1975). 'The varying intensity of pain felt by different individuals is often viewed by the physician as an indication of the patients attitude, giving rise to judgements like "brave" or "complaining" ... Intensive pain is often classified as "imaginary"' (Delius 1975). Popper and Eccles (1977) point to the danger 'that we can be mistaken about the localization of pain. When someone says, my leg hurts, this can be a wrong "causal hypothesis", a "wrong diagnosis", even if I do feel the pain which I erroneously believe comes from an amputated leg.' Physical pain as a 'presentation symptom' (Balint 1984) becomes a dimension of the doctor-patient relationship. In its chronic form, pain makes it possible to receive human affection and sympathy, and in fact also allows regression along with relief from responsibilities and care in the form of early disability pensions. The expanded possibilities of pain alleviation in various specialized medical disciplines can create a new neediness based on the patients wish to relate to the doctor; this neediness changes the nature of the pain and the subjective pain perception through intensified organ cathexis (Freud 1926). Popper and Eccles (1977) suggest that toothache may have changed in intensity and quality since there have been dentists who can offer effective treatment against it. Thus pain perception becomes a psychophysiological process determined by a wide range of factors. Intrapsychically speaking, pain means cathexis and concentration of attention as possible ways to relativize or repress conflicts; interactionally speaking, pain provides a possibility for the patient to communicate by receiving medical care and human sympathy. Unlike pain perception in animals, who are governed by instinct, human pain perception can be modified by awareness, knowledge about illness, maturity, sociocultural experience and tradition (Janzen 1966).

Pain and Personality

As far as its pathophysiological course is concerned, pain is a specific phenomenon, whereas with respect to its manifestation, it is an unspecific psychophysiological phenomenon whose psychosomatic component varies, depending on its original cause, from psychogenic conversion pain to somatopsychic states of pain and to non-self-inflicted physical trauma. Pain perception is also modified by different individual conditions and causes, which is why in the final analysis pain perception is a question of personality. Engel (1959) describes a pain-prone personality who has sadomasochistic character traits, intropunitive tendencies and a strong inclination towards guilt feelings for whom the pain symptoms have become a means of communication. Conversely, there are also pain patients who cannot accept their role as a sick person.

Pain intensity also seems to be determined by inborn factors. Pain sensitivity measurements in the Libman test (Libman 1934) were able to distinguish three pain behaviour variants on the basis of different pain reactions to pressure on the styloid process. The hyposensitive pain patient usually goes to the doctor too late in case of a critical illness such as a heart attack, and, moreover, complains of atypical symptoms. In contrast to the normally sensitive person, the hypersensitive patient misleads the doctor into making the wrong somatic diagnoses and into labeling the patient as a hypochondriac. Hyposensitivity is assumed to play a role in 'asymptomatic myocardial ischaemia' and the 'silent heart attack.' In three methodically different pain tests, Droste and Roskamm (1983) and other authors found asymptomatic patients to have significantly higher pain thresholds and tolerance levels than did symptomatic patients with myocardial ischaemia. It seems that endorphins are responsible for the bodys own pain regulation, since after injection of the opiate antagonist naloxone, the angina pectoris pain reappears.

Many neurological pain phenomena cannot be explained neurophysiologically. The hypochondriac feels pain where there is 'nothing' while the seriously ill person can remain free of pain in spite of extensive organ damage Pain sensations can continue after damaged tissue has healed and can become a therapeutic problem, as for example in Ramsey Hunt syndrome (Kütemeyer and Masuhr 1981).

Cohn (1983) says that, in the present state of knowledge, there is no justification for speaking of a 'pain personality'. For each patient the individual psychich significance and the extent of the somatic limitations must be examined anew. Thus, the conflict specificity assumed by Alexander (1951) makes way for individual specificity. Physical pain often represents an effort to repair a psychic injury, to compensate for an inner loss or to solve an unconscious conflict, with the aim of self-healing (Beck 1981). The personality structures known since Freud seem to have certain similarities in their individual conflict backgrounds. This will be illustrated by means of actual clinical examples.

In neurotic depressive patients, loss of object or security seems to be the major problem. According to the theories put forward by Freud (1917, 1926) as well as by Engel and Schmale (1967), these patients fall ill upon the imagined, impending or actual loss of key persons to whom they are usually symbiotically attached. The physical pain become the equivalent of the emotional pain. The pathological mourning reaction results in a retreat to the body for 'processing the loss' (Beck 1981). Furthermore, it often - by way of the secondary gains derived from the illness - leads to regression involving being passively cared for. Moreover, the physical illness allows the ego to gain a new emotional experience. 'Passivity, self-awareness or experiencing the limits of self are qualities of feeling that are otherwise experienced primarily in object relationships' (Beck 1981).

A 50-year-old patient complained of headaches which resisted treatment despite interdisciplinary diagnostics and therapy and had led to his early retirement. He fell ill when he was left by his wife while he was away at a health spa and his only daughter, aged 18, found her first boyfriend. In psychotherapy, he gradually became aware of the repetition of the situation when, as a 2-year old illegitimate child, he had been deserted by his mother.

In a neurotic compulsive patient, the pain can be an expression of inner aggressive tenseness along with important rage. Physical tenseness as an expression of inner emotional tension might well be an important partial cause of a multifactorial phenomenon, especially in nonarticular rheumatism (Bernhard 1983). Here a vicious circle results from the fact that the most conversion neurotic myotenopathies secondarily lead to an increase in tenseness because they are so painful.

A 67-year-old retired technical college professor complained of severe leg pain that became even worse after a knee operation. He had been a competitive athlete and had climbed numerous high mountains, including in the Andes. His whole life was oriented towards achievement, which he demanded of himself as a prerequisite of being liked, just as relentlessly as his strict father had done in the past. He tried to cope with the waning of his strength by 'pulling himself together' and by filling the time he had on his hands after retirement by finishing his doctoral degree. When both of these efforts failed, his leg pain allowed him to 'slow down' so as to compensate for the conflict between his powerlessness and his need to prove himself.

The neurotic background of hysterical patients is as many-faceted and equivocal as the illness itself; conversion neurotic oedipal conflicts seem to predominate.

A 25-year-old student had slept in her parents' bed until her father had dies 2 years before; during the last years, intimacies had occurred such as her cancer-stricken fathers touching her breasts. After his death, she suffered inexplicable breast pains that made her continuously insist on medical examinations as an expression of her subconscious wish for repetition of that experience.

Borderline structures, due to the early defence mechanisms with exceedingly strong primeval aggressive and sexual drive impulses (Kernberg 1979), lead to phenomena that are hard to empathize with.

During psychotherapy, a 30-year-old patient had to jab herself in the arm with a pair of scissors whenever she experienced depersonalization fears, so as to 'feel that I still exist'. Psychodynamically speaking, she was making an attempt to reverse her intrapsychic division by trying to bring the pain she felt emotionally in her reality conflict back to a physical level so as to feel 'while' again.

In cases of narcissistic disturbances, a pain symptom mainly serves the purpose of 'self-repair' (Beck 1981).

After the subsequent defeat, a 40-year-old former Olympic gold medal winner in a track event developed a meniscus problem with severe knee pain of unknown origin. This forced him to end his career, thus sparing him any further disappointment. After attempts failed to retrain him in another field, the patient now receives a pension.

From the point of view of differential diagnostics, physical pain is hard to pinpoint in cases of masked depression, whereas coenaesthesic experiences in schizophrenic psychoses are easier to recognize because of the delusional interpretations of the patient.

What these largely psychosomatic pain conditions have in common is their integrative function for the self-image and for the disturbed object relationships. By means of the physical pain, neurotically altered emotional distress can be depicted in physically comprehensible terms as an attempt at self-healing and can be converted into an interactional process. Pain is particularly suitable for this purpose since no demonstrable lesion need be present and many specialized disciplines can be consulted diagnostically and therapeutically.

This is especially true of chronic psychogenic pain that - since it serves as an appeal - is not allowed to be 'cured'. The life histories of patients with chronic pain often reveal a constant fixation upon key persons, even after apparently final separation, because of the inability to come to terms with separation and mourning (Kütemeyer and Masuhr 1981). Somatopsychic pain states are symptoms which accompany almost all severe organ lesions. They are also influenced by the patients ability to adapt and to resolve psychic conflicts and are furthermore a crucial factor in the healing process. As long as a patient is not free of pain, he or she feels ill.

Pain and Feeling

Pain is involved in the development of body boundaries and in the formation of the body ego, the division of inside and outside and the feeling of 'being in the world'. Pain does not only report a physical threat, but it also, in case of object loss, makes possible a palpable reverse cathexis of the body as a replacement object and thus a chance of psychic self-healing. 'Unpleasant affects such as anxiety, fear, shame, guilt, aversion, anger and rage may occur in changes in the sphere of ones own body, e.g. during an illness, or in the sphere of the psyche, e.g. during a threatening fantasy or in an environment that confronts the person with a problem situation for which he has no ready-to-use program (Adler 1974). Physical pain and feelings are closely related to all three psychic structure systems: to id or drive impulses such as rage and aggression, to ego feelings like fear, and to superego feelings like guilt. The psyche, on a regressive level, seems to make use of the body through converted or resomatized drive energy (Freud 1894a; Schur 1974) in order to dissociate drive conflicts and fears from the intrapsychic interconnections.

Pain and Aggression

A connection has been established in the literature between forceful aggression and pain development, whereby the latter serves as a general mechanism for the overall repression of aggression (Cohn 1983). This has been repeatedly confirmed for tension symptoms such as, for example, nonarticular rheumatism (Alexander 1951; Beck 1971; Bernhard 1983). Freud (1924) describes the psychic mechanism of 'turning aggression against oneself', in which, because of the culturally enforced necessity of drive repression, the 'sadism of the superego and the masochism of the ego join forces'. In masochism, pain and lust join together such that pain and other feelings of discomfort are transferred to sexual excitement. This is reminiscent of the pain-prone personality described by Engel (1959). Inhibited and inward-directed aggression, guilt feelings and punishment wishes are assuaged and objectivized by the pain.

Pain and Fear

Fear seems to be especially closely linked to pain perception. Benedetti (1973) sees a parallel between pain and fear and cites Meyer-Holzapfel (1955): 'The nervous processes which form the basis of these reactions to threats and the accompanying subjective sensation of fear apparently have the same function in the psychic realm as pain does in the physical realm: they warn the organism of danger.' Fenichel (1946) also saw - particularly in psychogenically triggered painful muscle dystonia - an equivalent of fear. In neuro-anatomical and electrophysiological studies, it has been possible to demonstrate topographical interconnections between fear and pain centres and paths. Pain is seen in evolution as the developmentally older reaction form in the development of life; fear as the more recent reaction form, that of the psyche (Benedetti 1973). Davidson and MacDougall (1969) demonstrated in a clinical study of the correlation between pain and fear that 'the pressure (pain) tolerance and electroshock (pain) tolerance had a negative correlation to the manifest fear', in contrast to the case of pain from heat and cold where there is no correlation. They draw the conclusion that less fearful test subjects can withstand a stronger dose of electroshock and pressure pain. There is a clear correlation of fear and pain as a function of consciousness. Pain proves to be a 'phenomenon of attentiveness' (Melzack 1970). Fear in the form of anticipated fear 'intensifies harmless and perhaps even beneficial pain to a point where it becomes unbearable or even elicits a psycho-autonomic reaction (Carrière 1983): for example, a patients fear before an operation. Clinical studies have confirmed what experienced surgeons have observed: that informing patients about the operation reduces their fear (Bischoff and Luderer 1981).

While acute fear seems to reduce pain sensitivity, to the extreme point of insensitivity to pain in cases of wound shock (Carrière 1983), chronic fear increases it. In the form of exaggerated fearful worry about ones own body, hypochondria is an expression of highly differing syndromes, ranging from hysteria to psychosis.

There can be numerous causes of fear, such as the fear of bodily injury, fear of object loss of fear of guilt and punishment.

Pain and Guilt

Guilt and punishment in connection with the arbitrary aggressive impulses during the oppositional phase and the hurtful limitations set by the parents start a far-reaching pricess of conditioning beginning already in the anal phase of a childs development. In the form of punishment and expiation, the pain involved with unburdening guilt is usually an intrapsychic regulative mechanism aimed at maintaining or re-establishing the object relationship and the love of the object. Human beings prefer abuse to loneliness, prefer pain to depression.

The connection of pain perception to all of the psychic structure systems is made possible by fear. Drive impulses, reality requirements and the demands of the superego all mobilize fear which can make use of nonspecific pain symptoms as a more regressive solution option and which, once again, narcissistically cathects the body organ involved. The pain perception, however, is not identical to the pain that can be expected as the result of an objective body lesion. In the same way as 'signal fear' (Freud 1915b, 1926) serves as a defence against actual psychic danger, psychogenic fear can prevent an impending emotional crisis as well as psychosomatic organ lesion. The perception of pain, like fear, is essential for life and protects it. As Balint (1984) says, 'How much easier it would be for the doctor if cancer and hypertonia were painful'.

Summary

As a starting point, pain perception with its many determining aspects is developed from a pathophysiological and psychoanalytical point of view. 'Normal pain' is of use in the construction of the body ego and the recognition of impending danger. At the level of the individual, pain perception is closely related to fate and to personality structure. By means of an integrative function, physical pain, as a nonspecific somatic state of alarm, can represent emotional distress interactionally by converting it complementarily to physically palpable suffering. In this context, pain perception is closely related to feelings, including in particular aggression, fear and guilt.

References

Adler R (1974) Schmerz. In: Uexküll T v (ed) Lehrbuch der Psychosomatischen Medizin. Urban and Schwarzenberg, Munich, pp 489-508

Adler R (1975) Das Phänomen 'Schmerz'. In: Weintraub et al (eds) Psychosomatische Schmerzsyndrome des Bewegungsapparates. Schwabe, Basle, pp 1931-1942

Alexander F (1951) Psychosomatische Medizin. De Gruyter, Berlin

Baar HA (19982) Diskussionsbeitrag in: Fortschritt und Fortbildung in der Medizin. Deutscher Ärzte-Verlag, Cologne, p 316

Balint M (1984) Der Arzt, sein Patient und die Krankheit, 6th edn. Klett-Cotta, Stuttgart

Beck D (1971) Psychosomatische Aspekte des Weichteilrheumatismus. In: Beck D (ed) Fortbildungskurs Rheumatologie, vol 1: Der Weichteilrheumatismus. Karger, Basle, pp 168-177

Beck D (1981) Krankheit als Selbstheilung. Insel, Frankfurt

Benedetti IG (1973) Psyche und Biologie. Hippokrates, Stuttgart

Bernhard P (1983) Chronische funktionelle Schmerzzustände des Bewegungsapparates aus psychosomatischer Sicht. Therapiewoche 33: 3837-3843

Berning D (1980) Sigmund Freuds Ansichten über die Entstehung und Bedeutung des Schmerzes. Psychosom Med 26: 1-11

Bischoff C, Luderer HJ (1981) Arztverhalten, Schmerzerwartung und Schmerzwahrnehmung bei ärztlichen Eingriffen. Med Psychol 7: 1-26

Carrière B (1983) Schmerz. In: Luban-Plozza B et al (eds) Der Zugang zum psychosomatischen Denken. Springer, Berlin, pp 74-87

Cohn N (1983) Psychologische Faktoren und Prozesse bei der Entstehung und dem Verlauf von psychogenem Schmerz. Psychother Med Psychol 33: 13-19

Davidson PO, MacDougall CEA (1969) The generality of pain tolerance. J Psychosom Res 13: 83-89

Delius L (1975) Mehrdimensionale Beurteilung des sogenannten psychogenen Schmerzes. In: Weintraub et al (eds) Psychosomatische Schmerzsyndrome des Bewegungsapparates. Schwabe, Basle, pp 142-147

Droste C, Roskamm H (1983) Experimental pain measure in patient with asymptomatic myocardial ischemia. J Am Coll Cardiol 1/3: 940-945

Engel GN (1959) Psychogenic pain and the pain prone patient. Am J Med 26: 899-918

Engel GN (1969) Pain. In: MacBryed CM (ed) Symptoms and signs. Applied Physiology and clinical interpretation, 5th edn. Lippincott, Philadelphia

Engel LG, Schmale AH (1967) Psychoanalytic theory of somatic disorders. J Am Psychoanal Assoc 15: 344-365

Fenichel O (1946) The psychoanalytic theory of neurosis. Routledge & Kegan, London Henley

Freud S (1894) Die Abwehrneuropsychosen. Gesammelte Werke, vol 1. Fischer, Frankfurt, pp 59-74. Standard edn, vol 3, p 41

Freud S (1909) Bemerkungen über einen Fall von Zwangsneurose. Gesammelte Werke, vol 8. Fischer, Frankfurt, pp 381-383. Standard edn, vol 10, p 151

Freud S (1915a) Die Verdrängung. Gesammelte Werke, vol 10. Fischer, Frankfurt, p 256. Standard edn, vol 14, p 141

Freud S (1915b) Das Unbewußte. Gesammelte Werke, vol 10. Fischer, Frankfurt, p 282. Standard edn, vol 14, p 159

Freud S (1917) Trauer und Melancholie. Gesammelte Werke, vol 10. Fischer, Frankfurt, p 427-446. Standard edn, vol 14, p 237

Freud S (1920) Jenseits des Lustprinzips. Gesammelte Werke, vol 13, pp 28-30. Standard edn, vol 18

Freud S (1923) Das Ich und das Es. Gesammelte Werke, vol 13. Fischer, Frankfurt, pp 237-289. Standard edn, vol 19, p 1

Freud S (1924) Das ökonomische Problem des Masochismus. Gesammelte Werke, vol 13. Fischer, Frankfurt, pp 369-383. Standard edn, vol 19, p 155

Freud S (1926) Hemmung, Symptom und Angst. Gesammelte Werke, vol 14. Fischer, Frankfurt, pp 203-205. Standard edn, vol 20

Hallen O (1956) Zur biographischen Genese des Phantomschmerzes. Z Psychother Med Psychol 6: 3-7

Hassler R (1960) Die zentralen Systeme des Schmerzes. Acta Neurochir 8: 353-423
Janzen R (1966) Über den Schmerz. In: Janzen R (ed) Schmerzanalyse. Thieme, Stuttgart, p 1-8
Kallinke D (1981) Psychologische Ansätze zur Schmerzbekämpfung. Verh Dtsch Ges Rheumatol 7: 228-230
Kernberg OF (1979) Borderline-Störungen und pathologischer Narzissmus, 3rd edn. Suhrkamp, Frankfurt
Kütemeyer M, Masuhr KF (1981) Psychosomatische Aspekte in der Neurologie. In: Jores A (ed) Praktische Psychosomatik. Huber, Bern, pp 353-370
Larbig W (1982) Schmerz. Kohlhammer, Stuttgart
Libman E (1934) Observation of individual sensitiveness to pain. JAMA 102: 335-341
Mahler MS, Pein F, Bergman A (1972) Symbiose und Individuation, vol 1: Psychosen im frühen Kindesalter. Klett, Stuttgart
Mahler MS, Pein F, Bergman A (1978) Die psychische Geburt des Menschen. Fischer, Frankfurt
Melzack R (1970) Pain perception. Res Publ Assoc Nerv Ment Dis 48 242-285
Melzack R, Scott TT (1957) The effects of early experience on the response of pain. J Comp Physiol Psychol 50: 155
Meyer-Holzapfel M (1955) Unsicherheit und Gefahr im Leben höherer Tiere. Schweiz Z Psychol 14: 171-194
Popp FA (1983) Neure Horizonte in der Medizin. Haug, Heidelberg
Popper KR, Eccles JC (1977) The self and its brain. Springer, Berlin Heidelberg New York
Reischauer F (1957) Wirbelsäulen und Bandscheibenschäden. Therapiewoche 8: 130-139
Schur M (1974) Zur Metapsychologie der Somatisierung. In: Brede K (ed) Einführung in die psychosomatische Medizin. Athenäum-Fischer, Frankfurt
Sternbach RH, Tursky B (1965) Ethnic differences among housewifes in psychophysical and skin potential responses to electric shock. Psychophysiology 1: 241-246
Struppler A (1975) Pathophysiologie der Schmerzsyndrome des Bewegungsapparates. In: Weintraub et al (eds) Psychosomatische Schmerzsyndrome des Bewegungsapparates. Schwabe, Basle, pp 15-30
Witkin HA, Dyk RB, Faterson HF, Goodenough DR, Karp SA (1962) Psychological differentiation studies on development. Wiley, New York

Skin and Body Experience

U. Gieler

The Skin As 'Mirror Of The Soul'

'Love is the harmony of two souls and two epidermes' (A. Montagu 1980)

To report on body experience with particular reference to the skin actually means to talk about an individuals everyday experience. Without the protection of his epidermis, the human being is practically in capable of living. Thus, to reflect upon psychic influences on the surface of the body means to pay attention to an everyday event which individual human beings experience every moment of their lives, although unconsciously. However, it seems not so easy to become aware of ones own surface - the skin - let alone awake to ones feelings at the borderline of contact. And yet, who does not remember the comfortable feeling of tender touches, the relaxation when bathwater washes around the body, the tingling feeling under the shower, or the daily reflection of ones own physique in the mirror?

Freud (1923) writes in his essay 'Das Ich und das Es': 'The ego is ultimately derived from bodily sensations, chiefly from those springing from the surface of the body. It may thus be regarded as a mental projection of the surface of the body besides, as we have seen above, representing the superficies of the mental apparatus.'

The skin thersefore, not only filters external influences and makes them accessible to the interior of the body, but also acts as the representative of inner experience.

Montagu (1980) describes the significance of the skin for the development of the human being in much the same way as Freud writes about the external perception in the projection onto ones own body feeling. On the other hand, psychodermatologists (e.g. Obermayer 1970) are occupied rather with the centrifugal approach, namely the consequences of internal perception for the borderline of contact.

In psychotherapy with skin patients this splitting-off shows itself again and again when the patients 'shut out' their own body surfaces: they regard their skin as not belonging to themselves. Statements like 'Todays one of those days when can't stand my own skin' show this. Sometimes the therapist does not want to 'get under the skin' of a case; that is, he does not want to get too close to his patient. Psychic influences on the skin have often been described: just thinking of the sensation of cold gives practically everyone goose pimples. The skin, as a physical and psychic organ of contact, provides the borderline between the self and the environment. Nevertheless, it stays mainly concealed from consciousness, even if body-oriented psychotherapies are used. The 18000 cm^2, of skin per adult human being are exposed to various influences, namely temperature, pressure, atmospheric humidity and chemical substances, as well as psychic stimuli. We know the skin as a 'mirror of the soul' from various colloquial expressions: we 'blush for shame', our flesh 'creeps' when we are afraid, or we 'jung out of our skins' when startled. One could easily continue this list.

According to Borelli (1967) the skin as a psychic organ of reaction has five main functions in the development of the self:

1. Borderline organ between person and environment
2. Organ of contact with the environment
3. Sensory organ
4. Organ of impression (aesthetic point of view)
5. Organ of expression, facing the environment

There is surely no need to explain that the skin, together with the nervous system and the other sense organs, is numbered among the most important systems of communication between human beings and their environment. According to Jürgens (1978), the first impression given by the outward appearance of a human being determines the behaviour of others towards him or her. The human ego is formed personal body image, which is mainly derived from the perception of the surface (Panse 1970; Ringel 1960). The development of a consciousness of ones body is dated from the psychoanalytical point of view in the 6th-8th month of life (Mitscherlich 1983, quoted in Rechenberger 1983), and this is a stage at which tactile stimulation especially is of great importance.

Importance of Psychological Aspects of the Skin for Development of the Self

Since publication of the study by Harlow and Zimmermann (1959), the importance of tactile stimulation for the development of personality has been generally acknowledged. Harlow and Zimmermann proved that in rhesus monkeys, being warmed and touched by a dummy mother is more important for the young than a food-providing dummy made of wire. Montagu (1980) and Joraschky (1983) describe more experiments with animals, showing lack of tactile stimulation causes developmental retardation in the maturation of organs and affects the immune system.

These conclusions are completely transferable to humans. Solomon and Moos (1964) show how a childs immunity is strengthened by early stimulation of his skin; contact, touches and caresses provide a calming basic experience for a human being. Montagu (1980) reports that the introduction of 'mothering' of hospitalized American children lowered the death rate from 35% in 1939 to less than 10%.

Another well-known phenomenon is the so-called Kaspar-Hauser complex, an expression of defective contact and inadequate communication, including tactile.

Despendence on tactile stimulation is especially evident in blind people who lost their sight very early and thus lack a sense organ as a means of communication from childhood on; in particular, the case of Helen Keller (quoted in Joraschky 1983), who was blind, deaf and dumb, demonstrates the possibility of primary communication by means of skin contact. Conversely, therapy of seriously schizophrenic or autistic patients uses body contact as therapeutic communication (Maurer-Groeli 1975). Montagu (1980) also describes the influence of tactile stimulation on an embryo in the uterus: when the area about the upper lip or the side of the nose was caressed, the embryo, which was 2.5 cm long and 8 weeks old, reacted by retracting its neck and body. At this stage of development, neither eyes nor ears has yet developed as a further sense organ.

The skin is the first organ to develop in the embryo: at the very beginning, the ectoderm (outer germ layer) develops, and out of this the epidermis will be formed later. The close connections of the skin with the central nervous system result from the common development of both out of the ectoderm and from the 7-135 tactile corpuscles per square centimetre, and about 1.5 million sensitive nerve fibres from the papillae to the spinal cord. Recently, structures similar to synapses have been found even in the basal cell layer of the epidermis, which underlines this close association with neuronal processes. This explains why Brocq and Jacquet (1891) describe atopic dermatitis (one of the most frequent dermatoses) as neurodermatitis, although this term has since been proved inappropriate. Alexander (1971) numbers atopic dermatitis among the seven classical psychosomatic illnesses.

Giss et al. (1977) even suggest naming the first phase of human extrauterine development the 'dermal' phase, thus taking into account the special significance of the skin at this stage. Riemann (1969) calls this earliest period of development the 'sensory phase', and talks about the skin as a specific phase key organ, describing this phase as dominated by sensations which are at first objectless. Mahler (1968) calls it the 'symbiotic phase'. It is not surprising that those skin-diseases which begin early, such as the afore mentioned atopic dermatitis, are regarded from the psychosomatic point of view as so-called basic disorders in an early nonverbal phase of development (Rechenberger 1979; Schechter 1972; Thomä 1980).

Recently, prenatal aspects of psychosomatic symptoms have also been discussed (Hau and Schindler 1982); however, the question of premature births and skin diseases has not yet been investigated. G. Ammon and K. Ammon (1982) report on a female patient born prematurely who later developed cancer of the skin, and describe the early disorder with psychotic elements. In the postnatal phase, it is imperative that a child set up boundaries. Spitz (1957) speaks of a 'cavity mode of perception' which differenciates between inside and outside; a child has to learn about the differences between the inner and the outer world. Disorders at this preverbal stage of development, which often occur in the important first hours after birth, when skin contact is regarded as absolutely necessary, may manifest themselves in skin diseases. Early disorders with narcissistic problems, which occur by no means seldom in psychodermatology, point to ambivalent borderlines of the self; Marty (1969) describes this as pseudopsychosis. Pines (1980) showed that particularly the early interactions between mother and child have a decisive influence on object relations when she described the example of a child with atopic dermatitis. She demonstrated that the patient suffering from this disease experienced his skin not as a protection but as an object which made him itch, hurt, feed unwell, feel cold, and gave him a fever. These aspects show that early dermatoses in particular have an important influence on body feeling and body image. This becomes evident when people with skin diseases are asked to draw their body and its surface the result is usually; only a two-dimensional line drawing without sharp outlines (Rechenberger, 1983). Moreover, no sensory perception other than that of the skin provides an experience of the self as well as objective sense stimulation. In other words if one's skin is touched, one feels like a touched subject, too. Thus, being touched has a double character: by being fondled and caressed, a small child comes to differentiate between his own body-self and that which is not self. This shows the significance of the skin as sense organ for finding ones identity. Body and outer world are connected like drive and drive object. The body surface becomes the organ of self-perception.

Body Surface as Organ of Self-Perception

In addition to the developmental psychological aspects, there is evidence of the skins function as an organ which reacts psychosomatically. Schur (1980), who integrates psychosomatic disease into the context of self-development and sees it as a specific form of disorder of basic self-functions, supports this by giving the example of an atopic patient.

The skin is of double importance for the human body image. On the one hand, a somatic change can have a secondary effect on the personality: for instance facial scars resulting from an accident can cause disfigurement problems, as shown by Bosse and Hünecke (1980) and Teichmann and Bosse (1974). On the other hand, intrapsychic processes can manifest themselves through the skin; the most expressive example is provided by patients with factitious disorders or self-induced skin damage (van Moffaert 1983; Rechenberger 1976). The skin is the organ through which pain is first experienced, as well as tender touches. As a picture of our perception, the mirror shows us our relationship to our self. A female patient with acne once quoted a popular saying: 'Don't look into the mirror for too long, or you'll lose yourself.' Nearly all patients with skin diseases have an intensive contact with their mirror image; this may point to an early disorder in the perception of the borderlines of the self. A child who does not authentically experience the touches of his mother as tender or caressing undergoes from the beginning a psychic development which differs from that of a child with a sound skin, or an 'intact' surface. Later, close contact arouses an inner ambivalence which shows itself in the transference relationship with the therapist (Pines, 1980). Indeed the 'allergic object relation' described by Schur (1980) and others is nothing else but this ambivalence.

According to Paulus (1982), touching causes reductions personal distance, the private area known in esoteric cults as the aura. This area, which surrounds the person, is experienced as personal space belonging to the individual; when borderline disorders occur, the nearness of someone else is experienced as a threat, and aversions or somatic reactions can result. Thus, the unconscious function of acne or herpes labialis is often to bring about a distancing from the external world and to avoid body contact. The more or less direct relationship between psychic experience and the skin is described by many authors, but only some can be mentioned here. Probably the most widely known is the development of blisters under hypnosis or following hypnotic suggestion (Borelli 1967; Chertok 1978). The suppression of allergic reactions by hypnosis (Whitlock 1980), as well as stress, causes a reduction in the conductive resistance of the skin (quoted in Overbeck 1984), and so-called pseudosunburn can be triggered during hypnosis (Bellis, 1966). The influence of stress on the immune mechanism is also known with regard to herpes simplex (Leise et al. 1974; Teshima et al. 1983) and alopecia areata (Perini and Bettin 1983). Shanon (1970) demonstrated that survivors of concentration camps suffered from skin diseases more frequently than a comparable group.

The importance of the sensory perception of the skin as a cause of psychosomatic skin-disease symptoms was described by Vogel (1979); its influence on the body image has often been analysed (Shuster et al. 1979; Whitlock 1980). The study by Porter et al. (1980) of the psychosocial processes of vitiligo patients showed that those patients with a more stable ego caped with their disease more easily, and my own analyses of patients with atopic dermatitis confirmed this (Gieler et al. 1984). In addition, there are reports on burn scars and their effect on social acceptance (Molinaro 1978), on the body image of haemangioma patients (Kalick et al. 1981) on the importance of disfiguring skin diseases in social and preventive medicine (Uhlmann 1969). Even the influence of psychic mechanisms on the prognosis of malignant melanoma has been demonstrated (Rogentine et al. 1979; Temoshok et al. 1984). Hughes et al. (1983) are of the opinion that psychiatric diseases occur more frequently among skin patients than in the normal population.

Leichtmann et al. (1981) showed the consequences for the body image of the visibility of the skins abnormality. Similarily, Lux et al. (1983) described the nonacceptance of the female role by hirsute female patients; the independence of subjective stress and the physical findings in hirsutism was demonstrated by Strauss and Appelt in 1984. The latter analysis is the more impressive as it shows that psychic attitude and conflicts have an enormous effect on subjective emotional stress, and that neither purely somatic therapy nor visibly good morphological results guarantee subjective improvement.

The influence of skin diseases on sexuality and shame is sufficiently well known (Buckwalter 1982), although it is constantly underestimated. The so-called nondermatological diseases, i.e. subjectively disfiguring symptoms without actual identifiable or serious findings on the skin itself, also represent a change in body image, which can be an important prognostic sign in cases where there is a danger of suicide (Cotterill 1981). Dysmorphophobia is yet another illness of this type (Bishop 1983; Hardy 1982; Mester 1983): here the experience of the (negative) body image often causes serious depressions or psychoses.

Pathological abnormalities of the skin make its importance for the body image especially clear. In most cases, people become aware of their skin only when it deviates from the norm in structure, form or smell. Jourard's (1966) analysis of the accessibility of a person's own body revealed the connection between touch received and ego. In a way, the surface of the body as an organ of psychosomatic reaction provides a physical signal to draw attention to possible, in some cases pathological abnormalities. Thus the skin and its diseases can provide an opportunity to become aware of the signals of the unconscious body-self (Teegen 1983). In more than a few cases, this 'use' of a disease (Beck 1981; Oberbeck 1984) has a symbolic meaning: when a patient, for example, 'ties his hands' by eczema of the hand (Hansen et al. 1981), or when genital pruritus points to a patients troubled attitude towards his or her own sexuality.

Since in most cases the skin is indeed not consciously accessible, and a human being can hardly, express his unconscious conception of his own body, he is often dependent on somatization - unless we can indirectly get hold of the unconscious processes of reaction, by analytical techniques, for example (Rechenberger 1984). Consciously or unconsciously, abnormalities of the skin have an influence on relationships with other people; the example of skin diseases makes body experience processes especially clear.

Body Experience and Disorders of the Body Surface (Skin Diseases)

In the following, disorders of body experience will be exemplified by a few skin diseases. Psoriasis, atopic dermatitis, acne and factitious disorders, the best-analysed examples of psychosomatic reactions at the body surface, will be described.

Psoriasis Vulgaris

Occurring with a frequency of 2%-5% in the general population, psoriasis is known as a mostly chronic skin disease which is genetically determined and depends on a multitude of factors (Braun-Falco et al. 1984).

The conflict caused in the patient by this disease inevitably leads to psychically caused attacks of psoriasis, or at least to secondary psychosocial assimilation of the disease, which is experienced as disfiguring (Bosse and Hünecke 1982; Bosse and Teichmann 1972; Schröpl 1982). Specific personality structures of psoriatic patients could not be demonstrated in multiple empirical psychological studies (Bojanovsky et al. 1981; Farber and Nall 1974; Gilbert et al. 1973; Wittkower and Russel 1953). Considering the manifold morphological manifestations and the variable degree of expression, one indeed cannot expect otherwise. However, psychic stress is generally accepted as a consequence of the disease (Falk 1982). In times of emotional stress, psoriasis patients suffer from new attacks; this was shown by Farber and Cox (1971) with 5600 patients, and by Braun-Falco et al. (1972) with 536, Seville (1978) reported that, when patients were aware of psychic stress factors, the relapse rate decreased over a period of 3 years.

Psychoanalytical studies have demonstrated that the skin as a means of regression provides a protection, so that unconscious ambivalence conflicts are avoided, especially in the oedipal phase (Rechenberger 1982). Concerning patient's contact with other people, Molitor and Seibt (1984) report on the fear of disappointment and the simultaneous desire to be accepted physically. Figure 1, a drawing by a psoriatic patient, shows a strong hint at desire for contact. 'The scale armour protects me', said one patient. if a conflict cannot be intrapsychically solved, skin and body experience are used as unconscious function of protection.

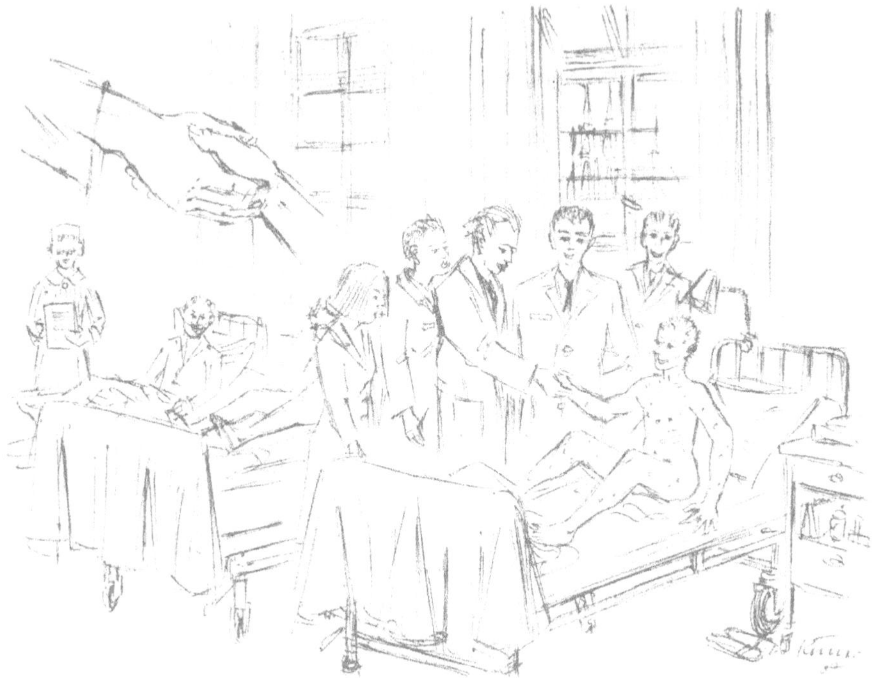

Fig. 1. Drawing by a talented psoriasis patient
(I thank Prof. Dr. H. C. Friederich of Marburg for making this drawing available)

Atopic Dermatitis

Atopic dermatitis, also called neurodermatitis, belongs to the group of atopical ailments, together with allergic asthma, allergic rhinitis and possibly also hemicrania and irritable colon.

The manifestations on the skin usually start in early childhood, and there efore disorders in psychic development can be expected during this phase. Pines (1980) pictures the ambivalent affection of a mother whose child suffers from this skin disease. Through his mothers affection, the child experiences not only tenderness but also pain and irritation because of its damaged skin; thus the development of the object relation causes ambivalence. The later personality, which is described in particular by Schur (1980), Marty (1969) and Rechenberger (1979), is characterized to a great extent by the so-called allergic object relation and is further marked by the lack of opportunity to do justice to the borderlines of the self. In extreme cases, as described by Marty (1969), pseudopsychoses can be caused (see above). These patients especially often experience their skin as not belonging to their own body; the skin is felt to be a separate object, and is treated as such. Dermatologic therapies applied here tend to support the method which treats the surface only, and to confirm the patient in his estranged body experience (Gieler and Effendy 1984). Here the experience of one's surface as a part of one's self though via the body, could be a chance to realize ones inner feelings. A patient said after some years of psychotherapy: 'My skin evokes my inside.' Often itching, an affect equivalent and characteristic of eczema, ebbs immediately when the situation causing fear has been avoided. Eczema mostly occurs under circumstances which Schröpl (personal communication) called 'it doesn't work' situations.

The skin openly presents one's body experience, which shows itself morphologically more by eczematous or pruriginous reactions than by aggression inhibitions.

Acne Vulgaris and Factitious Disorders

Acne is numbered among the diseases which are dependent on genetic or constitutional factors as well as on hormonal influences, but it can become worse in times of emotional stress (Koblenzer 1983). According to Sulzberger and Zaiddens (1948), acne vulgaris in particular causes general insecurity and feelings of inferiority. This connection is made use of by advertising psychologists, as caricatured in Fig. 2.

Not only the effects of the body image on the psychosocial situation but also psychodynamic reactions with effects on the acne are known: Obermayer 1970) reports on the increased productivity of the sebaceous glands in circumstances of emotional stress. Molinski and Rechenberger (1978) differentiate between several variants of acne from psychodynamic points of view, and point out that persistent acne in adulthood accompanies signs of regression to the puberty stage.

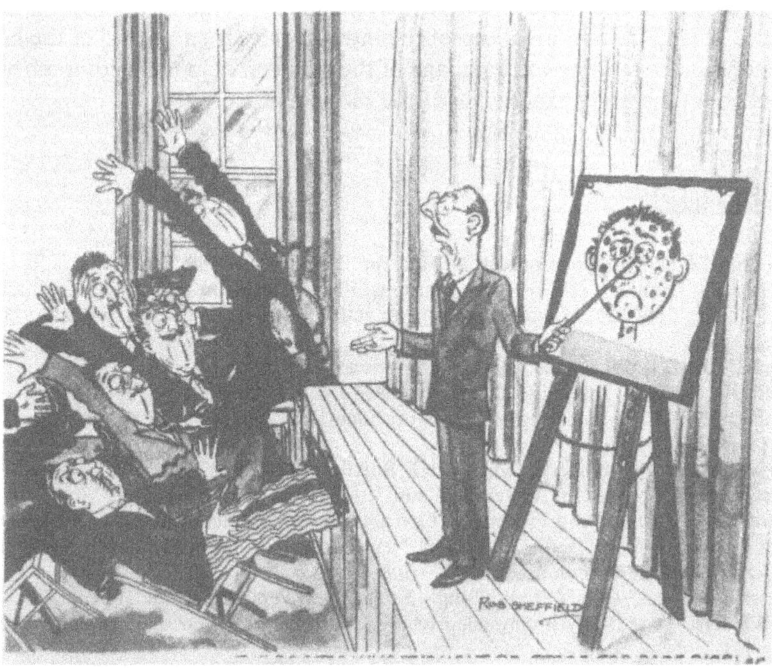

Fig. 2. Graphic advertising of an English medicament for acne

According to Gloor et al. (1978), acne makes a patient feel quite ill. The disease is used to facilitate with drawal into the development of the self.

The otherwise unconscious necessity to keep distance shows itself in the abnormal body image and corresponds to the unconscious motivation to avoid sexual drive impulses. In this connection, Overbeck (1984) says that, very frequently, those adolescents suffer from acne who believe that they have to take part in everything without being allowed to withdraw, and points out that, for reasons of adaptation, they overcharge themselves psychically as well as physically and show prematurely adult behaviour. As Overbeck sees it, in the end it is the skin disease which protects them from entering into relationships which might ask too much of them. Not surprisingly, symptoms often change during acne therapies, and even attemped suicide can occur because the body image has become changed while the personality remains unaltered (Studt et al., 1984). Individual ways of dealing with the body image differ considerably: while there are patients who do not suffer in spite of serious morphological acne efflorescences, for others minimal abnormalities cause massive personality disorders which can even result in suicide, as mentioned above (dysmorphophobia).

Excoriative acne shows a clear transition to the factitious disorders and neurotic excoriation by handicapping the body-self. Braun-Falco et al. (1984) describe this as maximal scratching with minimal acne. The transition to the factitious disorders (for example, stubbing out cigarettes on the skin) is fluid; the body surface is used here as a symbol of the perceived self.

Being satisfied with ones outer appearance is a purely subjective phenomenon which can only be understood through the psychodynamics of the individual. The skin, as one of the most important psychosomatic organs, often reveals morphologically tangible abnormalities of the intrapsychic structure and of the body experience. Understanding the language of the skin can help us to comprehend a great deal about the body experience of the individual.

References

Alexander F (1971) Psychosomatische Medizin. De Gruyter, Berlin

Ammon G, Ammon K (1982) Zur Psychosomatik von Frühgeburt und psychosomatischer Erkrankung. In: Hau TF, Schindler S (eds) Pränatale und perinatale Psychosomatik. Hippokrates, Stuttgart

Beck D (1981) Krankheit als Selbstheilung. Insel, Frankfurt

Bellis JM (1966) Hypnotic pseudo-sunburn. Am J Clin Hypn 8: 310-312

Bishop ER (1983) Monosymptomatic hypochondriacal syndromes in dermatology. J Am Acad Dermatol 9: 152-158

Bojanovsky A, Schöninger B, Kugler HG, Bojanovsky I (1981) Persönlichkeitsstruktur und 'life events' bei Psoriatikern. Aktuel Dermatol 7: 17-19

Borelli S (1967) Haut und Psyche. In: Gottron HA (ed) Grundlagen und Grenzgebiete der Dermatologie. Springer, Berlin Heidelberg New York, pp 264-568 (Handbuch der Haut- und Geschlechtskrankheiten, Supplementary vol 8)

Bosse K, Hünecke P (1980) Entstellung - Erleben und Verarbeitung der äußeren Erscheinung. In: Whitlock FA (ed) Psychophysiologische Aspekte bei Hautkrankheiten. Peri-Med, Erlangen, p 251

Bosse K, Hünecke P (1982) Krankheitsabhängiges Verhalten von Psoriasispatienten, Ärzten und Pflegepersonal im Krankenhaus. Aktuel Dermatol 8: 163-166

Bosse K, Teichmann AT (1972) Der Krankheitswert der Psoriasis. Hautarzt 23: 122f.
Braun-Falco O, Burg G, Farber E (1972) Psoriasis. Münch Med Wochenschr 114: 1105-1110
Braun-Falco O, Plewig G, Wolff HH (1984) Dermatologie und Venerologie. Springer, Berlin Heidelberg New York
Brocq L, Jacquet L (1891) Notes pour servir a l'histoire des neurodermatites. Ann Dermatol Syphiligr 97: 193
Buckwalter KC (1982) The influence of skin disorders on sexual expression. Sex Disab 5: 98-106
Chertok L (1978) Psychosomatique experimentale. La vésication. Ann Med Psychol (Paris) 2: 1-13
Cotterill JA (1981) Dermatological non-disease - a common and potential fatal disturbance of cutaneous body image. Br J Dermatol 104: 611-619
Farber EM, Cox AJ (1971) Psoriasis. Stanford University Press, Stanford
Farber EM, Nall ML (1974) The natural history of psoriasis in 5600 patients. Dermatologica 148: 1-18
Falk G (1982) Probleme des Psoriatikers in der Gesellschaft aus der Sicht des Patienten. Aktuel Dermatol 8: 167-169
Freud S (1923) Das Ich und das Es. In: Freud S (ed) Psychologie des Unbewußten. Textbook edn, vol 3. Fischer, Frankfurt, p 273. Standard edn, vol 19, p 1
Gieler U, Effendy I (1984) Psychosomatische Aspekte in der Dermatologie. Aktuel Dermatol 10: 103-106
Gieler U, Schulze C, Stangier U (1985) Das Krankheitskonzept von Patienten mit endogenem Ekzem. Z Hautkr 60: 1224-1236
Gilbert A, Rodgers D, Roenigk H (1973) Personality evaluation in psoriasis. Cleve Clin Q 40: 147
Giss G, Rothenburg W, Weigand P (1977) Über Zusammenhänge zwischen Psyche und Haut. Z Hautkr 52: 50-54
Gloor M, Eicher C, Wiebelt H, Moser G (1978) Soziologische Untersuchungen bei der Akne vulgaris. I. Mitteilung: Über den Krankheitswert der Akne vulgaris. Z Hautkr 53: 871-880
Hansen O, Küchler T, Lotz G-R, Richter R, Wilckens A (1981) Es juckt mich an den Fingern, aber mir sind die Hände gebunden. Z Psychosom Med Psychoanal 27: 275-290
Hardy GE (1982) Body image disturbance in dysmorphophobia. Br J Psychiatry 141: 181-185
Harlow H, Zimmermann R (1959) Affectional responses in the infant monkey. Science 130: 421f.
Hau TF, Schindler S (1982) Pränatale und perinatale Psychosomatik. Hippokrates, Stuttgart
Hughes JE, Barraclough BM, Hamblin LG, White JE (1983) Psychiatric symptoms in dermatology patients. Br J Psychiatry 143: 51-54
Joraschky P (1983) Das Körperschema und das Körper-Selbst als Regulationsprinzipien der Organismus-Umwelt-Interaktion. Minerva, Munich
Jourard SM (1966) An exploratory study of body accessibility. Br J Soc Clin Psychol 5: 221-231
Jürgens HW (1978) Der Mensch und seine Umwelt. Die menschliche Körperform im sozialen Umfeld. Ärztl Kosmetol 8: 61-75
Kalick SM, Goldwyn RM, Noe JM (1981) Social issues and body image concerns of port wine stain patients undergoing laser therapy. Lasers Surg Med 1: 205-213
Koblenzer CS (1983) Psychosomatic concepts in dermatology. Arch Dermatol 119: 501-512
Leichtman SR, Burnett JW, Robinson HM (1981) Body image concerns of psoriasis patients as reflected in human figure drawings. J Pers Assess 45: 478-484
Leise EM, Lesane F, Chambers RW, Gray I (1974) Lymphocyte and polymorphonuclear enzymes in stress. V. Changes associated with viral infection: Herpes simplex. Biochem Med 9: 214-224
Lux E, Gimes R, Csoemoer S, Rusz E (1983) Die Persönlichkeits- und Sozialbedeutung des Hirsutismus. Zentralbl Gynäkol 104: 1100-1105
Mahler MS (1968) Symbiose und Individuation. Klett, Stuttgart
Marty P (1969) Notes cliniques et hypotheses à propos de l'économie de l'allergie. Rev Fr Psychoanal 33: 243-253
Maurer-Greoli YA (1975) Die Haut als Medium in der Therapie depressiv und schizophren Kranker. Psychosom Med 6: 67-78
Mester H (1983) Die Dysmorphophobie: Klinische Bilder und die ihnen gemeinsame Psychodynamik. Extracta Dermatol 7: 113-135
Molinaro JR (1978) The social fate of children disfigured by burns. Am J Psychiatry 135: 979-980
Molinski H, Rechenberger I (1978) Psychosomatik der Akne. Fortschr Med 95: 2149-2153

Molitor P, Seibt G (1984) Zur Psychosomatik der Psoriasis: Affektivität und Konflikt. Z Psychosom Med Psychoanal 30: 247-269
Montagu A (1980) Körperkontakt. Klett-Cotta, Stuttgart
Obermayer ME (1970) Psychodermatologie. In: Gottron HA (ed) Handbuch der Haut- und Geschlechtskrankheiten, supplement and index. Springer, Berlin Heidelberg New York
Overbeck G (1984) Krankheit als Anpassung. Suhrkamp, Frankfurt
Panse F (1970) Pathopsychologie der Entstellung durch Hautkrankheiten. In: Gottron HA, Schönfeld W (eds) Dermatologie und Venerologie. Supplementary vol. Thieme, Stuttgart
Paulus P (1982) Zur Erfahrung des eigenen Körpers. Research reports. Beltz, Weinheim Basle
Perini U, Bettin A (1983) Eventi stressanti ed alopecia areata. Rassegna Psychiatr Siena 72: 503-511
Pines D (1980) Skin communication: Early skin disorders and their effect on transference and countertransference. Int J Psychoanal 61: 315-323
Porter J, Beuf AH, Nordlund JJ, Lerner AB (1980) Psychological reaction to chronic skin disorders: A study of patients with vitiligo. Gen Hosp Psychiatry 1: 73-77
Rechenberger H-G (1976) Die Auffassung der dynamischen Psychiatrie zum Krankheitsmodell der Trichotillomanie. In: Bosse K, Hünecke P (eds) Psychodynamik und Soziodynamik bei Hautkrankheiten. Vandenhoeck and Ruprecht, Göttingen
Rechenberger I (1979) Tiefenpsychologisch ausgerichtete Diagnostik und Behandlung von Hautkrankheiten. Vandenhoeck and Ruprecht, Göttingen
Rechenberger I (1982) Zur Psychodynamik des Psoriasiskranken. Aktuel Dermatol 8: 157-159
Rechenberger I (1983) Haut und Körperbild. In: Hahn P, Herdieckerhoff E (eds) Werkstattgespräche zum Thema Körperbild. Materialien zur Psychoanalyse und analytisch orientierten Psychotherapie, vol 9, part 1. Vandenhoeck and Ruprecht, Göttingen, pp 31-34
Rechenberger I (1984) Die gestörte Imago des Mannes. Sexualmedizin 13: 717-719
Riemann F (1969) Über den Vorteil des Konzepts einer präoralen Phase. Z Psychosom Med Psychoanal 15: 27-40
Ringel E (1960) Psychotische Reaktionen nach kosmetischer Operation. Wien Nervenheilkd 18: 51-63
Rogentine GN, Van Kammen DP, Fox BH, Docherty JP (1979) Psychological factors in the prognosis of malignant melanoma: A prospective study. Psychosom Med 41: 647-655
Schechter MD 1972) Psychoanalysis of a latency boy with neurodermatitis. Monogr Ser Psychoanal Study Child N Y 27: 529-564
Schur M (1980) Zur Metapsychologie der Somatisierung. In: Brede K (ed) Einführung in die Psychosomatische Medizin. Syndikat, Frankfurt
Schröpl F (1982) Praktische Lebenshilfe für den Psoriatiker. Patientenführung in der dermatologischen Praxis. Aktuel Dermatol 8: 170-172
Seville RH (1978) Psoriasis and stress II. Br J Dermatol 98: 151-153
Shanon J (1970) Psychosomatic skin disorders in survivors of Nazi concentration camps. Psychosomatics 11: 95-98
Shuster S, Fisher GH, Harris E, Binnell D (1979) The effect of skin disease on self image. Br J Dermatol [Suppl 16] 99: 18-19
Solomon GF, Moos RH (1964) Emotions, immunity and disease. Arch Gen Psychiatr 2: 657-674
Spitz R (1957) Die Entstehung der ersten Objektbeziehung, Klett, Stuttgart
Strauß B, Appelt H (1984) Psychologische Einflüsse auf die Beurteilung körperlicher Symptome am Beispiel des Hirsutismus. Psychother Med Psychol 34: 179-185
Studt HH, Richl A, Gollnick H (1984) Acne conglobata Persönlichkeit und seelische Folgen einer 13-*cis*-Retinsäure-Therapie. Paper presented at the 60th meeting of the North-West German Dermatological Society, 22 Sept 1984, Hanover
Sulzberger MB, Zaidens SH (1948) Psychogenic factors in dermatology disorders. Med Clin North Am 32: 669f.
Teegen F (1983) Krankheit: Was will uns der Körper damit sagen? Psychol Heute 11: 65-72
Teichmann AT, Bosse K (1974) Hautkrankheit und Kommunikation. Hautarzt 25: 427-429
Temoshok L, DiClemente RJ, Sweet DM, Blois MS, Sagebiel RW (1984) Prognostic and psychosocial factors related to delay behavior in patients with cutaneous malignant melanoma. Prog Clin Biol Res 156: 169-179

Teshima H, Kubo C, Kihara H, Imada Y, Nagata S, Ago Y (1983) Psychosomatic aspects of skin diseases from the standpoint of immunology. Psychother Psychosom 37: 165-175

Thomä H (1980) Über die Unspezifität psychosomatischer Erkrankungen am Beispiel einer Neurodermitis mit zwanzigjähriger Katamnese. Psyche (Stuttg) 24: 589-624

Uhlmann WJ (1969) Die Sozial- und Präventivmedizinische Bedeutung sogenannter entstellender Hautveränderungen. Zentralbl Arbeitsmed 17: 133-136

van Moffaert M (1983) Psychosomatik für den Dermatologen in der Praxis. Extracta Dermatol 7: 19-38

Vogel PG (1979) Hautsinneserleben. Seine Bedeutung für die Symptomauslösung psychosomatischer Hauterkrankungen. Ther Ggw 118: 46-65

Whitlock FA (1980) Psychophysiologische Aspekte bei Hautkrankheiten. Peri-Med, Erlangen

Wittkower E, Russel B (1953) Emotional factors in skin disease. Cassell, London

B. Body Experience in Therapy

Body Experience and Alienation: Psychoanalytically Oriented Concentrative Movement Therapy as an Introduction to Psychotherapy for Psychosomatic Patients

H. Becker

The theoretical and clinical material in this contribution applies only to those patients who present psychosomatic symptoms but show no manifestation of primary mental distress. The majority of these patients are from lower middle-class backgrounds; perhaps because of their socialization they seem to be rather overadjusted, have little capacity for intrapsychic conflicts and find it hard to give expression to their feelings on a verbal level.

To demonstrate the ambiguous relationship between psychoanalysis and the body and action which may be regarded as part of a more general social trend - I shall begin by quoting a member of the intellectual upper class who was in analysis and had experience both of classical analysis and of more nonverbal therapeutic methods: 'I fear that the oedipal individual not only never experiences that which he knows already; he does not even become acquainted with it when it is killing him. His thorough knowledge about his past origins goes hand in hand with an equally thorough ignorance about himself - that is what happened to me in analysis. I needed manipulation, i.e. a helping hand, so that my erudite ignorance, my unknowing knowledge could begin to turn into experience, self-experience and encounters with others; into a practical, useful kind of experience. Since then I feel it is no longer justifiable to talk about our bodies without using our bodies, to discuss life without living it; it seems to me no longer permissible to allow the head to stand in judgement over the body, to make false insinuations about it, not even in the context of Dr. Freud's scenario. Before our body's needs can be perceived, our body needs to have its say; and for it to have its say, it needs first to be perceived; but perceiving it takes practice, practice together. Psychoanalysis, once so notorious for its sexual fixation, is far from being really body-oriented. It does not need the body in order to know all about it; and it makes no use of it that might interfere with its knowledge about it. Let id become ego: so speaks the super-ego, which does not do us the favour of noticing its relationship with the central id - its secret identity which only in its repressed form is given to tyranny and blackmail' (Muschg 1982).

Although these words of Muschg already point in the direction of the necessity of psychoanalysis concerning itself more seriously with body experience in the future, the question still remains of why one should deal with body experience as a separate issue at all. Seeing the 'psycho-market' as part of a free market economy, could it be that we as psychoanalysts feel our livelihoods threatened by the indiscriminate supply of body-oriented therapies and self-awareness techniques being offered, partly even without proper qualification, on this market today? Do more patients nowadays suffer from symptoms which make it necessary to include body experience more explicitly in their treatment? Or has psychoanalysis, in line with a general social tendency but in contradiction to its own theory and origins, become further removed from the body than it has realized the very fact that body experience is being discussed as a separate issue is surely a symptom in itself. Many psychoanalysts are all too ready to consider themselves as independent of broader social trends and so appear to be somehow timeless. In my view the danger is all the greater that just these norms infiltrate themselves unnoticed and that psychoanalysts, failing to perceive their own drift from 'heart to head', conform more and more to social norms.

When interpersonal relationships become increasingly problematical, every possible branch of communication science flourishes; when we begin to become increasingly aware of our alienation from our bodies, publications and therapeutic offers on the subject multiply accordingly; when world peace and human rights are threatened and transgressed daily, commissions are set up to talk about peace. This is understandable, legitimate and necessary. Nevertheless, the facts seem to favour the interpretation that these activities, seen in the light of their compensatory function, actually have the effect of encouraging or perhaps even of rendering possible the very developments which they are intended to counter. The connection between communication, body experience and world peace or destruction appears at first glance arbitrary and absurd, but I would like to put forward the hypothesis that there is a close inner link between these things. The history of European culture and civilization has for centuries been following the path of alienation from the body, partly on religious and superstitious grounds but also for manifest socioeconomic reasons; this was brought about under the banner first of deliverance from evil and later of enlightenment, liberty and progress. 'The sciences which have dealt with the vicissitudes of the body in the course of history so far are almost unanimous in their agreement that historical progress, as it has been realized in Europe since the Middle Ages, was rendered possible at all by a specifically Western dichotomy between body and mind. From there it continued as a progressive "intellectualization" of life, as rationalization and abstraction at the price of the human body, i.e. a process of dematerialization, has taken place. "..." In bringing about this progress - as one could call the sum total of the scientific results - a distancing, or removal, from bodily life has taken place, to the point of hostile alienation. The body, with its veritable multitude of senses, passions and desires, was forced into a control system of rules and regulations and, through a whole network of repressive measures, turned into an imbecile "dumb waiter". It lost its public role and became forced to follow its own laws by underground means.' (Kamper and Wulf 1982)

Kamper and Wulf describe how the gulf that separates individuals from their own bodies and the bodies of others has grown in the course of a process of progressive abstraction, with prohibitions towards present needs and injunctions relating to abstract morals - all with the objective of securing a controlled social peace. Typical examples are the disciplining functions of the Church, army and education; but the area where the true 'mass abuse of the body' has taken place has been in economic life. Ultimately, it comes down to a question of power.

These authors see the greatest danger in an 'extensive internalization of external control, where the controlling and the controlled self become identical.' This is where, in their opinion, the fundaments of civilization are crumbling. The final result could be that there is no opposition left to counter 'the delusion of omnipotence entertained by the social forces of destruction.' This parallels Mitscherlich's (1962/63) ideas on the links between authoritarian upbringing structures and what he calls the 'prejudice disease'. He argues that authoritarian upbringing procedures lead to frustration and powerlessness. Subjugation may lead to good behaviour and obedience, but it also results in identification with, and glorification of, the aggressor. Drives remain presocial, i.e. they are only suppressed by defence mechanisms but not integrated into the social part of the personality; there they stay, not bound to an object, ready for eruptive forms of expression. Grunberger (1962/63) refers in this connection to a super-ego that is based not on introjected objects but on drilling. Here the suppression of drives is equated, with all reservations, with the suppression of bodily life through the exercise of power.

The phenomena that have been described so far from a more sociological philosophical point of view in connection with the increasing hostility of our culture and civilization towards the body, are reproduced in a surprising manner in the personality characteristics observable in psychosomatic patients. Terms such as 'infantile personality' (Ruesch 1948), 'pensée opératoire' (Marty and de M'Uzan 1963), 'psychosomatic phenomenon' (Marty et al. 1963; Stephanos 1973) and 'alexithymia' (Sifneos 1973; von Rad 1983) have been employed to describe a syndrome of communication phenomena and internal mental states which is to be found primarily, but not exclusively, in psychosomatic patients and which can also be seen as a form of adjustment to the demands of our civilization. There is mention of a mechanistic, instrumental manner of thinking and experiencing, of a marked lack of imagination in spite of high intelligence, of success in work or career and a pragmatic, action-oriented attitude to life. 'A further essential aspect of their dependency upon a partner, who is needed to guarantee their own mental and physical balance, is a very obvious insecurity when it comes to asserting their own sense of values, and a high degree of social conformity. They offer few contradictions, tend to the "golden mean", seek orientation in what is "the done thing", and through their inconspicuous social adjustment demonstrate a style of behaviour which is generally considered socially desirable and has been described as "pseudo-normal" or "super-normal".' (McDougall 1974, 1978, 1980; Ahrens et al. 1979; Brede 1971, 1972 quoted in von Rad 1983). One could say that ego performance is socially overadjusted whilst the id remains pre-social.

The clinical picture of anorexia nervosa is a good example for demonstrating the link between body experience, communication and destructiveness. In the biographies of female anorexia patients one often comes across the phenomenon of a home background consisting on the one hand of a very rigid family atmosphere with a great many rules and regulations (drilling), whilst on the other hand the patients themselves are described by their parents as having been not at all badly behaved or rebellious but rather good and obedient as children. The symptoms include breaking off communication with important key figures, a very achievement-oriented intelligence and a deficient, distorted perception of their own bodies, to the point of self-destructiveness. One could put forward the hypothesis that, due to identification with the drilling they experienced as children, their efforts towards autonomy primarily serve to strengthen their defences against bodily and instinctual urges. The degree of alienation from their bodies that is achieved in this way brings with it an illusory sense of triumphant liberation and lightness, but also represents a root of self-destructiveness. Drives, or body experience, are not an encumbrance that has to be overcome but are rather indispensable elements of life that have to be integrated, if they are not to have uncontrolled, eruptive and destructive effects.

The psychoanalyst working in the field of psychosomatics is confronted with a great many patients who present their suffering on a purely somatic, symptom-oriented level; they express no manifest emotional distress nor articulate any sort of intrapsychic conflict potential. They thus do not seem to fulfil the classical indication criteria for a psychoanalysis. Referring to psychosomatic patients, Schur (1955) postulates a regression to a preverbal, pre-ego stage of development. De Boor and Mitscherlich (1973) suspect that our analytical treatments, already so long-drawn-out, have still not penetrated far enough into the nonverbal and preverbal area of experience. Mitscherlich (1967) reports that with up to 40% of psychosomatically ill patients, psychoanalytic treatment is not undertaken due to a lack of communicative potential between doctor and patient. This he attributes to the fact that in these patients all those elements which have been kept out by defences have remained unverbalized.

Cremerius et al. (1979) have described a group of lower-class patients who came to the out-patients department of a clinic for internal medicine with symptoms that were diagnosed as functional, psychosomatic or neurotic. On the basis of certain criteria which were defined after psychodiagnostic interviews, the patients in this group were judged unsuitable for treatment by psychoanalysis. All came from more working-class backgrounds and all remained fixated on the idea of their organic illness, holding external factors responsible for its development; they appeared to have no intrapsychic conflict potential and, due to strict moral ideas, could not talk about sexuality and aggressivity, let alone such things as instinctual urges; they tended on the whole to a passive, receptive attitude. One must not forget that these observations were made on the basis of one initial psychoanalytic interview. Cremerius explains these phenomena observed during the dialogue as the consequence of an exceptionally severe super-ego and an extremely repressive upbringing in early childhood, which was clearly expressive of a strong hostility towards instinctual, imaginative or spontaneous elements. Instinctual impulses were met with threats of punishment at such an early age that they never even had a chance to develop properly. In their first interpersonal relationship (with their mother), these patients had as children experienced certain interactions either not at all or only as affective actions which were not accompanied by any sort of appropriate verbalization. From this he concludes that their verbal interaction potential is deficient. Cremerius continues: 'This also explains the predominance of acted-out forms of transference which cannot be translated into language. What never has been put into words will never be able to be put into words. It remains blind action, vegetative reaction, bodily symptom, a physiological state of readiness - as we know them in the psychosomatic diseases. Ferenczi (1921) was the first to point out that there are unconscious, pathogenic mental contents dating back to early infancy which never became conscious because they originated in the period of "unco-ordinated" or "magical" gestures. They can, as he says, never be remembered but only reproduced, by being brought back to life through repetition.' (Cremerius et al. 1979)

Theoretically, all those authors writing about psychosomatic patients agree on the assumption of a fixation or regression onto a very early developmental stage - a stage in which communication on a preverbal, sensori-motor level predominates, in which the capacity for symbolization and verbalization is only insufficiently developed and where the need for the real-life presence of the central object is in the foreground. Although the aetiological research in the field of psychosomatics can boast tremendous advances, amazingly few suggestions have been forthcoming about corresponding modifications in analytical technique. The few indications that have been made all point in one direction however. Ruesch (1948) suggests that modification is necessary in the direction of a psychotherapeutic approach similar to that used with children. He considers it important, especially in the initial phase of therapy, to establish a symbiotic relationship between therapist and patient. De Boor and Mitscherlich (1973) limit themselves to their suggestion that in our therapies we psychoanalysts have not yet penetrated far enough into the nonverbal and preverbal area of experience. Balint (1970), who includes the psychosomatic diseases in his theoretical model of the 'basic fault', stresses the need to be sparing with verbal interpretations, since adult language is often useless and misleading and no longer possesses its conventional meaning for these patients. Interpretations are often seen as ungrounded demands, attacks, criticisms, seductions or stimulation. He argues that it is necessary in the first phase of therapy to give the patient time and the right milieu and to offer oneself as a primary object.

Concentrative movement therapy, with its emphasis on the preverbal and nonverbal areas, which it reaches by means of free body associations and action associations, attempts as far as possible to meet the recommendations for therapy that have been made on the basis of the theoretical and empirical considerations mentioned above. It follows the tradition represented by Ferenczi (1921), Reich (1933), Balint (1970) and Winnicott (1971). So-called 'blind actions', 'vegetative reactions', 'somatic symptoms', 'physiological states of readiness', 'unco-ordinated gestures' and what have been termed 'magical gestures' are all seen as primary forms of expression for the patient and the attempt is made to integrate them into the therapeutic process.

Before going into the details of the theory and technique of concentrative movement therapy, I would like first to point to the abundance of inflexible taboos and prejudices prevailing amongst psychoanalysts nowadays; with these - partly for historical reasons but also because of its own rigid institutional structures - psychoanalysis is restricting itself and becoming further and further removed from its own origins. The set rules and taboos are most apparent in the way in which many analysts deal with the rule of abstinence and in their attitude towards acting-out, somatization and primary process thinking; this often amounts to an undifferentiated 'psychopathologization'. The implications of the concept of acting-out have been extended on an inflationary scale, to the point of including even socially reasonable behaviour, with no attempt at differentiating between where it really inhibits the emotional memory process and where it is actually beneficial to it. When Schur (1955) spoke of desomatization he did not mean it in the sense of alienation from the body. Where a somatic symptom has developed, the path of progress does not lead like a one-way street towards desomatization, but rather via a process of resomatization towards the ability to dispose more freely over de- and resomatization processes. The same applies to the area of primary and secondary process thinking, where it is largely also a question of attaining freer access to these things and so reaching greater autonomy, and not of a one-sided linear maturation process. To put it rather ironically and provocatively, we can only hope that all our patients and aspirant analysts have managed to retain their capacity for resomatization, their access to primary processes and their ability to act out, in spite of the often overintellectualized, verbal elaboration of conflicts. Could it be that the early experiences of Breuer and Freud (1895) led to a theory and technique of abstinence and frustration, which was subsequently interpreted by their grandchildren and great-grandchildren in a more and more rigid way? Was this, reactively, the price which had to be paid to the society of the turn of the century for the enlightenment achieved by psychoanalysis? A somersault done by an analysand during a session or a moment of physical contact with the therapist can be therapeutically necessary and beneficial or can have a defensive function (Balint 1970).

During a supervision session a trainee analyst reported that his patient had expressed the wish to offer him his hand in the middle of a session. The trainee/therapist had agreed to this but spent the rest of the session in a state of restless activity hitherto unknown to him, that evidently had the purpose of undoing what had been done. It took the supervisor several sessions to convince his student that with this patient, in this situation, it was technically correct to step outside his therapeutic abstinence and act out with his patient. It seemed important for the supervisor to discover and illuminate what it was that had happened after this scene, namely, the strong, unconscious defensive behaviour on the part of the therapist, that was unquestionably based on a trainee analyst's anxiety about having violated fundamental taboos, rules of technique. Inflexible rules relating to technique in psychoanalysis tend to transcend the interests of the individual and become an end in themselves, far removed from practical realities. I do not wish to bring up the issue of the necessity and reasons for having a rule of abstinence at all but it must be open to question again and again, in each individual case, and it must be permissible to give it up where this seems necessary and useful for the therapeutic process.

If one considers the developmental models upon which the psychoanalytical theory of illness is built, it is striking that they are largely based upon somatic phenomena. With the introduction of the terms 'oral', 'anal' and 'genital', Freuds phasic theory of psychosexual development remained unequivocally in the sphere of the body zones. Taking up and elaborating upon this approach, Erikson (1974) introduced the concept of organ modes, corresponding to the individual phases. To the oral phase he adds the organ mode of incorporation, of grasping and ingesting things; to the anal phase the retentive-eliminative, adjusting and relaxing mode; to the genital phase the mode of penetration and enclosure - each mode relating to the relevant area of the body zone in question: the skin, muscles or genitals. Erikson rounds this off with his concept of a psychosocial modality involving atmospheric feeling, hearing, seeing, smelling, receiving and enclosing, locomotion and self-assertion, holding on and letting go, rebellion and submission, which find their equivalents in the senses of basic trust vs basic mistrust, intimacy vs isolation, autonomy vs shame and doubt, initiative vs guilt. On the basis of their empirical observations of the mother-infant relationship, Margaret Mahler et al. (1974) have further supplemented Freuds model of psychological development by adding another, mainly communicative, level. As part of the 'normal' development of infants and young children they have identified the phases of autism, symbiosis, separation and individuation. With the help of this new conceptual plane, certain pathological manifestations in adulthood can be located and their possible meaning better understood, so that a decision as to the most suitable therapeutic course, e.g. concentrative movement therapy, can be reached. The terms introduced above to describe individual developmental phases represent basic situations in concentrative movement therapy as well. In the biographies of patients with psychosomatic diseases, but also in the situation triggering off their illness, a pronounced disturbance is seen in the areas of body self and interpersonal relations, as well as a special sensitivity towards object loss. Concentrative movement therapy stresses two aspects in particular:

1. It makes no assumptions as to the patient's abilities in those areas where a developmental deficit is suspected; this applies most of all to the areas related to the internalization of the object world and of symbolization and phantasy. In other words, a capacity for abstraction through language is not a precondition to therapy.
2. In just those areas where our Western civilization makes particularly high demands - desomatization, secondary process thinking and drive control, all processes which are closely associated with symptom formation - concentrative movement therapy is concerned with regaining access to our own bodies, in the sense of recovering our capacity for resomatization, primary process thinking and the instinctual elements of behaviour, as well as with integrating these areas into social reality. This initially requires the real-life presence of the object world which can then, via internalization processes, gradually lead the patient towards symbolization and language.

Concentrative movement therapy is a psychoanalytically oriented method of treatment which makes special use of our knowledge about the importance of preverbal and averbal, i.e. sensori-motor, elements in early infantile development. Through 'concentration' on the body self, an intensified spatial body image is achieved and the body is experienced subjectively instead of purely as an object. Thus, an attempt is made to overcome the patient's alienated attitude towards his own body, with the aim of achieving a maximum degree of autonomy - in the figurative sense as well. A further essential aspect is the process of coming to grips with, of perceiving, the animate and inanimate object world, which is seen as a precondition to the healthy development of the self and the growth of relatedness to the environment: concrete perception through tactile, manual, visual and motor exploration of space and its objects in a state of 'concentrated awareness', confrontation with one's own body boundaries, oneness and separateness, demarcation from the environment, giving and taking, controlling and being controlled, penetration of space, exploration, turning one's attention to things and other people. Through investigating and perceiving the object world on a concrete plane processes of internalization, symbolization and reality-testing are set in motion. A further central element is the area of communication, in the sense of social relatedness to other group members. Intimacy, distance, own needs, others' needs, being supported by and supporting others, feeling, being felt, shared responsibility - all these things demonstrate how, through concrete action in the psychodynamic field, processes of imitation, identification and social learning are initiated and so can be worked through.

The therapist tries to create a mainly preverbal and averbal space by using the introductory phase of therapy to prepare the ground for potential motivational areas, whether intentional, oral, anal, aggressive or sexual. The therapist's active role does not mean, however, that he shapes the therapeutic process himself; it is rather his task to prepare the therapeutic space in an almost protective manner, and to make a basic therapeutic 'offer', particularly in the initial phases. Later on, things should be turned over more and more to the patient, to shape the course of events - his passive and active experience - in his own individual way, using free associations on the level of bodily expression. This means that in one sense the therapist is 'offering' to help new patients overcome their initial inhibitions, break through the repetition compulsion and actively enter into an anxiety-arousing situation, but not in the sense of prescribing exercises that are to be performed with a given collective goal. What is meant by this basic offer coming from the therapist is, for example, opening up to the patient the possibility of closing his eyes, lying on the floor, being fully aware of his body, turning his attention to the space around him, etc. Particularly the action of closing his eyes enables him to eliminate those areas of perception which usually predominate and so are generally subject to a certain automatization and habituation, also to preconceptions; instead he can turn his full attention to less accustomed areas of perception. Verbal suggestions made by the therapist in the direction of focusing perception onto one's own body experience, experiencing one's own body in relation to the environment, experiencing whilst lying, standing, walking, exploring the surrounding space and the objects in it, are basic elements of the therapist's offer. Objects like balls, sticks and ropes, which are actively presented by the therapist, can also serve as stimuli for processes of abstraction and symbolization, for example through their possible significance as transitional objects, symbols or media of communication, through their shape and material, or through the fact of their being used for giving and taking. Scenic situations created in action stimulate an emotional process of remembering genetic material and often reinforce an emotional capacity for experiencing the present situation to a far greater extent than is usually possible by verbalization (Becker 1981). Our own observations, as well as studies by Carl et al. (1982), suggest that in this body- and action-related area, material can enter consciousness sooner than is possible in the verbal area. One could say that free body associations and action associations, alongside dreams, are another *via regia* to the unconscious.

The following case study is intended to demonstrate the connection between drilling in a family and social context, presocial drives, alienation from ones own body and destruction. It is also an illustration of a psychoanalytical approach to treating those patients who present a primary fixation on their symptoms and who, through dehumanizing processes in the family and society, could never develop, or have lost, the capacity for autonomous disposal over their body experience.

Herr E., a patient from a lower middle-class background, was brought by his family to the out-patient department of our clinic on the advice of their general practitioner. He suffered from a persistent noise in his ear which had begun after he had gone away on a journey, against the express will of his father who wanted him to stay behind and help as usual on the family farm. Before he left, his father had commented, 'You won't come back alive.' In the period following, Herr E. had succeeded in getting a great many doctors to perform active diagnostic and therapeutic interventions, which culminated in a dangerous secondary haemorrhage following a stellate block, necessitating a tracheotomy. This led the neurologist then in charge to diagnose Alzheimers disease (in the patient's own words, 'brain consumption'). Before beginning psychotherapy he had been unable to work for 9 months. On account of his growing suicidal tendencies and excessive anxiety, his family felt they could no longer cope with him at home.

In the first diagnostic interview his 'passive receptive' attitude fitted Cremerius'-description exactly. He appeared to be completely fixated on his somatic symptom, made external factors primarily responsible for his illness, appeared to have no intrapsychic conflict potential at all and showed all the signs of a rigid superego with a strong hostility towards drive-directed behaviour. Sexuality consisted for him largely of tortuous, mechanistic masturbation rituals, mainly for the sake of discharge of tension, that were accompanied by religiously motivated ideas of guilt and penance. Aggression was expressed in often grotesque, extremely right-wing, dramatic, military-type outbursts which occurred regularly under the influence of alcohol and were accompanied by images, dissociated from affective experience, of execution scenes and mass destruction. These destructive, aggressive outbreaks were directed primarily towards women and 'good-for nothings' and evidently served his defences against his own instinctual urges (dissociation, projection and identification with the aggressor, i.e. with the parental driller).

In his biography it was surely significant that the patient, a first child, was born shortly after his father's release from a Russian prisoner-of-war camp. Both parents stated that they had felt completely overwhelmed by their responsibilities at the time and the father, physically very weakened, was still totally under the influence of his war experiences. The mother, religious to the point of bigotry, had kept an unspoken hold on her son at the same time as maintaining her deference to the father. According to the patient, his relationship with his father consisted entirely of listening to endless accounts of wartime experiences which were accompanied even in his early childhood by militarist games and drilling. For example, the patient would salute as his father drove by on the tractor. Later on, the patient would give his father a book on weapons or war reminiscence every year for Christmas, which never failed to fill him, a man otherwise not given to showing any feelings, with strong emotion. Otherwise, the patient mainly felt that his father consistently tried to put him down. At work, the patient was overadjusted, a great believer in authority, would do unpaid overtime and was generally recognized by his superiors as a good employee in the finance department where he worked. His subordinates he treated with unbending severity. Only at weekends, when he drank, was he given to his recurrent impulsive, usually aggressive, outbursts. Until his illness, (the appearance of his physical symptoms), Herr E. was a socially respected and, not counting his occasional outbreaks, an average peaceable citizen.

This patient's background is exemplary for the alienating and dehumanizing processes that have been described already as occurring in the interplay between society, family and the individual. It helps us to understand what Kamper and Wulf (1982) mean when they speak of disciplining through the Church (religious mother) and in military life (father's militarism) and of the mass abuse of the body through the economy (work situation); or Mitscherlich (1962/63), when he says he sees a connection between authoritarian models of upbringing and the so-called prejudice disease, between good behaviour, obedience and glorification of the aggressor; or Grunberger (1962/63) when he talks in this connection about a super-ego arising not from the introjection of objects but from drilling (religious and militarist drilling). In such patients, sexuality and aggression have remained presocial, unintegrated, drive-ridden elements, which only appear in outbursts and then mainly in a destructive and self-destructive form, dissociated from affects. His pregenital, harsh super-ego, the consequence of childhood drilling, encouraged this tendency to dissociation and projection (scapegoat theory) and to identification with the aggressor. Grunberger (1962/63) describes these mechanisms in a sociopolitical dimension in his article *Der Antisemit und der Ödipuskomplex.*

At that time we recommended for Herr E. psychoanalytical in-patient psychotherapy, a combination of individual, group and concentrative movement therapy. The emphasis in the individual sessions was placed first of all on making interventions that were largely ego-supportive and relieving to the super-ego. The primarily preverbal and averbal therapeutic offer in the form of group concentrative movement therapy was intended to provide a medium for the re-enactment of elements that had so far remained unarticulated. To begin with Herr E. complained in an aggressive and demanding manner of his persisting physical symptoms and the inadequate therapeutic help he was receiving. He re-enacted his right-wing, militarist outbursts and composed a number of letters worded in a highly formal, official style (dehumanized language) which were addressed to me as therapist and to the director of the clinic and contained orders for executions, signed with the names of well-known SS generals; he evidently saw these as representing his therapists, who were ordering his execution or the elimination of the entire clinic.

In our team meetings, the first indications of the beginnings of a therapeutic process came through the reports of the female therapist in charge of his concentrative movement therapy group. The patient, who had lived in complete social isolation until then and had never had any form of sexual relationship, experienced in the group – first of all by observation – how other participants and the therapist talked among themselves about the ways in which they perceived and communicated with their bodies and what feelings they had in the process. In a next step, he had the experience of his own body being touched and accepted by others. He experienced how intra- and interpersonal conflicts and above all aggressive feelings could be perceived and expressed in words, without a breakdown of communication or the introduction of drilling resulting. He himself reported 18 months later, during individual, analytical out-patient therapy, that for him the decisive therapeutic breakthrough had come when a fellow patient advised him to try concentrating his mind on his somatic symptom (the noise in his ear) for a change, physically feeling his way into it, instead of constantly trying to push it away from himself as he had done so far. A vital factor here was surely that Herr E. found a way for himself, outside of authoritarian structures, not, significantly, through a therapist, that helped him take a first step towards integrating an aspect of his bodily life and so also his instinctual urges. The initially nonverbal field suitable for acting out that was offered in the group situation during concentrative movement therapy suited the patient with his background and its deficits at the beginning of his therapy ('what never has been put into words will never be able to be put into words', Cremerius et al. 1979). By means of imitation and identification, through this corrective new experience with respect to his own body (e.g. his body being accepted by others as well) and, last but not least, through affects and conflicts being articulated for the first time, a belated maturation process was initiated which constituted an indispensable preliminary phase for the reflective process (in the psychoanalytical sense) that was to begin later and was finally to lead to a growth of autonomy. The path to desomatization thus led via a process of resomatization.

In concentrative movement therapy one observes repeatedly how patients have what are known as key experiences, such as that described by Herr E. These are usually scenes and/or affects which have so far been warded off by the patient's own defences and which emerge in a certain situation in the course of therapy. In retrospect they are best understood atmospherically, rather like screen memories. However, the really effective therapeutic agent is the ego-supportive and super-ego relieving situation, the atmosphere created by the therapist and other participants, that enables a patient, often for the first time, to find a way through to his own bodily and instinctual life, making dissociation and projection more and more superfluous as predominant defence mechanisms. By means of initially primitive forms of identification, such as imitation, and later by identification, symbolization and verbalization, a growth of autonomy in the area of emotions and relationships becomes possible.

Some basic postulates on the significance of integrating body experience during the psychoanalytic process are listed below:

1. The concept of 'mind over body' can have as its parallel an economically desirable process of dehumanization and alienation, which can serve power interests and lead to individual and collective destruction.
2. The rediscovery and reintegration of primary process thinking and feeling, which enable the individual subsequently to dispose more freely over these aspects, and the encouragement of a resomatization process, can be vital to the healing process.
3. Patients with pronounced body schema disorders of varying origin often find that a mainly pre- and averbal offer of therapy provides them with their first ever means of access to their disorder.
4. The experiential quality of concrete actions and psychosomatic forms of expression promotes the recollection of material relating to the genesis - which directly contradicts the postulate of 'acting-out instead of memory'.

5. While in the verbal area defences and instinctual wishes usually tend to be ego-syntonic, in the nonverbal area patients often have their first ever confrontation with ego-dystonic experiences. Thus, the nonverbal approach often reveals instinctual and affective aspects whilst the verbal area is still completely dominated by the defence aspect.
6. The nonverbal and especially the preverbal areas appear in the initial phases of a therapeutic process to be invested to a far greater extent with affects, to be closer to the unconscious and primary processes and thus to be less subject to censorship than the verbal area.
7. Differences in social class background among the patients or between patient and therapist lead in the pre- and averbal area, particularly in the initial phase of therapy, to markedly less difficulties in communication than in the verbal area, since one can assume that on the nonverbal level one is working with basic collective forms of expression.

Besides certain basic features which they have in common, concentrative movement therapy differs in some very important respects from other more body-oriented psychotherapy techniques, most of which, like the more verbal methods, are usually also very dependent on the qualification of the therapist. It seems to me to be especially necessary to differentiate between this approach and those techniques which have a more exercising, covering-up character, which pay no attention to resistance, transference and counter-transference phenomena and which do away with all conflict and developmental theories. In such approaches the cathartic character is clearly to the fore, giving rise to spontaneous emotional outbursts and 'artificial situations through group games with a strong tendency to encouraging acting-out' (Schmidtbauer on encounter groups 1973). The bioenergetics groups, which have their roots in the ideas of Wilhelm Reich, come closest to concentrative movement therapy, particularly in their theoretical approach. The therapeutic technique for dealing with character resistance that was described first by Reich (1933) and later by Lowen (1967) is a basic element of concentrative movement therapy as well. Also, the possibility and necessity of verbal elaboration is stressed both in bioenergetics (at least by Lowen) and in concentrative movement therapy. Basic differences come out, however, particularly in the area of social orientation and in the manner of dealing with aggression – areas which are closely interwoven. We regard the group process, especially when seen in relation to its broader social context, as a microcosm reflecting the macrocosm of the outside world. This inevitably involves placing special emphasis on a more general social orientation in the group. Bioenergetics groups, on the other hand, attach far more importance to the idea of working with the individual in the group. What is more (and to be viewed in relation to the aforsaid), the therapeutic process in bioenergetics groups does not go further than to aim at attempting a general acceptance; aggression, rivalry, demarcation between individuals appear in the light of things that are to be overcome. Lowen (1967) describes the ultimate aim of this sort of acceptance and recognition in terms of freedom, pleasure, joy and the sense of unity. In many cases this has its equivalent in the basic elements constituting the initial phase of the therapeutic process in concentrative movement therapy: but here, in contrast to bioenergetics groups, these things are seen as a necessary foundation for the growth of basic trust. However, concentrative movement therapy goes a step further in that it regards particularly the expansive, aggressive areas of motivation as vital prerequisities for individuation. The danger in bioenergetics groups lies in my opinion in the fact that the transference process and the individual's bond to the group (and this applies to the therapist as well) cannot as such be worked through, so that a subsequent translation of the group process into terms of outer reality - the social relatedness of therapy - is impeded. Bioenergetics groups negate the productivity and creativity of aggressive motivational areas (Becker 1981).

References

Ahrens S, Gyldenfeldt H von, Runde P (1979) Alexithymie, psychosomatische Krankheit und instrumentelle Orientierung. Psychother Med Psychol 29: 173-177

Balint M (1970) Therapeutische Aspekte der Regression. Klett, Stuttgart

Becker H (1981) Konzentrative Bewegungstherapie. Integrationsversuch von Körperlichkeit und Handeln in den psychoanalytischen Prozess. Thieme, Stuttgart

Brede K (1971) Die Pseudo-Logik psychosomatischer Störungen. In: Lorenzer A et al (eds) Psychoanalyse als Sozialwissenschaft. Suhrkamp, Frankfurt

Brede K (1972) Sozialanalyse psychosomatischer Störungen. Fischer-Athenäum, Frankfurt

Breuer J, Freud S (1895) Über den psychischen Mechanismus hysterischer Phänomene. In: Freud S, Gesammelte Werke, vol 1. Standard edn. vol 2

Carl A, Fischer-Antze J, Gaedtke H, Hoffmann SO, Wendler W (1982) Vergleichende Darstellung gruppendynamischer Prozesse bei Konzentrativer Bewegungstherapie und Analytischer Gruppentherapie. In: Stolze H (ed) Die Konzentrative Bewegungstherapie. Mensch und Leben, Berlin

Cremerius J, Hoffmann SO, Trimborn W (1979) Psychoanalyse, Über-Ich und soziale Schicht. Kindler, Munich

de Boor C, Mitscherlich A (1973) Verstehende Psychosomatik: Ein Stiefkind der Medizin.Psyche (Stuttg) 27: 1-20

Erikson E (1974) Kindheit und Gesellschaft. Klett, Stuttgart

Ferenczi S (1921) Weiterer Aufbau der 'aktiven Technik' in der Psychoanalyse. In: Ferenczi S (ed) Schriften zur Psychoanalyse, vol 2. Fischer, Frankfurt

Grunberger B (1962/63) Der Antisemit und der Ödipuskomplex. Psyche (Stuttg) 16: 255-272

Kamper D, Wulf C (1982) Die Wiederkehr des Körpers. Suhrkamp, Frankfurt

Lowen A (1967) The betrayal of the body. Macmillan, New York

McDougall J (1974) The psychosoma and the psychoanalytic process. Int Rev Psychoanal 1: 437-459

McDougall J (1978) Plea for a measure of abnormality. Int Univ Press, New York

McDougall J (1980) A child is being eaten. Contemp Psychoanal 16: 417-459

Mahler MS, Pine F, Bergmann A (1974) The psychological birth of the human infant. Basic Books, New York

Marty P, de M'Uzan M (1963) Das operative Denken ('Pensée opératoire'). Psyche (Stuttg) 32: 974-984

Marty P, de M'Uzan M, David C (1963) L'investigation psychosomatique. PUF, Paris

Mitscherlich A (1962/63) Die Vorurteilskrankheit. Psyche (Stuttg) 16: 241-265

Mitscherlich A (1967) Krankheit als Konflikt. Studien zur psychosomatischen Medizin 2. Suhrkamp, Frankfurt

Muschg A (1982) Manipulation und Psychoanalyse. Paper presented at the annual meeting of the Deutsche Gesellschaft für Psychosomatik, Psychotherapie und Tiefenpsychologie, Freiburg

Reich W (1933) Charakteranalyse. Selbstverlag, Vienna

Ruesch J (1948) The infantile personality. Psychosom Med 10: 134-144

Schmidbauer W (1973) Sensitivitätstraining und analytische Gruppendynamik. Piper, Munich

Schur M (1955) Comments on the metapsychology of somatisation. Psychoanal Stud Child 10: 119-164

Sifneos PE (1973) The prevalene of 'alexithymic' characteristics in psychosomatic patients. Psychother Psychosom 22: 255-263

Stephanos S (1973) Analytisch-psychosomatische Therapie. Jahrbuch Psychoanal [Suppl 1]. Huber, Bern

von Rad M (1983) Alexithymie. Springer, Berlin Heidelberg New York

Winnicott DW (1971) Playing and reality.Tavistock, London

Body Therapeutic Techniques in Disease-Oriented Psychoanalytic Group Therapy with Asthma Patients

H. C. Deter and C. Heintze-Hook

Psychotherapeutic treatment of patients with bronchial asthma has a long tradition. However, in recent years this form of treatment has undergone a crisis also to be found in the treatment of other so-called psychosomatic illnesses such as ulcerative Colitis or rheumatoid arthritis; this was in part due to the demand that psychotherapy should heal the illness completely. Giving up the so-called psychogenic concept and restricting the treatment goal to adaptation to the illness could be one way of circumventing the problems of treatment. The other possibility, discussed in the present paper, lies in modification of the psychotherapeutic procedure with regard to the psychopathological and situative conflicts which are considered to be causes of asthma.

The psychoanalytic difficulties specific to the treatment of asthma patients are due on the one hand to the therapeutic procedure in patients with so-called early childhood disturbances and on the other to the abstinent analytic-therapeutic approach.

Therapeutic Procedure in Patients with 'Early Childhood Disturbances'

However one rates the severity of early childhood developmental deficencies in patients later afflicted by bronchial asthma, it may be assumed that some of them have developmental problems similar to those described by Spitz (1965) in children with eczema.

The postulated trauma can probably be dated to the period prior to or at the beginning of the development of self and object representation, a vulnerable phase of the physiological development of body functions. A normal development of object relations may thus have been made more difficult. No assumption of stable object relations can therefore be made in psychotherapeutic or psychoanalytic treatment of these patients. From an analytic point of view, this disturbance is assumed to originate in the preverbal developmental phase (Spitz 1972); language may therefore not be the appropriate means for description of the disturbance; the disturbance can therefore only be approached carefully and in part therapeutically in the transference of diffuse emotional states.

For patients with an early childhood developmental disturbance, the necessity arises for a supplement of the psychoanalytic treatment technique. This supplement should keep the previous concepts of the psychopathogenesis of psychosomatic disturbances in mind.

When considering the development of psychosomatic illnesses in infancy, the analytic concepts of development of the earliest psychophysiological self, setting up stable object representations and production of lasting object libido cathexis within the ego system are of fundamental relevance. A further development in this connexion is the emergence of self representations, i.e. of unconscious, preconscious and conscious intrapsychic representations of the physical and psychic self within the ego system (Jacobsen 1978, p.29). Within these differentiation processes, our body sensations (inner stimuli, tactile awareness, deep sensibility and temperature exchange) mediate the feeling of individual identity and finally lead to an integration of our body feeling. They form the foundation of the psychic representations of the body ego as a body schema (Mahler 1968, p.42).

Psychosomatic disturbances may be the result, for example, of an intensified cathexis of certain organs with an 'emptying of the neutralized cathexis of object ans self representions' (Mahler 1968). Spitz (1965) describes this process in children with eczema: libidinous and aggressive instincts of healthy children are usually purged within the context of a physiological interrelationship between mother and child (cf. Hoffer 1978). The child with eczema, however, does not have this opportunity because of the mothers's behaviour, so that an 'agressivization' (Mahler 1968) within the body schema results (in psychoanalytic concepts this is comparable to disintegration of drives), leading to a fragile ego (Mahler 1968) or a retardation of ego development (Spitz 1965).

Within this context, regular contact awareness plays an important role in the development of representations of a person's own body (i.e. body schema) and thus in the further development of the ego and its object relations.

If the need for bodily contact is not satisfied (Montagu 1971), then children may possibly develop aggressive psychic energies which they cannot adequately control psychically and therefore somatize them. This process is, however, reversible (i.e. desomatization; Schur 1978).

Some Psychoanalytic Concepts of the Body Image of Adults (Federn 1978, Reich 1975)

Federn (1978) has applied the term 'ego feelings' to self representions of adults. He differentiates between a psychic ego feeling and a physical ego feeling; the latter entails all motor and sensory memories and yet is not identical with the body schema (the totality of the properly evaluated awareness of one's own body), but rather 'the physical feeling of the ego'.

Federn points out that in a healthy ego, in contrast to a psychotic, there exists evidence of perception of the physical ego limits which must be overcome by impressions from the outside world. Whereas the physical ego limits are intensified in fear, in shock the ego loses its narcissistic cathectic limits; the outside world may also be alienated by narcissistic cathexis.

The intensity of physical cathexis varies between individuals and is dependent on frame of mind. In hysteries, the physical feeling was reduced during symptoms but intensified immediately before these set in. Federn assumes clear qualitative differences in the physical ego feeling.

Reich (1975) has emphasized the connection between physical ego and psychic ego; he spoke of 'character armour' and suggested that character armour and muscular armour are functionally identical. The character formation is the result of a bonding of vegetative energy, which could be distilled (i.e. reactivated) from the character and muscular armour using certain techniques (i.e. character analysis).[1] According to Reich, severing the vegetative excitation from its bonding in the tension of the musculature of head, neck, pharynx and larynx is a prerequisite e.g. for solution from oral fixations: 'Without solution (in analysis) one only abtains memories, not agitations.'

In the muscular armour (as in the character armour) affects are tied up, if the ego is continually confronted with the same or similar conflicts between its own needs and fears conditioned, by the outside world; a chronic, automatically functioning reaction, i.e. character, is the result. This armour allows insensitivity to unpleasure, limits the libidinous and aggressive mobility of a person and reduces the capacity for achievement and pleasure. Character armour uses up energy because it constantly consumes libidinous and vegetative strength.

Aggression, fear and sexuality are bound by the armour. One could therefore say that rigid muscle tone is proof of vegetative excitement, fear or sexuality having been intercepted and bound. In constant fearful expectations, the musculature remains under constant tension, if not loosened by some kind of motoricity. Whereas the musculature relaxes in 'terror paralysis', in 'terror rigidity' it remains inflexible and a feeling of fear is not present or only partially developed. This would lead to the assumption that muscular rigidity can replace the vegetative anxiety reaction and therefore a functional unit exists formed by neurotic character and muscular dystonia.

The Therapeutic Approach

An abstinent therapeutic approach (as in a mirror function) will, in a psychically early disturbed patient with ego-function deficits and primary libidinous and aggressive impulses, stimulate uncontrollable processes which can lead to a destructive experience and aggravation of symptoms if not structured to a certain extent by the therapist. It is probably the combination of severity of the symptoms, weak ego and conflicts with an aggressive content which permits only a few asthma patients to endure the more neutral atmosphere of treatment over a long period. One prerequisite for this would be early childhood experience of a caring, trusting relationship, which is probably lacking in these patients.

The introduction of a first treatment phase, which Schöttler (1981) applied in severely disturbed psychosomatic patients, would seem of great importance here. According to her, acceptance of the corporality of the patient, common perception and verbal realization of this perception, and an approach of primary maternalism (Winnicott 1960) stand uppermost in this phase. This first treatment phase probably has an important therapeutic status for those patients not suited to psychoanalysis, not yet ready for treatment on the couch.

[1] Besides the character analysis used by Reich, Groddeck (1966) refers to the therapeutic possibilities of massage in influencing individual elements of the body, especially the movement apparatus.

Body awareness during psychoanalytic treatment has been systematically researched and further developed in theoretical as well as practical therapeutic approaches by M. Mitscherlich (1971, 1973, 1977). One sign of developmental disturbance which Mitscherlich saw in the psychosomatic patients she investigated (patients with spasmodic torticollis) was that the narcisstic, childish-magical omnipotence phantasies of these patients could not be shifted by means of a transitional object to a more realistic approach to reality. For these patients, therefore, the developmental stage of symbiosis still existed, which meant that the patients could not experience their body as autonomous and independent of the mother. These patients had not yet discovered their own (body) boundaries and even in their unconscious phantasies they could not experience their body as autonomous. It is therefore important that in time the patients experience their own body as belonging to them and being a part of their self.

Because of a disturbance in the early mother-child relationship, a specific interaction behaviour exists. The child has never had the experience of its body signals being correctly interpreted and responded to. It is therefore important in an analytic treatment to realize gestures, facial expressions, posture - all the patient's movements, in fact - and to draw these into the verbal dialogue. Instead of symbolization of the conflict on a physical level, as in the case of psychosomatic symptoms, the conflict should be raised to the verbal level and kept 'in suspension', i.e. in a corporeal emotional context. According to Shulte-Herbrüggen (1983), with such an approach one easily discovers an disturbance of the body schema and realizes that the way patients approach their own body determines to a considerable extent how they relates to themselves.

With the ego-disturbed patient, the therapist must, according to Fürstenau (1983), assume at the beginning of therapy certain ego functions as a substitute for the patient, so that the patient 'may gradually dissolve defensive structures and replace them with healthier ones'. However, mere perseverance in such a dual substitutive interaction does not suffice in order to attain satisfactory, stable treatment results; to persist would again result in a further life-long inner dependence on a providing and supportive object, which would in turn conjure up once more the danger of renewed psychic or psychosomatic decompensation. This assessment of Fürstenau applies especially to the so-called exercise approaches, also applied in asthma patients not suited to couch treatment. Autogenic training (Schultz 1979) and breathing gymnastics (Curtius 1965; Jores and Kerekjarto 1967) come to mind here, which from a psychoanalytic viewpoint represent a suggestive treatment with the possibility of positive transference (which through the use of a relaxation technique contains a self-hypnotic or auto-suggestive component). On the other hand, this form of treatment opens up a physical-emotional approach, which in part can renounce verbal interaction and which in a hypnotic 'maternal' manner appeals to the physical awareness of the patient. One could therefore, in an analysis of such an interaction, speak of a repetition of the mother-child relationship with a possible reparative character. The concentration on the physical awareness and the arbitrary guiding of the autonomic physical functions, e.g. in autogenic training, but also in concentrative movement therapy (Stolze 1977) or functional relaxation (Fuchs 1979), could be seen as a possibility of reliving early traumatic mother-child interactions (having occured during the formation of physiological body functions during the first weeks and months of life) and to relive them more positively. At least one effect of relaxation therapy is very evident and that is the awareness and strengthening of the body self. This leads to a strengthening of the ego and thus an improvement of self-confidence, both of which we as therapists assume to be particularly poorly developed in asthma patients during the first phase of life.

It is of interest that patients with early disturbances have particular difficulties with body awareness and body perception. It is almost as if a non-awareness of feelings, in the sense of a two-phase repression (Mitscherlich 1970), existed as well as a non-awareness of body sensations, with the exception of illness in the narrower sense. All other areas of experience and body awareness seem to be remarkably shallow.

Within such a situation, psychoanalytic treatment may bring diffuse early childhood states of emotion into the transference in those patients who have a favourable prognosis and are capable of introspection. In the area of secondary-process thinking, these may then be applied and worked through on an abstract level, as demonstrated in psychoanalytic case reports (e.g. Schöttler 1981).

The basic physical-psychic processes, however (in the sense of a psycho-physical interaction), especially in patients who are chronically ill and those less capable of introspection, demand additional techniques which will revive awareness and the experiencing of the body sphere by means of the newly implanted emotional recall.[2]

For some of the psychosomatically ill, a modification of the psychoanalytic technique or a complementation with body therapeutic procedures is recommended (Bräutigam 1978; Diederichs 1985), because 'in certain cases, besides the working up of remaining (because traumatic) infantile innocence, the mediation of new experiences - in the relationship to the analyst, but also in body therapy - represents an important prerequisite for successful treatment' (Fürstenau 1983).

The question to us was whether functional relaxation could be useful in the treatment of patients with bronchial asthma and what their experience would be with this body therapeutic technique.

Contrary to exercise techniques, offered more or less schematically in the form of breathing exercises or goal formation in the course of autogenic traing, functional relaxation according to Fuchs (1979) attempts a more differentiated approach: first of all patients are given the opportunity at the beginning of therapy to preoccupy themselves with their body and autonomous breathing rhythm; thereafter, they verbalize their body awareness or body experience with the corresponding sensations. The therapist incorporates these systematically, acts as a mirror and adds depth to the experienced sensations.

[2] In more intensive uncovering techniques, e.g. bioenergetics or gestalt therapy, it is sometimes very difficult adequately to work through the psychodynamics resulting from the technique and integrate them in to the mature ego of the patient without risking flooding by primary process maternal and thus evoking unforeseen consequences for the ego integration of the patients.

Method

Ninety selected asthma patients from the University Medical Hospital, Heidelberg, who had been in-patients between 1 Januar 1977 and 31 July 1980 were offered analytic disease-oriented group treatment Deter and Allert 1983). Thirty-one patients were set up in three groups according to the order in which they signed up: one treatment group with the additional offer of autogenic treatment, one group with the offer of functional relaxation and a control group (treatment was offered to the latter group 1 year later).

Laboratory tests were carried out for each patient, as well as pneumological, clinical and psychodiagnostic examination before and after treatment; they kept complaint and medication progress reports. The mean age of the 31 patients (14 men and 17 women) was 43.5 years, the mean duration of illness was 16.8 years. Nine patients had moderate asthma and 12 patients severe asthma. In 64% of the patients, the cause of the asthma was assumed to be allergy induced, in 87% an infection was assumed. Ninety-three of the patients showed psychic conflicts in varying degrees which in 48% of the patients led to asthma attacks.

The results of this investigation have been published previously (Deter and Allert 1983; Deter 1986a, b). Of interest for this present investigation was that there was a distinct difference between the three groups after 1 year of group therapy (1 h/week) as shown in a standardized questionnaire (15 questions) to body awareness. Whereas the control group replied to an average of 6.8 of the suggested responses, the group with functional relaxation as additional treatment showed twice that (13.6). Of interest is also that, in comparison, the group given autogenic training were noticeably less able to verbalize their body sensations (on average 8.1 responses).

This inquiry into body awareness will now be supplemented by reports from the functional relaxation therapist and the analytic group therapist of what they observed during the course of the combined functional relaxation group.

Observations of the Functional Relaxation Therapist

My first impression of the participants was an extremely rigid, armour-like, and drawn-up posture, especially in the men. In two overweight patients a certain awkwardness and heaviness was apparent, and in most patients an audible breathing sound. In contrast to this, most of the women seemed depressed, reserved and strikingly pale.[3] The patients seemed to be isolated, i.e. they hardly spoke to one another, and in a monotonous voice described in great detail their somatic disease and treatments in hospital and at health resorts. While speaking the turned primarily to the therapists or reacted only to their questions or interventions. The

[3] Fuchs has made similar observations: 'The pathological functional structure of the asthma patient shows itself in functional relaxation as reserved, closed and tense. Specific emotions and affects of the patient are expressed in this behaviour which is part of the pathogenesis of bronchial asthma, and it is the goal of functional relaxation to alter this.' (Fuchs 1979, p. 95).

men turned more to me (the female therapist) than the women, who were oriented more towards the male therapist. This differing approach played an important role for the group dynamics throughout. It was noted in general that over the 2 years of treatment an obvious improvement of communication between the participants took place, while the transference observed at the beginning continued throughout, although less pronounced.

The men's flow of speech often began as if someone had pressed a button, and was very difficult to interrupt. This overflow of speech did not, however, however alleviate their difficulties with interaction. Their profound bodily disturbance obviously influenced their interpersonal relationships. At this point in time, the meaning of their behaviour or of their symptom was not apparent to the patients. This changed, however, with the growing ability to be aware of the various body sensations and to verbalize.

An understanding of the symptom and of themselves came about during treatment; in general the capacity for interpersonal relationships developed. Slowly the patients became interested in the new ways of interacting and the support they could give themselves for their own stabilization. Here again the men were more open in accepting and applying the approaches of functional relaxation; the women were more resistent, and hesitant. In this first phase of functional relaxation, they preferred massage, baths, and also transcendental meditation, yoga, and zen, as just as good if not better methods of therapy.

The first approaches to functional relaxation concerned the perception of the patient's own body weight and the changing pressure relations in the body when "letting go" on the mat, on "solid ground". during the first sessions I did not talk about breathing; at the most I would ask the patients to let themselves fall onto the mat or into a chair with an unaffected moaning or growling inwards-outwards. We tried out and talked about the possibilities of letting go. We took our time in talking about the phantasies associated with the words "letting go" and "letting". As in individual therapeutic treatment, the first reactions to the words "letting go" were more or less negative. To begin with it meant nonchalance, negligence, loss of composure and instability. The worst association was loss of control of oneself, thus exposing oneself to uncertainty, without knowing what this would lead to. The possibility or the danger of behaving aggressively, uncontrollably and for no good reason, was extremely disquieting.

Functional relaxation has the advantage of reliving invented, imagined, phantasized words and pictures. I asked the patients to act for just one moment as if they mistrusted the mat, the carrying, holding and supporting base: it could possibly collapse. The patients went into a "watch out" position; they pulled themselves together and became quite obviously rigid and tense: a slight drawing-up of the posture markedly altered the unpleasant and restrictive side of such a physical imagination. After a short try, they let go, let themselves plop down and fall, realized that the mat held and carried them, and that nothing unexpected or terrible would happen. They felt lighter, did not threaten to dissolve, but retained their shape and their boundaries. In short, externally, visibly, hardly anything had changed, but their physical awareness contrasted sharply to the controls. The advantage of the described body experience within a homogeneous group lies in the individual experience which each group member can experience for and with himself, e.g. how the he perceives, feels and experiences himself in his interactive contact with the mat. That is his reality; it is his own experience and perception, comparable with but not the same as that of the other patients.

A differentiated body awareness is striven for, which will allow the development and consciousness of a distinctive body perception from the sick body perceived as "foreign". The physical perceptions at the beginning of group therapy as stipulated by the patients were for the most part the following: the body is tense, hard as a board, clumsy, heavy, wooden and immobile. We differentiated between those parts of the body which could be let go more easily, which were felt to be softer, yielding, warmer, wider and permeable. The increasing ability of differentiating perception, acquired in a patient learning process - "I am like this: the others are like that" - was the basis on which differentiation between perception of self and of others became possible.

The invitation of functional relaxation to use space, to expand according to one's own needs, to use the space where one is sitting, lying or standing, to weigh it down, to take control of it, led to different reactions. For example, the feedback that the floor is hard, solid, supportive or that the mat is fading away, yielding, uncertain, "I am falling into a deep hole", "I dare not", may be used diagnostically by the functional relaxation therapist.

It is not a specific experience that I have frequently had as a functional relaxation therapist, but it could be observed throughout in our group that the men stretched out more unreservedly, more naturally, and much more securely than the women, who hesitated, closed their eyes and in general were more on the watch. A similar distribution could be seen in the conversation: again the women were more hesitant, were silent, or only spoke when asked to do so.

After by a long and patient process found the solid ground during the first sessions, and after everyone could decide whether they felt securer sitting or lying down - thus having the freedom to chose what is right for each person - we then turned to the individual body regions: the joints, the sacral region, the spine and the internal cavities.

To begin with we looked at the unnoticed blockades of the oral cavity and the oropharynx. Again and again the tongue which closed the oropharynx "hundreds of times a day" had to be released from the palate. It was now no longer difficult to approach the inward-outward flow of expiration. Two patients had accepted the "opening" especially well because a tense mouth, with frequent nocturnal grinding of the teeth, had led to painful jaws. It was easy to feel the faulty tension here and just as easy to do something about it immediately, to withdraw oneself from the excess of tension, to become open and permeable towards one own's centre. The minimal expiration in the mostly tense thorax was at first not felt there, but in the abdominal-pelvic region, by which the connection and direction of the autonomous downward rhythm could be traced. We frequently began the sessions, having let go on the mat, with a brief checking of the oropharynx and the connection between head-neck and trunk. The loosening of this region could soon be done at home without any difficulty and was felt to be very helpful and comforting by all. It was especially important before falling asleep to relieve oneself of unnecessary tension and to thus reduce the fear of nocturnal attacks. Some patients were already able to take a quiet "inner" break unnoticed by anyone during work or during the course of the day. Functional relaxation was turning into a better medication, or as one patient put it, "a safer pill".

All participants, asthmatics as well as therapists, had to be patient with the upper sacral region and the thorax. To begin with we tried to mobilize the "stick-like" thoracic spine into various initial positions, and with great cautiousness and care we were able to sense that the tense and armour-like thorax had become more compliant, yielding. There is no one sequence or prescribed method of procedure in functional relaxation; one should be guided by one's physical condition and individual needs. The approach functional relaxation offers to goal-oriented, will-power-oriented as well as slightly compulsive patients was at first disconcerting: there was no training, no formation of rules or resolutions, one did not have to start at a certain point, but rather at the point where tension, a narrowness existed, and, again, one only had to remain there as long as one wanted to. Such alleged freedom of movement and freedom of method had to be emphasized again and again. However, despite this playful handling, the patients must play by the rules established on a distinct methodological concept.

'"Waggling" the lower sacral region, the upright position, mobility of the spine, lying down as well as sitting, again and again the fathomless thorax open to the abdominal-pelvic region - this was our material, what we had to work with. The patients came looking for help, they were suffering. This meant that they determined the pace of therapy, the course of the sessions. The complaints, faulty behaviour, were the material which the functional relaxation therapist had to handle. For this purpose, patience and perseverance were necessary; it was especially importanct not to feel pressure, not to want to see results after each session: something always happens anyway, because "the patient knows best what will help him" (von Weizsäcker 1951), i.e. he may complain as long as he needs to, or rationalize or offer resistance in the psychic as well as physical sense, whereby we can understand the physical tensions as materialized resistance. Only when the gamble of loosening up became possible were the patients capable of working through their conflicts in the psychotherapeutic sense. This phase of working through set in after about 8 months.'

Observations of the Analytic Group Therapist

While writing the protocol, but also of course during the group sessions, it became evident that our experiment of a psychoanalytically oriented group therapist and a functional relaxation therapist working together in a homogeneous group of asthma patients would lead to language problems, as well as to problems in associating with one another. As described above, dissociation processes in transference developed, which were probably due to the psychodynamics of the patients treated.

One striking fact was that the men had a positive transference and the women a more negative transference towards the female functional relaxation therapist, whereas this transference, although not quite as strong, was reversed where the male therapist was concerned. The therapeutic technique applied seemed to lead to a symbiotic constellation in which the men being treated felt comfortable, whereas the women demonstrated ambivalence, a distinct distance and nonverbalized criticism. Nevertheless, the physical work was continued. The female therapist experienced this form of resistance towards treatment as a disturbance of the intensive body therapy taking place within the positive transference and had the wish to remove the female patients from the group, since they seemed to show no interest. The male group therapist, however, experienced these transference situations more as an aggressive, distant latency of all group members, which he therefore verbalized in order get to grips with the latent group dynamics. The women especially took this up with great relief. On this level, therefore, there was a dissociation within the group concerning the libidinous and aggressive transference to the therapists; the therapists, for their part, had to communicate quite often and very intensively, so as not to fall prey to these dynamics.

On another level, there was dissociation in an early preverbal symbiotic dimension, allowing for similarities with primary process thinking, and a level of verbalized dynamic object relations corresponding to a later development stage, in which a rival "oedipality" (between the therapists) became evident. Comprehending and resolving these dynamics seemed to be a important prerequisite for the integration of the psychic strivings and the conflict dynamics of the individual patient.

It was very clear to me that within the first group session the rigid thinking patterns of the patients and their social adaptation could be related to, individualized and therefore partially overcome by means of their own body awareness. This also meant an influence on the attitude towards the illness. We talked about everyone being responsible for their own illness and the treatment measures; in the case of mistreatment, they would be the ones to suffer. Thus a stronger consciousness of their individual situation arose with the feeling of responsibility ("There is no one right thing for the treatment of the illness, but rather all measures and attitudes must be related and checked for each individual": there is an individual body awareness and an individual managing of the illness).

What the "letting go" or the search for a basic physical confidence meant may be shown using the following example. A 30-year-old female patient concentrated so hard on letting go that she had an asthma attack during the group session. On the basis of her life history, her letting go had ambivalent connotations. She experienced it as being very dangerous because she had to a certain extent to give up control over her personal situation, as well as over the illness; the latter entailed a danger to her life, an asthma attack one could also, with Reich, speak of the development of fear on loosening the character armour).

Parallel to the body therapy, the group sessions showed that the thematic accents within the treatment period had changed. At the beginning, medication, the weather, coughing, mucus, and general illness problems were the topics, but within the course of therapy, patients' own, personal and familiy events, moods or emotions were at the centre of attention. However, in certain phases of the group, these were also supplemented by description of new symptoms of illness.

At the end of the group it seemed important to thematize this separation continously. However, the body experience of separation and the delineation from the others and the group could be intensified by working on patients' own body borders (Federn) using functional relaxation. This new way of handling the body worked; the participants developed a sense of sureness towards unknown and dangerous situations with less development of fear and less muscular tension. They now had the possibility of handling everyday events. They now accepted the body more as being a part of themselves and experienced it more: a body they could handle, a body that was sometimes ill, but which also had positive sides. The patients appeared to be more sensitive and, at the same time, noticeably more self-confident.

In addition, they showed more possibilities of communicating and a more sensitive treatment of other group members, so that emotions could be verbalized within the group almost unnoticeably. By means of this treatment technique, group therapy remained not only cognitive, but led to differentiation with the patients' own corporality and intensive experience and emotional states, which could be treated psychotherapeutically within the body treatment.

It should be evident that it was not an isolated body treatment that was offered, but that new body experiences influenced the psychic situation of the patients and their verbalization abilities in the same manner; thus, a new personality dimension of the patient was treatable, which up to that point the patient had not been able to verbalize.

Besides the body awareness and the verbalizatiuon of states of well-being and emotions, transference developed towards the therapist and the functional relaxation therapist, which must be designated as symbiotic; depending on their early experiences, the male patients developed a positive transference to the female therapist, and a few female patients a positive transference to the male therapist (with distinct negative-colloured elements, e.g. in a patient with a hyusteric structure and a deeply distrusting attitude). One could speak here of a splitting-up of the transference into a good and a bad object. It is interesting that in this warming-up phase of the group there was competition only at a very superficial level; of more importance were the basic functions of trust and distrust.

The development of "safeness" with the emergence of the feeling of being able to let go and the simultaneous experience of inner and outer security can be seen as connected with this.

We had the impression that the patients were beginning to give their bodily self-representation new forms and, with the help of their ego function (self-perception), emotional life, i.e. expanding their ego boundaries. They were investing in their body positively, with the result of wanting to use the newfound mobility. This whole process was accompanied by a rise in self-esteem which in chronic asthma patients is often very low. Parallel to this there was also an investment displacement of their own physical feeling; up to that point, the asthma patients had concentrated their attention for years on breathing and lung function. The extreme desire to control bronchial function had taken away all interest in possible other body perception and for the most part paralyzed perception of all free activity.

Kuhn et al. (1981) have described the attitude of asthma patients at the beginning of an asthma attack: the feelings of helplessness, anger at being confronted with a situation they have no control over and which they can not dominate. This basic experience (but also perhaps the possible initial position in early childhood before the development of asthma or its forerunner)could now be taken up again and mastered by means of physical observation and perception exercises; the positive transference to the therapists (espicially to the female functional relaxation therapist, who intensified this effect by means of her behaviour) seemed to be the motivating and supportive strength needed for this new body awareness.

The combination of a new physical investment and positive transference seemed to allow a new physiological-psychic experience, in which the male group therapist, because of his rational support and professional competence, seemed to represent the dissociated part of reality in the reorganization of the mother-child symbiosis; this allowed the adult ego of the patient to reattempt a working out of traumatic early childhood experiences.

This emotional maturation was possible within the context of the 2-year group therapy; besides a certain emotional stability achieved during this time span, other factors surely aided this: the cathartic moments of exchanging views during group treatment, the existential experience of realizing one is alone with one's illness (but so are the others), the adaptation to the reality of handling the illness as well as mastering it medically.

The extensive mastering of the psychic maturation, as described by Schöttler (1981) in psychoanalytic treatment lasting up to 8 years, with correspondingly complete working out of the psychic disturbance, could of course not be demonstrated within our group therapy. The question is whether in long-term chronic asthma, such as most of our patients had, such working out is possible and good policy. Our treatment technique described here was from the beginning restricted to a particular analytic treatment goal.'

References

Bischof N (1966) Stellungs-, Spannungs- und Lagewahrnehmung. In Metzger W (ed) Handbuch der Psychol. vol 1, part 1. Hogrefe, Göttingen, p 409-497

Bräutigam W (1978) Verbale und präverbale Methoden in der stationären Therapie. Z Psychsom Med Psychoanal 24: 146-155

Casper R, Halmi KA, Goldberg SC, Eckert ED, Davis JM (1979) Disturbances in body image estimation as related to other characteristics and outcome in anorexia nervosa. Br J Psychiatry 134: 60-66

Conrad K (1933) Das Körperschema. Eine kritische Studie und der Versuch einer Revision. Z Ges Neurol Psychiatr 147: 346-369

Curtius F (1965) Moderne Asthmabehandlung. Springer, Berlin Heidelberg New York

De Boor C (1965) Zur Psychosomatik der Allergie und des Asthma bronchiale. Huber, Bern, p 285

Deter HC (1986) Cost benefit analysis of psychosomatic therapy in asthma. J Psychosom Res 30: 173-182

Deter HC (1986b) Psychosomatische Behandlung des Asthma bronchiale. Springer, Berlin Heidelberg New York

Deter HC, Allert G (1983) Group therapy of asthma patients. A concept for the psychosomatic treatment for patients in a medical clinic. Psychother Psychosom 40: 95-105

Diederichs P (1985) Über den Versuch einer Integration narzissmustheoretischer und triebpsychologischer Aspekte am Beispiel der männlichen Miktionsstörung (Prostatopathie). 4th scientific meeting of the Deutsche psychoanalytische Gesellschaft, Frankfurt, 15 Feb 1985

Federn P (1978) Ich-Psychologie und die Psychosen. Suhrkamp, Frankfurt, pp 28-49

Freud S (1914) Zur Einführung des Narzissmus. Gesammelte Werke, vol 10. Fischer, Frankfurt, Standard edn. vol 14

Fürstenau P (1983) Einige Bemerkungen zur psychoanalytischen Behandlung basaler, leibnaher Störungen. Mater Psychoanal 9: 40-46

Fuchs M (1979) Funktionelle Entspannung. Hippokrates, Stuttgart
Groddeck G (1966) Massage. In: Clauser G (ed) Psychoanalytische Schrift zur Psychosomatik. Limes, Wiesbaden, pp 249-255
Hartmann H, Schilder P (1927) Körperinneres und Körperschema. Z Ges Neurol Psychiatr 109: 666-675
Hoffer W (1978) Die Entwicklung des Körper-Ichs. In: Overbeck G, Ovberbeck A (eds) Seelischer Konflikt, körperliches Leiden. Rowohlt, Hamburg, pp 185-194
Jacobsen E (1978) Das Selbst und die Welt der Objekte. Suhrkamp, Frankfurt
Joraschky P (1983) Das Körperschema und das Körperselbst als Regulationsprinzipien der Organismus-Umwelt-Interaktion. Minverva, Munich
Jores A, Kerekjarto M von (1967) Der Asthmatiker. Ätiologie und Therapie des Asthma bronchiale aus psychologischer Sicht. Huber, Bern
Kiener F (1973) Untersuchungen zum Körperbild, Teil I. Z Klin Psychol Psychother 21: 335-351
Kiener F (1974) Untersuchungen zum Körperbild. Teil II. Z Klin Psychol Psychother 22: 45-66
Kuhn H, Engel R, King U, Hörnig G (1981) Psychophysiologische Untersuchungen beim Asthma bronchiale. In: Zander W (ed) Experimentelle Forschungsergebnisse in der psychosomatischen Medizin. Vandenhoeck und Ruprecht, Göttingen, pp 129-141
Lickint K (1970) Die psychische Steuerung physischer Abläufe insbesondere bei der Konversion. Psyche (Stuttg) 24: 292-306
Mahler MS (1968) Symbiose und Individuation. Klett, Stuttgart
Meermann R, Fichter M (1983) Störungen des Körperschemas bei Pupertätsmagersucht. Psychother Med Psychol
Mitscherlich A (1970) Ein psychosomatisches Modell. Schritte der Forschung. Studien zur psychosomatischen Medizin. Suhrkamp, Frankfurt, pp 2-39
Mitscherlich M (1971) Zur Psychoanalyse der Torticollis spasticus. Nervenarzt 42: 420-426
Mitscherlich M (1973) Analytische Behandlung von Hyperkinesien. Med Welt 25: 1058-1062
Mitscherlich M (1977) Der interaktionelle Ansatz im psychosomatischen Denken. Weiterentwicklung der Psychoanalyse und ihrer Anwendungen. In: Condrau G, Hicklin A (eds) Individuum, Familie. Gesellschaft im Spannungsfeld zwischen Zwang und Freiheit. Vandenhoeck und Ruprecht, Göttingen
Montagu A (1974) Touching: The human significance of the skin. Columbia Universities Press, New York
Paulus R, Otte R (1979) Zur Erfassung der Zufriedenheit mit dem Aussehen des eigenen Körpers. Psychother Med Psychol 29: 128-141
Reich W (1975) Lust, Angst, Wut und muskuläre Panzerung. In: Reich W (ed) Charakteranalyse. Fischer, Frankfurt, pp 344-357
Schilder P (1923) Das Körperschema. Ein Beitrag zur Lehre vom Bewusstsein des eigenen Körpers. Springer, Berlin
Schöttler C (1981) Zur Behandlungstechnik bei psychosomatisch schwer gestörten Patienten. Psyche (Stuttg) 10: 111-141
Schulte-Herbrüggen UW (1983) Die Bedeutung des Körperschemas für die Technik psychoanalytischer Behandlung von psychosomatisch Erkrankten. Mater Psychoanal 9: 27-31
Schultz IH (1979) Das Autogene Training, 16th edn. Thieme, Stuttgart
Schur M (1978) Zur Metapsychologie der Somatisierung. In: Overbeck G, Overbeck A (eds) Seelischer Konflikt, körperliches Leiden. Rowohlt, Hamburg, pp 83-142
Schwab J, Harmeling J (1968) Body image and medical illness. Psychosom Med 30: 51-61
Spitz RA (1965) The first year of life, 2nd edn. International Universities Press, New York
Stolze H (1977) Konzentrative Bewegungstherapie. In: Eickc D (ed) Psychologie des 20. Jahrhunderts III. Kindler, Zürich, pp 1250-1273
Weiner H (1977) Psychobiology and human diseases. Elsevier, New York, pp 223-317
Weizsäcker V. von (1951) Fälle und Probleme. Enke, Stuttgart
Winnicott (1960) Primäre Mütterlichkeit. Psyche (Stuttg) 14: 25-28

Exercises in Concentrative Body Perception: A Psychophysiological Therapy Technique

W. Dahlmann

An Approach to Treating Diseases of the Locomotor System with Disturbances in Body Perception

On the following pages we shall be dealing with disurbances in body perception and how they can be treated with exercises in concentrative body perception. Two types of disease where this is especially relevant will serve as examples: first, multiple sclerosis, where especially the spinal efferent tracts have been disrupted by defects in the central nervous system and, second, forms of backache in which the objective pathological findings in the lumbar vertebral column and the paravertebral muscles cannot adequately explain the excessive degree of pain subjectively experienced by these patients. Clinically speaking we are dealing here with spinal-ataxic gait disturbances occurring in chronic progressive (benign) multiple sclerosis (diffuse encephalomyelitis) and chronic backache of psychosomatic origin with predominant subjective pain.

Disturbances in Body Perception

Body perception disorders in the locomotor system arise above all when the sense of posture and movement (kinaesthesia), which as a rule works below the threshold of consciousness, is impaired in its functioning as a result of disturbances in the sensorimotor system and - actually or potentially - enters consciousness as an impairment.

All finely co-ordinated movement, whether voluntary or involuntary, and the changes in muscular tension this involes, depends on a complex sensorimotor regulatory system. From superficial and deep sensibility receptors there is a continous flow of afferent information coming from the skin (pressure and position sensations), tendons, joint capsules and muscles (postural and movement sensations) for central evaluation, so that the precise position of every part of the body can be ascertained at any moment in time. For every fine voluntary or involuntary movement, this afferent information can be called up at lightning speed to establish the initial position. The movement itself is regulated by efferent information but also brings with it new afferent information, and so forth.

Thus the central nervous system is constantly processing afferent information and using this to regulate and monitor motor efferents. The motor system is a sensorimotor system (Ebbecke 1959). Within the sensorimotor system it is possible to perceive the motor and the sensory aspects consciously as being both separate and related and to influence them as such. Motor sequences can be planned in the imagination and carried out by the muscles on the periphery. Every movement or postural change taking place in the locomotor system can be identified in detail 'from within', i.e. without optical control and purely on the basis of centrally registered information about pressure, posture and motion coming from peripheral receptors situated in the skin, tendons, joint capsules and muscles. In this manner the central interplay of motor sequences and sensory information can be followed consciously in the finest detail. Furthermore, this incoming sensory information is subject to constant alteration by every new motor movement, making even more intensive perception of sensory processes possible.

Impairment of the motor system (paralysis) upsets one's perception of one's own posture and movement just as much as defects in the sensory sphere, even though body perception disorders are caused primarily by disturbed or defective afferents. In cases of peripheral or central paralysis, the disturbances in body perception are due to asymmetric alterations in the afferent information. The changes in muscle tone (atonic or spastic) associated with the paralysis influence perception of the affected area. Defects in the afferent sensory system give rise to very considerable disorders in body perception because they have the tendency to spread their influence beyond the actual region of the defect. Thus, relatively minor defects in the spinal afferents can, for example, make a whole extremity feel numb and alien. Around an afferent defect, additional functional disturbances arise in body perception which make themselves felt whenever the person affected tries to perceive his or her body more consciously.

Undisturbed perception of our own posture and movements and of the functioning of our locomotor system in general is for most of us a matter of course. Many people are not even able to become consciously aware of their bodies at rest and in motion, and of the constant changes in muscular tension that are involved, without external help. This is probably also why sudden changes in our perception of our bodies are so disconcerting. Disturbances in body perception have a detrimental effect on the co-ordination of motor sequences (e.g. in spinalataxic gait disturbances) and, where they are also accompanied by chronic pain, on other things such as muscular tension as well (e.g. in chronic backache).

The functional aspects of disorders in body perception can be treated with body perception exercises. Improved perception of posture and motion in the locomotor system has a beneficial influence on motor co-ordination and on the muscular functions.

Concentrative body perception exercises help patients to discover and become conscious of disturbances in their body perception. These are generally to be found where there are known to be defective efferents, as with paralysis involving changes in muscle tone, and with defective afferents, like ataxic conditions. In the course of the exercises, present as well as past areas of pain (e.g. chronic backache, an old fracture or shell wound dating many years back) can make themselves felt again as disturbances in body perception.

Patients with peripheral paresis of the facial nerve report a subjective sensation of strangeness and numbness on the side of the face affected. This disturbance in their perception of the facial muscles, which has its origin in an alteration in muscular tension on only one side, bothers the patients so much that they repeatedly touch the skin of their face and sometimes even pinch the muscle. Objectively what has happened is that the tone of the facial muscle supplied by the facial nerve has been reduced, causing an asymetrical alteration in the usual perception of the muscle tension in the face. The reduced tone of the paralysed facial muscles and the lack of motor activation produce the strange, alien sensation and the numbness, although the trigeminal nerve is quite intact. In a similar manner every peripheral or central paralysis is accompanied by disturbed body perception.

Wherever there are lesions of the peripheral, spinal or central tracts that carry information on superficial or deep sensibility (afferents), the accompanying perception disorders are brought out particularly clearly by the body perception exercises. These lesions regularly develop the tendency to extend beyond the original, organically limited afferent defect. Thus, even minor afferent defects such as hypo-aesthesia L5/S1 as a rule produce disturbances in body perception involving the entire leg, which is perceived as a numb, strange entity, disconnected from the trunk. The disturbances in fine motor control have spread to affect the entire extremity.

When patients with localized chronic pain conditions (e.g. chronic backache) do body perception exercises they too evince disorders in body perception. Either the painful area of the body is banned from conscious perception completely or the pains are initially felt even more acutely than before. It appears that in these conditions the central evaluation of the otherwise intact afferent information coming from the affected part of the body has been altered as a result of the excessive pain. At first, these patients are incapable of more conscious perception of posture and motion in this part of the body.

Exercises in Concentrative Body Perception

The method of concentrative body perception at rest and in motion makes use of body exercises originally taken from physiotherapy (Engeling 1966; Meyer 1961). The use of this sort of motion exercises goes back to the observation that, besides the control of motion sequences by optical means, there is another, very precise, means of access to fine motor regulation. With eyes closed it is possible to perceive very fine muscular tensions and motion sequences from within. These percepts are based on information coming from pressure, postural and motion receptors. Motion sequences can be controlled more exactly through this sort of concentrative, inner perception than is possible by visual means, e.g. via a mirror, partly because the muscular tension that initiates a movement is perceived immediately, at a stage when no movement is yet visible to the eye. In this manner, very finely regulated motor sequences can be performed and, if necessary, corrected and repeated. Patterns of movement that are impaired by defective body perception can be improved through repeated practice using this sort of concentrative body perception.

The therapeutic exercises themselves really amount to a series of concentrated mental and perceptual processes, whereby the pressure and tension conditions present in the skin, tendons, joint capsules and muscles when the body is at rest or in motion are sensed very acutely. In this way, the patients learn to become more consciously aware of how the senses of pressure, posture and motion function in the locomotor system.

To enable them first of all to become acquainted with this sort of mental and perceptual approach, it is best not to involve the areas known to be affected by perceptional disturbances straight away but rather to begin with exercises focusing on the respiratory system. Concentrative breathing exercises offer a good starting point for teaching the technique to beginners and should be repeated as part of the exercise repertoire throughout.

Breathing work is particularly easy to perceive and helps the beginner to develop the sort of understanding and concentration which is required for subsequent work with other areas of the body. Our breathing consists of a rhythmical in- and outflow of air which usually regulates itself without voluntary control but can also be directed at will. Learning to be more aware of the ways in which one can breathe in and out (doing it voluntarily or allowing it to happen involuntarily) is a good way of becoming acquainted with one's own capacity for consciously perceiving tension and relaxation states in the body. Once the person doing the exercises is able to experience how their own body perception functions here, then exercises involving other areas of the body will usually succeed as well. Concentrating on being able to perceive states of tension and relaxation in larger and smaller areas of the body is a recurrent theme throughout the exercises. Once the basics of the technique have been acquired, the actual therapeutic work with those areas affected by perception disorders can begin.

The exercises are performed with the patients lying on their backs on firm mats, quite relaxed, concentrating their whole attention on their bodies. In individual stages, the physiotherapist repeats aloud the mental and perceptual steps to be carried out and the patients follow these instructions by actively applying them in thought and perception to their own bodies.

For the initial breathing work the text spoken by the therapist could run as follows: 'Lie quite still and watch your breathing. With every wave of breath, feel how your chest and rib cage are raised up and how they slowly sink back down again. Breathe in deeply and feel how your chest and thorax expand and broaden out. Let the air out gradually and feel how your chest slowly relaxes. Allow your breath to continue gently flowing in and out and give yourself over to sensing how it does it; watch it in your mind's eye; turn your thoughts inwards, into your body ...'

An example of a shorter text related to a smaller area of the body could go something like this: 'Now concentrate your mind completely on your left leg; let your thoughts wander into your foot; feel the tips of your toes, one after the other; feel your way up the underside of your toes, along the arches of your feet and on into your ankles. Let go completely, relax and then go on feeling your way into your lower leg ...'

The method of concentrative body perception is a psychophysiological technique whereby the relative pressure and tension conditions in the skin, tendons, joint capsules and muscles are repeatedly sensed and consciously perceived. Little movement exercises requiring alternate tensing and relaxing of the muscles assist these perceptual processes. The heightened body awareness acquired through the technique means that the afferent information delivered from the periphery for central processing becomes more conscious than it was before. With more differentiated afferent information at its disposal, the sensorimotor system can improve its motor performance. At the same time a better, because more conscious, perception of one's own posture and motion as part of the locomotor system becomes established.

The exercises in concentrative body perception can be learnt and continued later on by the patients independently, without further help from a therapist. Thus, this form of therapy contains a further activating function in that it encourages the patients to alleviate their complaints on a symptomatic level themselves by means of the exercises.

For the spinal ataxic gait disturbances that result from the incurable chronic disease of multiple sclerosis, this method has the special advantage that the exercises can be repeated again and again without risk and still retain their effectivity. With ataxic gait disturbances the success of the method has been proved by objective measurements of walking ability. The main emphasis in the treatment of sensorimotor motion disturbances is usually on physiotherapy. Significant additional improvements can be achieved if this work is supplemented by concentrative body perception exercises.

With cases of chronic backache, it is preferable to begin by combining concentrative body perception work with gentle extensions of the muscles and tendons. Concentrative perception of muscular tension together with careful, step-by-step extension of the muscles in the region of pain make it possible for the patient to begin extending the muscles in the affected area without exceeding the considerably raised pain-reflex stimulus threshold. Extension stimuli are very important for the overstrained muscles, not least for the sake of improving their metabolism.

Concentrative Body Perception Exercises for Spinal Ataxic Gait Disturbances

Spinal ataxic gait disturbances are a form of handicap frequently resulting from chronic progressive diffuse encephalomyelitis as well as other diseases or post-traumatic lesions affecting the spinal cord. In contrast to mainly spastic ataxic gait disorders, for which drugs that relieve muscle spasm are available, there is no known therapy which can influence disorders of the spinal afferents.

We treated 39 patients suffering from spinal ataxic gait disturbances (22 of them with chronic progressive multiple sclerosis), offering them a course of exercises in concentrative body perception. The main focus of the exercises was on the region of the lower extremities. The physiotherapist's instructions to the patients to concentrate their thoughts on the pressure and tension conditions in the skin, tendons, joint capsules and muscles, were given in roughly the words below. These she repeated with calmness and concentration, inserting small pauses throughout. The whole exercise takes about 15–20 min. With daily sessions, about 15–20 sessions are necessary.

You are lying stretched out on the floor, eyes closed, your face muscles are relaxed; your arms are lying loosely at your sides, your hands resting palm down on the mat; your legs are a little apart, your feet turned slightly outwards with toes pointing down; your calves are touching the mat, the hollows at the back of your knees are quite relaxed and should gradually, little by little, sink down towards the floor. You can feel the underside of your thighs, from the back of your knees right up to your buttocks, resting gently on the mat.

Try to release the tension in both legs, direct the relaxation down into your feet, and try to sense your toes; relax them, letting them sink down slightly. Begin to feel your way along the soles of your feet, feeling their breadth and their shape, feel how they arch up in the middle; wander down towards your toes and once again picture in your mind's eye the sole of your foot. Inch your way along every bit of it again, from your heel to the tips of your toes. Now you can sense the bottom of your feet quite clearly. Feel your way gradually up the back of your heels to your ankles; release the tension there and let your feet and toes sink down a little further. Wander slowly up from your ankles into your lower leg and feel how the muscles in your calves make closer contact with the mat. In your imagination begin to work your way gradually up your calves, feeling the breadth of the whole area, and turn your mind to your knee joints. Both knees are quite loose and relaxed, the joints sink a little closer to the floor, and your attention begins to wander further upwards and into your thighs.

Go on climbing, feeling the whole breadth of your thighs, how they broaden as you get higher and reach the place where they merge into your hips. Let all the tension go out of your hips, let them sink towards the floor and try to feel the base of your spine between your hips. Feel the expanse of your lower abdomen stretching right down to the groin and across the whole area of your pelvis. Release all the tension there and let the small of your back sink down; feel the relief spreading right down into your legs, your thighs, your knees, your lower legs and into your feet. Feel the light, relaxed sensation from your abdomen down to your legs and feet and feel how heavily you are lying on the floor.

Now turn your thoughts to your breathing and concentrate completely on the region of your abdomen. A deep wave of breath makes your abdomen expand right down to the groin so that you become aware of the whole breadth of your lower abdomen. Follow the wave of breath further and feel how it fills your waist and spreads into your back on both sides of the base of your spine. Release the areas of tension in your abdomen and back, let go when you breathe out; always make your breathing come from the centre of your body, from your diaphragm, and allow it to spread down into your back and up into your chest. Loosen the tension in your back and shoulders, let your hips sink right down: give way, feel your hips and the small of your back resting gently on the floor. Feel how the whole length and breadth of your back, from buttocks to shoulder blades, is touching the mat. One wave of breath follows another. As the air flows in, it raises your diaphragm and chest, expands your whole rib cage; then it gradually flows out, making your rib cage and abdomen sink back down again, right down into your back. Feel the whole of your back as a single unit reaching from your shoulder-blades to the base of your spine. Let it sink down, right down to your knees; give way, loosen all tension. Feel the expanse of your chest and abdomen once again, right across your back, and feel the air flowing into it. Check again whether the region around the base of your spine and the small of your back is really relaxed, whether the area of your lower pelvis reaching right down to the insides of your thighs is really free of all tension, whether your abdomen is still loose and relaxed. See if your shoulders are both resting symmetrically on the floor and whether your neck and shoulders are quite relaxed.

Turn your attention again to both legs, feel them both lying stretched out, their whole length from heels to buttocks, on the floor, quite relaxed. Give way still more in your hips and the small of your back, letting everything sink down still further towards the floor. Become aware once again of how broad your abdomen and chest are as you breathe, sense how deeply you are breathing, how your body expands from groin to chest, right to your collar bones, and how everything stretches, from the bottom of your spine right up to your shoulder-blades. Give way to it, let everything go as you gently breathe out and lie quite calm and relaxed.

If it seems necessary, go back and repeat: 'turn back once more to your feet and try to sense your toes ...' (as above).

Before beginning treatment with these exercises, the speed with which each patient walked certain distances (5 m and 10 m), first with eyes open and then with them closed, was measured in seconds. During this period, no exercises involving closed eyes were done in physiotherapy. After 15-20 exercise sessions with concentrative perception of the locomotor apparatus at rest and in motion, the patients' walking speed was again measured under the same conditions as before. Nearly three quarters of the patients showed subjective and objective improvements. Subjectively they could, among other things, perceive their foot, lower leg or whole leg in outline and were better able to perceive fine motion sequences. With great relief they reported that the unnerving alien feeling had gone and that their legs were fully 'reunited' with the rest of their bodies. Many patients noticed that they did not need to control their walking visually so much as they had before. Walking performance was measured objectively before and after treatment. Particularly significant differences could be observed for the condition of walking with eyes closed. We also found that some of the patients who beforehand had not been able to walk at all with their eyes closed could now, after 15-20 treatment sessions, slowly and with crude control, manage a few metres without looking.

Systematically applied, the technique of concentrative body perception with focus on the legs represents a viable psychophysiological method of treatment for patients suffering from spinal ataxic gait disturbances, which has the added advantage that the exercises can be constantly reproduced. The subjective and objective findings indicate that irreversible defects in the spinal afferent tracts bring with them additional functional disturbances in the central registration and assessment of afferent information. Through its psychophysiological approach, the technique of concentrative body perception can eliminate these functional disturbances. For this reason, exercises in body perception of the sort described above can well be applied as a fruitful supplement to the usual, mainly visually controlled, movement exercises offered by the physiotherapist to this group of patients.

In a follow-up enquiry among the multiple sclerosis patients 2 years later, we discovered that about 40% of them were still actively working with the body perception method. This means that the exercises do indeed encourage an attitude of self-help.

Multiple Sclerosis Patients

Multiple sclerosis is one of the commonest of the incurable chronic diseases. However, most forms are benign and can go on for decades. For the emotional stability of these patients it is vitally important that they maintain their capacity for working and earning their living as long as possible. The special forms of physiotherapy, ergotherapy and drug treatment available are all aimed at alleviating symptoms. With strong personal involvement, the multiple sclerosis sufferers do their best to learn and perform the tasks set for them by the physiotherapist and ergotherapist. The special emotional problems stemming from the knowledge that they are incurably ill are seldom discussed. But in private, an attitude of hopelessness, resignation and withdrawal is often taking root. One of the consequences of their deep despair can take the form of magical expectations.

In learning the psychophysiological exercises described and repeating them at will, the patients experience their bodies directly. Conscious perception of their locomotor apparatus makes them more aware of their physical disablement, but also of the sensorimotor potential still available to them. It stimulates an active personal involvement with the physical problems with which they are confronted. If those with mulitple sclerosis can permit themselves to become more consciously aware of their bodily disablement, then they are more likely to be able actively to come to grips with their psychosocial handicap as well.

Many multiple sclerosis sufferers develop irreversible patches of demyelinization, mainly in the spinal cord, with ataxic disturbances in the arms and legs which are a serious handicap in everyday life and at work. Their mental faculties are not affected, although the motor disability may mean that these become less used. Multiple sclerosis sufferers can learn the concentrative body perception exercises without risk and apply them themselves at will, which can be a help to self-help.

The sort of medical and neurological care offered those with multiple sclerosis at present hardly entrusts them with the responsibility of coming to grips with the problem of their illness and their physical disability themselves or of coping with the resulting psychosocial stress.

Doctors and lay helpers have recently become overanxious that activating therapeutic measures could have a detrimental effect on the further development of the disease, with the result that sufferers are left even more alone than before, with a burden too heavy for them to carry. This may lead to magical expectations, since they have been robbed too early of the possibility of actively and personally coming to terms with their disease.

Concentrative Body Perception Exercises for Chronic Backache

Chronic backache is a very widespread problem nowadays. Years of treatment with painkilling drugs, massages, extensions, chiropractic procedures, braces, and not infrequently surgical interventions (intervertebral disc operations), as often as not leave the backache sufferer no better than before. The subjectively extremely severe pain cannot be fully explained by the pathological organic findings in the locomotor apparatus and the lumbar section of the vertebral column, so that ageing processes causing alterations in the intervertebral spaces and the vertebral joints are often taken to be the major cause. With the so-called therapy-resistant backaches, the time comes when doctor and patient resignedly agree upon the formula: 'Due to age-appropriate degenerative changes in the spinal column, the back troubles are no longer responsive to treatment.'

The statistics on premature retirement in West Germany are not encouraging. The figures published by the Verband Deutscher Rentenversicherungsträger (responsible for work-related pension insurance schemes) on pension claims made by insured employees, many of whom have a sedentary occupation, show that conditons affecting the bones, muscles and connective tissues take second place after cardiovascular disease as the reason given for early retirement. For the years 1982 and 1983 (respectively), 37.6% and 43.6% of the men and 28.8% and 32.6% of the women had to give up employment because of cardiovascular disease, whilst conditions affecting the bones, muscles and connective tissues were the grounds for the claims of 14.1% and 17.0% of men and 24.8% and 29.1% of women.

Among the conditions affecting the bones, muscles and connective tissues, those involving the back are particularly well represented. For men the figures are 9.2% and 11.3%, and for women 16% and 19%. Although women do not as a rule have to do heavy physical work, 19% of women going into early retirement in 1983 did so because of back trouble, which itself takes second place among all diseases causing men and women to give up working prematurely. A large proportion of these troubles take the form of chronic backaches that are assumed to be psychosomatic. Besides the somatic causes, these chronic backaches develop against a background of psychosocial stress and conflict, together with a staunch attempt on the part of the individual to see then steadily through, whatever the price.

In the locomotor system the lumbar section of the spine has very special functions. It enables us, among other things, to maintain our upright posture as well as the mobility of the entire upper part of the body. The intervertebral discs act like water cushions as a protection against continuous mechanical jarring. Both the mobility of the spinal joints and the functioning and metabolism of the intervertebral discs depend upon the work of the paravertebral muscles. If a state of muscular tension or an irritation of the nerve root, due to psychosomatic causes, gives rise to a lumbar pain complex, a reflex in the paravertebral muscles has the effect of increasing the tension further. Continuous tension in the paravertebral muscles due to this sort of pain reflex forces them into the unphysiological role of supportive muscles.

The important alternation between contraction and extension is lacking. The flexibility between the vertebrae is reduced and the intervertebral discs are put under great pressure. The intervertebral spaces diminish. Muscular and radicular pains are provoked further, creating a vicious circle which ultimately results in chronic, frequently 'therapy-resistant' backache. Metabolic disturbances gradually cause organic damage to the muscles and intervertebral discs (myogelosis, degenerative alterations with diminished distance between vertebrae, degenerative changes in the intervertebral joints). A psychosomatic clinical picture has developed, whose future course will be determined by psychic and social stress factors as well as by somatic disturbances and the damage arising in the paravertebral muscles, the intervertebral discs and the intervertebral joints.

The deep-rooted perception disorders associated with this process are already indicated by the subjective reports of chronic backache sufferers. Besides the pain - to which they have become more or less 'accustomed' - they often feel very troubled by a lack of support in the lumbar part of the spine (I am buckling under, my back is breaking, I am going to snap, my spine isn't holding me up, it is too loose.') Mechanistic phantasies about therapeutic possibilities are the result: operations that 'build in' some extra support are the great hope (stiffening the joints between the vertebrae, implanting bone chips, inserting metal plates, etc.) After years of suffering, many patients place almost magical hopes on new 'iron vertebrae'.

If patients with chronic backache do concentrative body perception exercises, considerable disorders in the way they perceive their bodies are revealed. Even though the afferent information systems such as the senses of pressure, posture and motion in the lumbar region of the spine are intact, the organically determined pain (nerve root irritation, metabolic disturbances in the muscles, etc.), together with the psychic experience of pain, apparently have a repressive influence on the central registration and utilization of information from this area. Perception exercises carried out with the body at rest, in combination with gentle extension of the muscles in the lumbar region, reveal two apparently contradictory perceptual disorders: the existing pain is either perceived more acutely or it is not perceived at all. The entire area of pain has been debarred from normal body perception. The organically intact afferents, such as the senses of pressure, posture and movement, are initially inaccessible to more conscious perception. It may reasonably be assumed that this afferent information is also not sufficiently available to central sensorimotor control processes. The highly sensitized perception of pain appears to disturb the sensorimotor system, possibly also impairing the central tone regulation of the paravertebral muscles. The muscular tension arising as a pain reflex may well become self-perpetuating at a spinal level and lead, among other things, to metabolic disturbances and reduced flexibility in the spinal column, which in turn give rise to the development of further pain.

In patients who have only recently undergone an intervertebral disc operation, concentrative body perception exercises tend as a rule to give rise to increased pain perception in the lumbar region of the spine. At the same time, the patients make the unnerving observation that their whole back seems to have been shortened or to have shrunk.

The concentrative body perception exercises for chronic backache patients are somewhat modified compared with those described for patients with spinal ataxic gait disturbances. Years of pain have given these backache patients a deep mistrust of any new form of treatment. It is therefore advisable to begin the exercises in areas far removed from the painful region of the back. The breathing exercises described above are a good starting-point.

After a few sessions, the focus can gradually be shifted from the legs or the upper part of the body towards the region of the chronic backache (cf. the body perception exercises for spinal ataxic gait disturbances). Cautious extension exercises in the form of rotary movements on the axis of the vertebral column are the crucial stimulus required by the cramped, painful muscle. The shortened, inelastic and metabolically disordered muscle system is vitally in need of extension as this improves its metabolic conditions. The muscles regain their elasticity and the intervertebral joints become more mobile, which assists the recovery of the metabolism of the intervertebral discs. The metabolism of the intervertebral discs comes about by diffusion through semipermeable membranes, the constant alternation between pressure and relief working on the intervertebral discs like a pump mechanism (the intervertebral disc as an osmotic system).

When the physiotherapist feels it is time to approach the painful lumbar region of the spine, the following could serve as an introduction:

'You are lying stretched out on the floor, eyes closed, your face muscles are relaxed; your arms are at your sides, with your hands resting palm down on the mat; your legs are a little apart, your feet turned slightly outwards with toes pointing down; your calves are touching the mat, the hollows at the back of your knees are quite relaxed and should gradually, little by little, sink down towards the floor. You can feel the underside of your thighs, from the back of your knees right up to your buttocks, resting gently on the mat ... [as for spinal ataxic gait disturbances]'

Later on gentle, springing extension movements are introduced. The spoken instructions could go something like this: 'Keeping your legs and feet together on the floor, bend your knees, drawing your feet up to your buttocks. Keep your knees bent and allow both legs to sink slowly down to the right; your feet are still together, one on top of the other, on the mat. Now, very slowly, move your left shoulder down towards the floor. The lower part of your back is now gently extended on the left side; hold it like that for a moment.' No great pain should arise. The patients are then asked to draw their breath quite consciously into the somewhat extended, usually rather painful area. Breathing in increases extension; breathing out reduces it. 'Every wave of breath that flows in flexes and extends your muscles slightly; when you breathe out they relax and come to rest. Allow your breathing to feel its way very gradually into the area that hurts most'; (these very finely regulated extension exercises can be repeated again and again for a few minutes at a time) 'your muscles give way a little, the pain gets less.' If, at any point, a patient should be suddenly overwhelmed by pain, their attention should immediately be diverted onto their breathing. After this exercise, the patients are given corresponding instructions to lay their legs to the left and lower their right shoulder.

With chronic backache sufferers, the most important focus of concentrative body perception is on the very painful, taut state of the paravertebral muscles, both at rest and whilst performing extending movements. As the patients learn how to give way by degrees and how to apply the inflow of breath as a very fine instrument for extending the paravertebral muscle system, the muscles which have been shortened because of the pain reflex very gradually begin to give way.

Clinical experience has shown that concentrative body perception exercises are able to help patients with chronic backache in various ways. The technique allows for very finely regulated movements which enable the patient to extend the muscle fibres whilst remaining below the raised pain threshold. Extension stimulates the muscular metabolism and alleviates pain. The paravertebral muscle system which has become so painful through continuous contraction can slowly start working physiologically once more. The almost immobilized (and painful) spinal joints gradually recover their mobility, the intervertebral discs can expand and once again take in water and nutrients by osmotic diffusion. The intervertebral spaces are widened. Mechanical nerve root irritation is less possible.

The exercises have the effect of making sensations of pressure, posture and motion in the affected area of the spine more conscious, so that they become available once more for central sensorimotor perception and evaluation, and counterbalance the oversensitized perception of pain. The region of the back which had been banned from conscious perception can be felt again and becomes a part of the body once more. The negative perception of the chronically painful lumbar region of the spine gives way to a more trusting perception of the body. The patients' sense of physical reliance on the lumbar region of their back returns; they feel it is supporting them again.

Therapy with concentrative body perception can only be successful if the chronic backache sufferer can recognize his own mechanistic phantasies about therapy and give them up, in order to make way for a new understanding of psychosomatic processes. With such patients, psychotherapeutic work on their intrapsychic and social areas of conflict only becomes possible once the pain symptoms have been treated successfully. The technique of body perception actively involves the patients in their treatment. The exercises in perception - combined with those stimulating muscular extension - can be applied repeatedly at will (self-help). If patients find they are able to alleviate their pain through their own efforts, it is less difficult for them to relate their pain to personal stresses and conflicts.

Chronic Backache Patients (Psychosomatic Disorder)

Chronic backache is treated medically with painkillers (usually injected), massage, extensions, chiropractic exercises and braces. The patient's role is that of the passive receiver of help. The method of concentrative body perception takes a more active body- and symptom-related therapeutic approach. The exercises can be repeated at will and so encourage patients to come to grips with their pain themselves in a more enterprising manner. Concentrative body perception of the lumbar region, at rest and in motion, allows for very fine control of movements, which enables the tautened, painful muscles very gradually to recover their elastic function. Later on, when the patient is alone, he or she can combine the perception exercises with gentle extending movements, thereby encouraging the physiological mobility of the lumbar section of the spine and preventing the pain from developing further.

Concentrative body perception exercises make it possible to introduce movement into the lumbar region of the spine by minute degrees and so create suitable conditions for chiropractic exercises and physiotherapy. A combination of concentrative body perception and chiropractic exercises offers the lumbar region of the spine the relief and painless support that it needs.

One of the problems confronting chronic backache sufferers is that they are basically prepared to do something active for the mobility of their spine, but that the sudden, overwhelming pain repeatedly forces them to fall back into a passive attitude of expecting pain-alleviating treatment immediately. The therapeutic path lying ahead of those with chronic backache consists of a series of minute patient, initially body-related steps.

The exercises in concentrative body perception described above have proved themselves in clinical practice to be an important form of therapy. Only later on does it become possible to reach the individual patient's underlying emotional and social conflicts.

References

Ebbecke U (1959) Psychologie des Bewusstseins in entwicklungsgeschichtlicher Betrachtung. Thieme. Stuttgart

Engeling J (1966) Die Entwicklung der Wahrnehmungsfähigkeit für Bewegungs- und Spannungsvorgänge. Krankengymnastik 10: 332-336

Meyer JE (1961) Konzentrative Entspannungsübungen nach Elsa Gindler und ihre Grundlagen. Z Psychother Med Psychol 11: 116-120

C. Sex-Specific Body Experience

Body Experience of Men with Prostatosis

P. Diederichs

Introduction

Prostatosis (chronic prostatitis) is a psychosomatic clinical condition in which urological examination may show an actual swelling of the prostate, but where neither bacteria in the expressed prostatic secretions nor any other organic disease can be found. Synonyms of this condition are: prostate neurosis, prostate congestion, urogenital neurosis, autonomic urogenital syndrome, chronic recurrent prostatitis and abacterial prostatitis. Clinically, prostatosis is characterized by a micturition disorder (for example, pollakiuria, dysuria or strangury) as well as discomfort or pain in the urogenital and anal areas (for example, burning in the urethra; pain in the inguinal region, which can radiate all the way to the testicles; or pressure in the perineal area). Günthert (1983) points out that, without being asked, many patients stress the fact that they do not experience actual pain, but rather a very unpleasant, disturbing feeling. Some of them cannot even sit comfortably. Over 50% of these patients also complain about sexual disorders, such as erection difficulties or painful or premature ejaculation (Günthert 1983; Janssen et al. 1983).

In the field of urology, this is probably the most common psychosomatic disorder among men (Diederichs and Günthert 1985). Analytical psychosomatic research into prostatosis began only very recently (Diederichs 1983; Janssen et al. 1983; Riedell and Brähler 1983): psychodynamically oriented case studies have been carried out by Günthert (1983) and Rechenberger (1979). In a rather stimulating study Junker (1970) limits himself to accounts obtained through psychological testing, even though he examined his patients psychoanalytically as well. Psychometric findings about men with prostatosis have also been reported by authors from Belgium (Mendlewicz et al. 1971) and Scandinavia (Keltikangas-Järvinen et al. 1981; Nilsson et al. 1975).

The reason why this urological-psychosomatic clinical condition is of such interest to fundamental research into psychosomatic illness is that it seems to have remained unchanged for centuries. For example, Christoffel (1944) found that Rousseau suffered from prostatosis: According to his confessions, written in 1767, he was plagued by the frequent urge to urinate, which disappeared after a visit to a Venetian brothel but reappeared in connection with hypochondriac fears of having a venereal disease. Today - in the age of antibiotics - this psychopathological phenomenon can still be found almost regularly, to a greater or lesser degree, in men who have prostatosis. This brings us to our theme, for hypochondria is the expression of a central disturbance of body experience, or the body image, or schema. Early body experience and resultant body image constitute a fundamental building block for a person's self-representations, the representation of one's own genital area probably being especially important for the development of ego or identity.

Moreover, the clinical picture of prostatosis may be of importance in controversy about alexithymia, since the extent of psychic and somatic symptoms is roughly similar in the latter. One might add that this urological-psychosomatic disorder is widespread cross-culturally; so far I have been able to diagnose it in an Algerian, an Egyptian, a Persian, an Italian, several Yugoslavs and Turks, and one African from Djibouti. It can be assumed that all these men come from patriarchically oriented cultures.

Methodology and Patients

I did not conduct systematic, empirically measurable investigations into the body experience of men suffering from micturition disorders, particularly since to the best of my knowledge no appropriate, practicable methods yet exist, or, if they do, they are still in the developmental stage. My accounts body experience of men with prostatosis are based upon the experience and observations gathered during psychoanalytically oriented investigation conducted since 1979 at the Department for Psychosomatic Medicine and Psychotherapy at the Steglitz Hospital of the Free University in Berlin.

The following is a summary of the psychodiagnostic methods I used (for more detail see Diederichs 1983):

1. Psychometric instruments
   (a) Freiburger Beschwerden-Liste, Gesamtform (Complaints List, Full Version) → Beschwerdemuster (Sample of Complaints)
   (b) Self-Rating Anxiety Scale (SAS) → anxiety measurement
   (c) Fragebogen zur Erfassung von Aggressivitätsfaktoren (FAF) → aggression measurement
   (d) Giessen-Test → Selbsteinschätzung (self evaluation) → Idealbild (ideal image)
2. Initial psychoanalytical interview (video)
3. Berlin documentation system for psychotherapy

The core of my diagnostic procedure was the initial psychoanalytical interview, which was evaluated and documented using the Berlin documentation system for psychotherapy (Dührssen et al. 1980; Rudolf 1981).

The 50 male patients I have examined so far were sent to me by the urological outpatient clinics of two university hospitals or by Berlin urologists in private practice. Prior to the psychoanalytical diagnostic procedure, each of the patients had undergone a thorough urological examination to rule out any organic pathological causes which could have triggered prostatosis.

The psychosocial, psychopathological and psychometric results in men with prostatosis were compared with those of an unselected male control group ($n = 37$) from a different outpatients' clinic at a university hospital (Glass 1983). The two groups were suitable for comparison since they did not differ significantly in age or in the most important sociological parameters; only one of the 37 men in the control group suffered from a disorder in the urogenital area.

Results

A detailed description of the results can be found in Diederichs (1983) and Glass (1983). Mention will be made here of only those data that are relevant to our theme.

The average age of the patients was almost 35 years; the frequency of symptoms peaked at around the age of 40-42. Even though almost 80% of the men claimed to be living in a steady partner relationship, about 50% had remained childless. The majority of the patients had experienced the symptoms for 1-3 years. Psychodynamically, the triggering conflict situation arose primarily in the area of striving for recognition. Psychopathologically, the most prominent factors were hypochondriac fears, depressions with passive tendencies, and inhibitions in the aggressive domain.

The majority of the men transferred to us with prostatosis displayed an obsessive-compulsive structure. A qualitative evaluation according to psychological criteria relating to the ego and the self revealed that behind the compulsive structure there were vast differences in the ego level, the coherence of self and the quality of object relations. Only about 20% of the patients examined possessed a relatively good ego level; they displayed a flexible personality, were capable of introspection and talked about lively and varied partner relationships as well as creative leisure activities. An additional 10% were still characterized by a relatively good personality level and also lived in stable object relations, but already appeared far more rigid. Among the rest of the men, namely two-thirds, there were indications of more serious personality disorders including mania, borderline syndrome, narcissistic disturbance and conspicuously compulsive character.

The kind and the extent of disturbed urogenital function displayed by our patients with prostatosis correspond for the most part to the frequencies documented by Junker (1970; Table 1).

The metaphors which some of the patients spontaneously use to describe their symptoms characterize the disturbed body experience in the urogenital area:

A 33-year-old scientist: 'There's no real stream any more; it (the micturition) has gradually become weaker and weaker. For the past 6 months I have only been able to urinate in a sitting position. The stream stops at a certain point, and then there is only a dribble'.

A 38-year-old postal clerk whose wife and three children had suddenly left him: 'As if she had thrown a club between my legs.'

A 40-year-old man whose admired father had died of prostatic cancer: 'I feel as if I were under an electrical current down there'; or, later on: 'as if I were sitting on a tennis ball.'

One patient described the pain in his testicles: 'As if I had stones in my scrotum.' A 42-year-old, very simply structured patient, who experienced a permanent burning in the urogenital area and pressure extending from the rectal area and the genitals all the way up to the navel: 'When it comes to intercourse, I finish in no time; I have already lost a large amount of sperm; women drain me; it feels as if there is a worn-out groove underneath my penis.'

Table 1. Symptoms of nonbacterial prostatitis ($n = 44$) (from Junker 1970)

	Percentage of cases
Repeated urge to urinate	81
Pain in the groin and bladder	78
Pain in the penis and testicles	78
Pain in the upper and lower back	75
Delayed onset of urination	67
Itching and tickling in the urethra	65
Pain during urination	62
Frequent nocturnal rising in order to urinate	60
Nocturnal urinary discharge	57
Premature ejaculation	57
Sexual over-excitability	57
Difficulties during urination	56
Feeling of heaviness in the rectum	55
Insufficient penile hardness	55
Pain in the perineum	55
Pain during defecation	50
Itching of the sexual organ	46
Sexual under-excitability	44
Discharge from the urethra	35
Worry about not being able to urinate	32

One narcissistically structured patient, distinguished by an attractive external facade (male model), complained of no longer having a physical feeling of self: he said that he was standing 'beside' himself, outside his own body. In addition to having prostatosis, he claimed that the tip of his penis was covered with a very thin layer of skin, which would tear during intercourse, and that therefore he could not 'afford' to have intercourse more often than once a month.

A 34-year-old 'borderline' patient related: 'Something starts to swell, then begins to cramp and gets plugged up.' Since he frequently experienced intense heat accumulation in the genital area, he treated himself with cold compresses. Sexually, he felt like a 50-year-old grandfather.

An older, once professionally successful patient, who had developed prostatosis after a heart attack, stated spontaneously: 'I have lost faith in myself; I am not a man any more.'

Yet another patient, who had pain on ejaculation as well as a micturition disorder, blamed this condition on the varicose veins in his scrotum, which, in turn, he regarded as a result of tonsillitis.

In this context it is interesting to notice that over 25% of all patients with prostatosis also mention disorders in the throat, nose, and facial areas. One might see this as a shifting from 'bottom' to 'top'. Additionally, it is not uncommon to find cardioneurotic symptoms in the medical histories of prostatosis patients.

The most important finding in relation to our topic lies in the frequent occurrence of hypochondria, which represents the central disturbance of the body experience and seems to be an extraordinarily characteristic feature of men with prostatosis. Its frequent occurrence in these patients is significant when seen against its frequency in a comparable group of psychosomatic male patients from a different psychosomatic outpatients' facility. Of the 50 men with prostatosis whom we examined, only two did not express any hypochondriacal anxiety. With regard to the clinical intensity of hypochondria, however, there is no significant difference between the two-groups: severe forms of hypochondria can also be found in other psychosomatic diseases, especially with cardio neurosis and colitis ulcerosa. As to content, the hypochondria in men suffering from a urogenital disorder usually centres upon the fear of having contracted a venereal disease or of suffering from an insidious, malignant illness which cannot yet be diagnosed.

The finding of hypochondriac fear typical for men with prostatosis is not completely new, although it has surely never before been so well documented with the aid of descriptive statistics. Even in the earlier and, of course, mainly organically oriented literature, the urologists noticed hypochondria in connection with this male micturition disorder. As shown by the reports of Frankl-Hochwart and Zuckerkandl (1906), this in turn set off negative feelings of countertransference: 'Everyone will have unpleasant memories of those patients who want to be examined over and over again, who describe their illness in never-ending detail and who, not satisfied with just verbal descriptions, finally take pleasure in handing over their memoirs containing exact descriptions of their feelings on a day-to-day basis. Quite frequently, the bladder symptoms are linked to sexual-neurasthenic conditions like premature ejaculation, pollution, spermatorrhoea and impotence.' (von Frankl-Hochwart and Zuckerkandl 1906, p. 79).

Discussion of Results

Before dealing metapsychologically with the topic of hypochondria as a central disturbance of the body experience, I would first like to relate a few observations about the psychosomatic aspects of micturition. Undisturbed development of the urethral apparatus is, after all, the prerequisite for a positive urogenital body experience.

Urethral Drive Experience

The peripheral urinary apparatus (urethra and bladder) is like the mouth or the anus, a zone of pleasure and drive. The mucous membranes of the urethra and bladder also have erotogenous characteristics, indicated by relatively common masturbation practices involving the urethra; in 1910, Sadger introduced the term 'urethral eroticism', analogous to anal eroticism. The pleasurable 'streaming' of lust associated with a full bladder, which can be felt all the way to the groin, is known to all. In his characteristically eclectic way, Schultz-Hencke (1927, 1951) summed up theoretical positions on the libido, including the theory of psychophysical parallelism and more general anthropological categories, in the term 'urethral drive experience'. The theory of psychophysical parallelism, or of 'coincidence correlative', says that bodily functions - such as micturition - are accompanied by specific feelings; an inhibition in the psychic area can also lead to a disturbance in the physical process. The urethral drive experience includes both the libidinal experience of 'pleasurable streaming' in the act of micturition and - especially in small children - the experience of total abandon to one's own will without regard to temporal or spatial conditions. (The aggressive side of the urethral experience is derived from limitations experienced during toilet training. It is also reflected in our language, for example, in the phrase 'Piss off!') Hence, the emotional security of confident 'pleasurable streaming' during urination provides, among another things, the basis for yielding oneself which is an essential prerequisite for the ability to establish relationships. It is not astonishing, therefore, that the urogenital area can become the site of symptoms of relationship conflicts in women as well as in men.

An additional important emotional aspect of the urethral drive experience has, according to Schultz-Hencke, a gender-specific anthropological meaning: perception of the difference in behaviour between boys and girls during micturition (boys guide their stream of urine up into a high arch and associate this act with feelings of pride, preference, and a 'reaching up high') leads this once neutrally experienced act into the area of striving for recognition. Boys, as opposed to girls, can urinate standing up right and guide their flow wherever they wish. Also, the proximity of the urethral area to the phallic area is greater in men. As early as 1900, Freud's interpretation of dreams gave examples of people's belief that the flow of urine can have powerful effects. Young children love to urinate into large puddles and then claim to have produced the entire result by themselves. The meaning of power, recognition and achievement is, associated with micturition, especially among men. Thus it can be assumed that the narcissistic cathexis of urethrality is the basis for a positive body experience in the urogenital area. The patients' spontaneous remarks about their symptoms made it apparent how the disturbed micturition can be accompanied by feelings of discomfort or pain in the entire urogenital tract. The interpretion of prostatosis only in relation to oedipal problems, for example, as an expression of castration fears resulting in regression to the urethral level, appears too simplistic to me, or disregards pregenital aspects. As the following theoretical discussion of hypochondria in relation to narcissism should make clear, this psychosomatic disorder should generally be placed earlier aetiopathogenetically. By the term 'narcissism' I mean the psychology of self according to Kohut (1973).

Hypochondria as the Expression of a Central Disorder of Body Experience

Until now, hypochondria has been left in the domain of psychiatry (Fischer-Homberger 1970); as the expression of disturbed body experience it has hardly been examined from a psychoanalytical point of view. Grunert (1977) rightly points out that bodily feeling and the sense of self, or physical integrity and narcissistic stability, are closely linked. A child learns the libidinous cathexis of his body through his first reference person: in most cases, his mother. 'In the case of a disturbed body image, a defective body schema, there cannot be a reliably cathexed feeling of self furnished with neutralized energy' (Grunert 1977, p. 11). The quality of personal hygiene and the way in which toilet training was handled are probably pathogenic here. The early ego is a body ego. A defective body ego or unfamiliarity with individual body parts thus provide the basis for unease in the observation of one's own body. Moreover, a disturbed body image will make on adequate passage through the oedipal phase more difficult, if not impossible.

Freud himself gave the first decisive impulses for interpreting the phenomenon of hypochondria based on theoretical considerations relating to narcissism in his *Introduction to Narcissism,* published in 1914. In this, points out the different distribution of libido underlying hypochondria. The hypochondriac withdraws his interest, or rather his libido, from the objects of the outer world and concentrates them on the organ which occupies his attention. One might say that, in his further explanations, Freud hints at first connections between hypochondria and a pathological body image by saying that the relation of hypochondria to paraphrenia (schizophrenia) is similar to that of actual neurosis to hysteria and compulsive neurosis; in other words, hypochondria in structural ego disorders corresponds to signal anxiety in functional ego disorders or transference neurosis. Where signal anxiety indicates the danger of a breakthrough of instinct, hypochondria signals the danger of the fragmentation of self.

According to Grosch, based on experience gained from analyses of hypochondriacs, the type and localization of the organic disease of these individuals is connected to their reference persons, who are admired but also hated. Occasionally, the men whom we examined mentioned that their fathers, too, had suffered from a prostatic ailment or even died of cancer of the prostate. 'The reference person, as seen by the hypochondriac, is always distinguished by a special greatness, by some kind of standing apart from the mediocrity of the rest of mankind' (Grosch 1958, p. 198). Kohut (1973) would call this phenomenon an idealized parent imago. It is caused by the hypochondriac's underlying conflict of striving for recognition, the desire to be great and unique himself. Formulated in Kohut categories: the fear or rejection of feelings of inferiority makes the patient withdraw to his 'grandiose self'. During the exploration of the family histories of men with prostatosis, it was noticeable that their fathers had either remained rather colourless or were vaguely idealized. In other words, the 'grandiose self' corresponds to the idealized parent imago. The relationship with the reference person, who is seen as especially great and powerful, is, of course, always ambivalent; the overcoming and settling of this ambivalence are accomplished by introjection. In this connection, Grosch points out that 'hypochondria' originally meant 'imagined illness'; here, the 'over-elevated image' of a person, or model, is incorporated into the self or imagined to be as one with the self. It should be remembered here that approximately two-thirds of the men with prostatosis displayed a kind of pathology of the self that had in numerous cases led to a narcissistic character defence.

Furthermore, Grosch (1958), who obviously anticipated Kohut (1973) in some very important lines of thought, hints at the mirror transference which he later describes in detail. Mirror experiences have indeed been observed to play an extensive role in the lives of all hypochondriacs. 'Their narcissistic structural constraint and disturbed contact lead them to seek a dialogue with themselves in the mirror image. The hypochondriac always experiences his own importance as so great that his surroundings sink into complete insignificance, and thus he seeks a constant echo experience in his mirror image ... The self-observation of the hypochondriac is always disguised self-admiration. The hypochondriac is the kind of person who, figuratively speaking, always directs the spotlight, onto himself, so that the rest of the world lies in darkness for him' (Grosch 1958, p. 205).

These somewhat theoretical explanations should be clarified using the case study of a man with prostatosis:

The 40-year-old unmarried policeman was referred to me by our urological polyclinic. At first contact, the conventionally dressed patient appeared latently distrustful: his posture was stiff, and he avoided any eye contact. He required an unusual amount of time for the completion of our out-patient questionnaire. He then talked slowly and long-windedly, but tried to answer my questions precisely revealing on the one hand his compulsive structure and on the other an arrogant and know-it-all attitude. Describing his symptoms, he stated having pains in the groin area. At first, the pain had been in his penis only, then there was a burning in the area of the groin, and the pains began to radiate around towards the back. Finally, the pains shot all the way into his legs. Since he also felt pain in his shoulder joints, he thought that he had an insidious rheumatic disease. He continued to insist on this diagnosis in spite of all negative somatic results. As to his micturition, he mentioned that he was suffering from an increased urge to urinate. Altogether, he had the feeling that his body was in a state of irritation. Recently he had been afraid that he would die of this insidious disease, which was why he had already consulted various specialists as well as hospitals. He had even succeeded in obtaining whole-body computed tomography. His condition had existed for more than a year and had been preceded by a conflict at his place of work, during which the patient had been attacked and humiliated by a colleague. He described his past history as outstandingly harmonious and satisfactory. Since various out-patient therapeutic attempts had failed (for example, with a neurologist and a non-medical practioner), and the threat of disability became apparent (he had been on sick leave for more than 3 months, he was interested in an attempt at psychotherapeutic treatment as an in-patient.

During the very first session, he gave a demonstration of his disturbed body experience in the urogenital area: without being asked, he let down his trousers to show me his genitals. Emphatically, and with a suffering expression, he explained that the whole area was burning, especially the groin, and that the pain radiated all the way to his buttocks. Upon my repeated statements that I did not notice anything unusual, neither about his genitals nor about his inguinal area, he insisted that the veins in the groin were swollen, maintaining that, after all, he knew his own body better than anyone. This shows the 'medical megalomania' of the hypochondriac described by Kehrer (1930). During the therapy session, he mentioned, while pointing to his urogenital region. 'It feels like one giant pus-filled pimple, everything has gone soft is swollen and burning. My sperm is still white but full of pus.' Throughout the session, the patient repeatedly insisted on an examination of his ejaculate. His narcissistic side or 'grandiose self' was soon revealed during group therapy. He continously drew attention to himself, especially the women's, and considered himself to be more intelligent than the others. 'I believe in myself as I believe in God; then I have so much strength that I can do everything myself!' His delusions of grandeur showed up most clearly during creative performance therapy: he drew a picture of himself in a doctor's cap with a book of wisdom in his hand, which, interestingly enough, he was carrying right in front of his genital area. He then signed the self-portrait with 'Baron, Nobleman, Professor von ...' followed by his name.

During concentrative motion therapy it became noticeable that he had hardly any access to his body experience, that he always required a lot of space for himself and that he avoided all bodily contact with others.

In the course of his therapy, it became apparent from his childhood history that he had grown up in a family atmosphere in which he did not get very much attention. In particular, a sister 6 years older than he must have been psychoneurotically relevant, since she was regarded as the good and intelligent one in the family and he felt constantly put down by her. However, he did not give up his idealizing defence against his parents.

The aetiology of hypochondria should be seen against the background of a pathology of the self. If one was not loved or paid attention to as a child, one must at least be admired. At the inception of a disturbed body experience there can certainly be unpleasurant or painful physical sensations which, in turn, lead to increased self-observation and may end in hypochondriac fear. As Grosch (1958) described it graphically, using the metaphor of the spotlight, the entire spiritual energy is concentrated on one's own body and thus the relationship to the environment becomes greatly diminished. The patient just described was also so intensely occupied with himself that he could not relate to other people, and his environment lost its and challenging character. The only time he felt at ease and free of physical complaints was when he received undivided attention and strictly positive feedback, as in the individual therapy sessions.

Psychodynamics of the Triggering Conflict Situation

As suggested earlier, the psychodynamics of the triggering conflict situation for men with prostatosis lie primarily in the area of recognition and the narcissistic side of micturition and of the phallus predisposes them in such a way that the insult allows their already primarily damaged body self to become obvious. It is therefore not surprising that a large number of men with disorders in the urogenital tract feel that they have been hurt down to the 'core'. In this connection, it is interesting that the mean age of our patient group is relatively high, with a peak at around 40 years. The threshold situation around the 40th year of life may be due to the fact that men are then approaching their professional and sexual limits of achievement, which, in turn, changes their body experience. Without trying to stereotype the phenomenon of mid-life or 'a man in his best years', I agree with Beck (1981) that, psychodynamically, we are dealing with the loss of hitherto narcissistically highly cathexed objects such as beauty or at least a positive body image, the onset of physical strength, sexual potency and career, caused by factors such as baldness or a flabby stomach, or children leaving home. A 40-year-old patients who arrived for the initial interview in a coloured sweater with the words 'Ice cream' written on it, expressed this problem - when asked to describe his symptoms - in the following way: 'I noticed that I was pissing like an old man.' The urological symptoms appeared after he had lost a fight for the first time in his life and had subsequently had to be hospitalized with a broken jaw. Even though he was of rather small stature, he emphasized the fact that he had never run away from a fight; his spontaneous comment was: 'When you beat a big guy, you are the greatest!' His primarily labilized body self had become cracked, so to speak. The crumbling of his narcissistic regulation, or the loss of recognition, corresponds to a disturbed micturition: the 'high arch' is weakened. He felt that there was no longer any real stream, the first observation of many men with prostatosis: 'The stream becomes thinner and thinner; finally it only comes in the form of a few drops!' Of significance in this connection are, in my opinion, Beck's explanations (1981) of the psychosomatic symptom as a 'repair reaction' to the narcissistic insults or injuries to the self. The insult results in regression, and the adaptive function of the illness is to repair the damaged self and thus also the physical self. Thus the pains in the prostate or the pain-determined hypercathexis of the body represent an attempt to restore the damaged borders of the self. The tendency to repair has shifted to the bodily sphere, since it can no longer be achieved in the mental area alone. The physical symptom is therefore a valuable stabilizer, whose preservation the patient will defend with all his forces against the therapeutic interventions of the physician (Beck 1981).

The Meaning of Aggression

The pathogenesis of hypochondria cannot be entirely explained by consideration of aspects of theories of narcissism: An essential part is played by aggression, a drive-dynamic component. One can assume that patients with a defective self or body self have a more difficult time integrating their aggressive impulses. Men with prostatosis are aggressively inhibited. Grosch (1958) stresses that the same applies to all hypochondriacs. However, in the case of the latter, it is a tenacious, lingering form of aggression revolving around slow dissolution and destruction: 'From a psychological viewpoint, all those experiences of apprehension have the common denominator of insidious organ destruction: a slow-moving destructive agent which works from within causes gradual disintegration of the body or the organ in question and thus brings on a state of lingering illness' (Grosch 1958, p. 198). This means that hypochondria can also be understood as an inadequate method of dealing with aggression. In our case study, too, it became clear that hypochondria served to conceal rejected feelings of hostility and hurt pride from oneself and others. On the basis of experiences gained during two long-term analyses with hypochondriac patients, Broden and Myers (1981) arrive at the opinion that hypochondriac symptoms are derivatives of unconscious phantasies of being beaten and abused. Like Grosch, they find that hypochondriac patients have prevailing aggressive conflicts with internalized objects that were admired. The patients themselves, however, see themselves as damaged, which results in the compensatory wish to become an admired child. At the same time, Broden and Myers believe that hypochondriac symptoms help in the rejection of guilt feelings, since the hypochondriac's rage is directed against important love-objects.

The biographical data of a proportion of men with prostatosis point toward strict fathers, some of whom inflicted physical punishment on their sons, which means that they repeatedly 'injured' or 'hurt' them. In spite of this, the patients attitudes towards these fathers were remarkably neutral or warm, even admiring.

Interactional and Therapeutic Aspects

Janssen et al. (1983) worked out a good assessment of the interaction between urologists and patients with prostatosis. The disturbance of self-esteem and identity of these men, or their disturbed urogenital body experience, forces them unconsciously to seek constant confirmation of their intact maleness. The neurotic repetition compulsion, however, causes them to push the urologist into the position of the damager by provoking him into conduction renewed diagnostic examinations and therapeutic measures. Ultimately, however, they are bound to be disappointed,disparage those treating them and look for new physicians. Any diagnostic intervention of an invasive character should therefore be precisely indicated, since it is unconsciously experienced as yet another genital injury and could contribute to making the symptoms or the disturbed body experience into a chronic condition. Unjustified measures, such as the prescription of chemotherapy without detection of bacteria, or the prostatic massage still performed by some urologists, should be avoided in order to prevent the patient's fixating on an organic illness. However, supportive urological measures such as Ichthyol suppositories, which promote the circulation of the small pelvis, or hot hip-baths (Günthert 1983) can definitely be helpful.

Altogether, these unattractive and querulous patients with their chronic conditions and their refractory ailments make the doctor keenly aware of the limits of his medical knowledge and ability, which often leads to feelings of countertransference (see the quotation above from von Frankl-Hochwart and Zuckerkandl

(1906). It should be mentioned with regard to psychotherapeutic measures that with prostatosis an analytically oriented (i.e. conflict-revealing) psychotherapy was indicated for about 20% of the 50 men referred to us. I was personally able to take on five of the men, or 10%, and include them in out-patient group therapy or an in-patient psychotherapy programme. The patient discussed in detail above had an unfavourable prognosis, partly because of his enormous character-neurotic defence and partly because his hypochondria had taken on the dimensions of an obsessive idea and was thus near to psychosis. Six months after our attempt to treat him, he had to be declared disabled and was consequently withdrawn from his position.

To the best of my knowledge, no experiences with specific somatic therapies for this symptom picture have yet been reported. A 32-year-old college graduate who had a favourable prognosis, and was also able to benefit from our in-patient therapy, told us during the follow-up interview that bioenergetic therapy had had a positive effect on the 'lower part' of his body. He rather proudly related that in the meantime his girlfriend had become pregnant by him.

Summary

Proceeding from a psychoanalytic examination of 50 men with prostatosis, the findings and clinical observations were centred around body experience. The spontaneous verbal descriptions the patients gave of their symptoms, clearly showed that they felt they had been injured or damaged in the urogenital area - or struck to the 'core'. Their 'narcissistic wound' was discussed from the angles of drive and the psychology of self. The hypochondriac apprehension regularly found in men with prostatosis was treated as the central point since, as a disguised form of self-admiration, it represents an attempt to repair the damaged body self and thus also the regulation of self-esteem.

References

Beck D (1981) Krankheit als Selbstheilung. Insel, Frankfurt

Broden AR, Myers WA (1981) Hypochondriacal symptoms as derivatives of unconscious fantasies of being beaten or tortured. J Am Psychoanal Assoc 29: 535-557

Christoffel H (1944) Trieb und Kultur. Schwabe, Basel

Diederichs P (1983) Zur Psychosomatik der Miktionsstörungen. Thesis, University of Berlin

Diederichs P, Günthert EA (1985) Psychosomatische Aspekte in der Urologie. In: von Ueyküll T (ed) Lehrbuch der Psychosomatischen Medizin, 3rd ed. Urban & Schwarzenberg, Munich

Dührssen A, Bodenstein D, Holitzner WV (1980) Das Berliner Dokumentationssystem für Psychotherapie. Z Psychosom Med 26: 119-157

Fischer-Homberger E (1970) Hypochondrie. Huber, Berne

Freud S (1900) Die Traumdeutung. Gesammelte Werke, vol 2/3. Fischer, Frankfurt. Standard edn vol 4/5

Freud S (1914) Zur Einführung in den Narzissmus. Gesammelte Werke, vol 10. Fischer, Frankfurt. Standard edn vol 14

Glass W (1983) Harnentleerungsstörungen ohne Organbefund. Dissertation, University of Berlin

Grosch M (1958) Über Hypochondrie. Z Psychosom Med 4: 195-205

Grunert J (1977) Körperbild und Selbstverständnis. Kindler, Munich

Günthert EA (1983) Prostatitis aus psychosomatischer Sicht. In: Brunner H, Krause W, Rothauge CF, Weidner W (eds) Chronische Prostatitis. Schattauer, Stuttgart
Janssen PL, Kukahn R, Spieler KH (1983) Psychosomatische Untersuchungen zur chronischen Prostatitis. Z Psychosom Med 29: 253-269
Junker H (1970) Sind Patienten mit chronischer bakterieller Prostatitis Sexualneurastheniker? - Ein psychodiagnostischer Beitrag. Z Psychosom Med 16: 264-278
Kehrer H (1930) Über Hypochondrie. Allg Ärztl Z Psychother Psych Hyg 3: 473-507
Keltikangas-Järvinen L, Järvinen H, Lehtonen T (1981) Psychic disturbances in patients with chronic prostatitis. Ann Clin Res 13: 45-49
Kohut H (1973) Narzissmus. Suhrkamp, Frankfurt
Mendlewicz J, Schulman CC, De Schutter B (1971) Chronic prostatitis: Psychosomatic incidence. Psychother Psychosom 19: 118-125
Nilsson JK, Colleen S, Mardh PA (1975) Relationship between psychological and laboratory findings in patients with symptoms of non-acute prostatitis. In: Danielsson D, Juhlin L, Mardh PA (eds) Genital infections and their complications. Almquist & Wiksell, Stockholm
Rechenberger HG (1979) Andrologie. In: Hahn P (ed) Die Psychologie des 20. Jahrhunderts, vol IX. Ergebnisse für die Medizin (1) Psychosomatik. Kindler, Zurich
Riedell H, Brähler E (1983) Prostatitis und Ehepaarbeziehung. In: Brunner H, Krause W, Rothauge CF, Weidner W (eds) Chronische Prostatitis. Schattauer, Stuttgart
Rudolf G (1981) Untersuchung und Befund bei Neurosen und Psychosomatischen Erkrankungen. Beltz, Weinheim
Sadger J (1910) Über Urethralerotik. Jahrb Psychoanal Psychopathol Forsch 2: 409-450
Schultz-Hencke H (1927) Einführung in die Psychoanalyse. Thieme, Jena
Schultz-Hencke H (1951) Lehrbuch der analytischen Psychotherapie. Thieme, Stuttgart
von Frankl-Hochwart L, Zuckerkandl O (1906) Die nervösen Erkrankungen der Blase. Hölder, Vienna

Male Body Image

D. Bongers

Men tend to define themselves more often through achievements in the intellectual and professional fields, and their relationship with their own bodies is rather utilitarian; while woman tend to define themselves more through their bodies, particularly their looks, or rather are defined that way by other people. For women, the body constitutes the 'basis of identity', not so for men.

(Mrazek 1984)

The quotation above reflects a widespread popular-scientific assessment of the relationship of men to their body. Does the popular wisdom still apply which says that a men does not need a beautiful body, only success in a career?

In this paper I will report some empirical findings about how men describe their bodies. They come from a larger empirical study of male self-images (Bongers 1984, 1985). The particular reasons for investigating this subject were as follows:

1. The crisis of traditional life patterns in marriage and family life.
2. The extraordinarily high proportion of sexual problems which comes up in therapy.
3. The alarming relationship of many men to their bodies and their health.

I will deal mainly with the last two of these problems. I will not concern myself here with the theoretical problems of psychological self-image research, which I have done elsewhere (Bongers 1985). Here it should suffice to explain that the term 'self-image' as used in this context derives from the conceptual framework of the cultural history school of psychology (see Leontjew 1982).

To obtain empirical material about male self-image some preliminary methodological considerations were necessary. Firstly, there have been hardly any ingvestigations as yet in the field of psychology about men and their views about their own manhood. So there were no developed theories, from which exact hypotheses could be deduced. Thus an explorative method was necessary. Secondly, feelings regarding women, sexuality and the relationship to one's own body were taboo, and men would rarely reveal them (see Jourard 1971). In this context questionnaires and standardized interviews risk producing only results which are socially acceptable, but which are not very meaning ful. The best research method proved to be a form of open interview where the relating of experiences and establishing positive contact with the interviewer were of critical importance (see Merton and Kendall 1979; Thomae 1968; Schütze 1977).

The interviews were subsequently carried out and partly evaluated on two research projects at the Institute of Psychology at the Technical University, Berlin. Thirty-six men between the ages of 20 and 40 years (average 26.5) were interviewed. Seventy-five percent of them had finished their education with the German *Abitur* (school-leaving examination qualifying one for admission to university). So, here we are dealing with a random sample of primarily young men with an above-average education. Even though only 10% of the interviewes were students of psychology, the composition of the sample remains heavily weighted towards a 'social science type of intelligence'.

Thirteen narrative interviews dealt with the theme 'My first great love'. The aim was to get to know as many details as possible about severing the family bonds and turning to one special woman for the first time. The first experience with sexuality also came to the fore.

Twenty-three interviews had the sole theme 'body self-image'. After the first interviews it became apparent that the interviewee often evasively took refuge in theoretical considerations and did not mention any body awareness or sensations. We tried to treat the theme of the body with the following questions as a guideline:

1. What kind of relationship do you have to your body?
2. If you feel a strong affection, how do you feel that?
3. If you have sexual feelings for somebody, how do you feel that? And how do you express that with your body?
4. If you had the chance to change everything that you want in your body (for example, through training, surgery, etc.), what would you want to change?

All interviews were taken down in writing. Recordings of the interviews were then played back to small groups of the research team, compared, and first of all analysed in terms of social interactions:

- What kind of contact developed between the interviewer and the interviewee?
- How were the guideline questions asked; what was the mature of additional questions asked?
- Did significant disruptions and breakdowns of communication occur?

At the end of this process an explicit characterization was made of the atmosphere of the interview. This focussed on the question of to what extent the interviewees had clearly revealed something about themselves. Some of the interviews could not be used for further evaluation because permission had been implicitly or explicitly refused.

The first question of the guided interview asked for an overall assessment of the interviewee of their relationship to their body. In the course of this a tendency towards a positive overall assessment became apparent: 11 out of 23 men made statements like: 'I like my body'; 'All in all, certainly, very good', 'Potentially an athlete's body; too fat, but attractive', Often the body was summed up like this: 'Yes, all in all, quite good!'

In six interviews men expressed a negative overall assessment. 'I have a poor relationship to my body'; It is just there and I use it, so what?'

In a further six interviews no clear overall assessment can be made out or it is clearly kept neutral: 'Well, it all depends, what is important is one's relationship to the environment.'

A similarly positive result regarding body-acceptance by men were also shown in investigations using questionnaires (see Mrazek 1984). Nevertheless, there are some indications in open interviews that a string of positive overall self-assessment tend to be conditioned by the social situation and have to be understood as an act of self-presentation.

Here are some verbatim statements by men with a positive overall opinion about their bodies: 'My body isn't worth putting on show'; 'I'm not exactly satisfied, but I just accept my body.' Others use metaphors like: 'My hand is a solid lump of meat': 'My body is just my partner, a means to an end'; 'My body is accepted and used; you could replace parts of it.'

These statements show a distancing from the body and a utilitarian attitude, but this is not borne out in the conscious overall assessment (see Bongers 1984, pp. 11 f.).

There was a widespread attitude which could be summed up like this:

'My body is just there, of course'

This attitude is found with in men with positive, neutral and negative overall assessment. You find it in remarks like, 'My body, well, I never think about it!'; 'In reality, I just an inside my body'; 'I accept it but I don't pay any special attention to my body'; 'In the end it doesn't matter what kind of body you have: if your soul isn't right nothing fits'; 'But that I am a health freak and only care for my body and look after it, no!'; 'It it just there and is - I don't know - taken for granted.'

Often the position of distancing is shown through rejection of another equally possible position: Don't be a health freak, don't be vain and don't spend time in front of the mirror. These statements often also show up a good deal of lack of interest on one's own body.

The Body as Opponent

This could be the fromulation of a different type of attitude. Without a question being directly aimed at the body's performance, this theme was addressed independently in 12 out of 23 interviews. There we are mostly dealing with 'going to the limits of one's own physical capabilities.' Some men are describing their experience in sports, where the aim is to conquer one's body, to overcome one's impulses. This aspect is shown very clearly in the following excerpt from an interview:

G.: There are the things which bother me about my body: that the mind is more efficient than the body, that the body reaches its limits too soon. That I often demand more from it than it can give.

I.: Does it make you dissatisfied then?

G.: Well, sometimes, yes, when the body deserts me at a time when one would actually need more performance, it does bother me sometimes. Then I often try to pull it out a bit, to increase the performance a little.

H.: (...) I just think you have to struggle with your thoughts quite a bit, you also have to struggle with your physical aspects quite a bit. Mostly you become aware of your body in extreme situations. If it just functions like that, goes on functioning, it's as if it wasn't there. Only at moments when it signals extreme desires, then you pay attention to it. (...) So my body showed me its limits several times, where I thought mentally I could go on enduring severe strain for longer. In these instances my body showed me its limits, as if it wanted to say, 'I won't take that any longer.' Then I treated my body ... affectionately by paying attention to it ... taking care of it and allowing it the rest which it demanded.

In these attitudes - the body as opponent - there is often a separation of head and body or mind and body. This attitude is addressed explicitly in nine interviews. This attitude corresponds strongly to Christian tradition, where the body is just a mortal shell for the immortal soul. One person interviewed expressed it like this: 'I guess my head is above my body.'

The relation between the two separate elements, mind and body, isn't just hierarchical: the mind is a kind of higher command centre above an insubordinate savage. One man reports that his ideal of a body is the emaciated, ascetic body.

To accept one's own body lovingly, or just to sense it constantly or pay attention to it, seems indeed unmanly. This attitude fits the ideology of manliness where a man has to keep his weaker self under control, particularly fear and the need for tenderness and security - all female aspects.

Before? - Yes, I've had Problems with my Body in the Past

There is a general tendency for many men to introduce problems with their body into the interviews, these being attributed to the past, especially the period of puberty.

G.: Yes, I have to say that my body has become important to me. In the past when I was younger my relationship was different. At that time I felt insecure, disturbed, often inhibited. Partly because of my body and my looks. Since then I have developed a pretty good relationship to my body.

In altogether 15 interviews people reported that in the past their relationship to their bodies was more negative; only two said that in the past it had been better. Some of the accounts of past problems are quite extreme: 'Well, in the past I was really fat and had what you would call an ugly body.' 'In the past I was terribly small, the smallest in the whole class, retarded.' 'My relationship was awfully bad, in the past. I was full of complexes and had no idea at all of sexual needs.' 'In the past my relationship to my body was somewhat strange, my nose too long or I blushed too easily, but now this dosn't bother me anymore; besides, my nose isn't too long.' Some of these men also explained how they came to a better relationship to their bodies - most of them through thinking!

P.: I noticed also that there were many people who looked like me, and that I'm not the only one, who looks like that (...) and I thought, well, ... it can't be your fault, and least of all your body's fault. And also because such a body is so vulnerable, that people, who look incredibly good, ... that they could be terribly disfigured by an accident, that the physical is secondary, as a matter of principle. Yes, that's the conclusion I came to. So, for me the physical is basically secondary, and in a way I'm happy that today I can think like this. I don't care if I have a chest like Tarzan, or whether I'm almost flat-chested, well this doesn't bother me at all. Many people who really looked great were later patched up, had scars all over, and that is even uglier.

Reading some interviews, one gets the impression that a powerful social rule is at work: 'Accept what's there!' (Or 'Happy are they who forget about what can't be changed anyway.') This rule pervades the whole account and leads to the positive result mentioned above. The small number of men who reported explicitly negative self-images support this with definite physical complaints: allergy, rheumatism, obvious overweight, hypernervousness.

This leads me to the associat that the others act according to the motto, 'As long as nothing falls off, we are healthy!' This confirms the theses found in the literature that men systematically ignore slight signals of indisposition (see Richter 1974; Jourard 1974). This ignorance is acquired through learning: at first the young boy learns that he will be praised if he does not show pain and does not make a sound. He also learns that his peers (sometimes even his parents) will jeer at him and call him a cry-baby if he gives his feelings free range. As an adult every man knows that it is unmanly to listen too intently into one's body - and after not having done it for many years, at the end of this development he has actually lost the ability to notice his own body signals. This does not necessarily contradict the observation that men often feel quite sorry for themselves when they are really sick. Because of ignoring pain for years, they have not developed the experience to cope with pain sensations.

Wishing to Change One's Own Body

We considered the request to name any possible wishes for changes to the body as an extra question to validate the other answers. One thing we learned in the interviews was that' the specific phrasing ('If you had the chance to change everything that you want to change about your body, for example, by surgery or training, what would you want to change?) made the interviewee rather wary.

P.: Hm, I wouldn't change anything. Well, if you ask me like that, by surgery or training, involving ... relatively great exertion, I wouldn't change anything.
I.: But?
P.: If you asked if I would wish for something ...
I.: Yes, that's how I meant it.
P.: Yes, perhaps I would say then not such a sticking-out nose or something.
I.: What else?
P.: I can't think of anything else.

In some cases the interviewer got outright refusals:

I.: If you had the chance to change everything that you would want to change about your body, what would you want to change? Just a sketch of your ideal self.
G.: My dear Mrs. Interviewer: it's in front of you. I feel like I am, that's really how I want to be. That's how I feel; that's me.
I.: And you don't have any parts on your body you don't like, which you would like to change?
G.: I need a haircut, that's true. I'm not satisfied with that.

Some interviewers tried to improve the question by letting the men express three wishes at will in order to penetrate to deeper aspects of their ideal body-image. There, too, however, they met most often with resistance. In the following excerpt the interviewer is relentless.

I.: If you had the chance to change something about your body - just imagine you had three free wishes or an operation or something like that - what would you want to change then?

J.: Body means face also, doesn't it?
I.: Yes (...)
J.: ... Okay, so, if you say the face is included now, so - if I could wish for something ... Would it be bad if I say initially I don't know? (Pause) No, I don't know.
I.: Satisfied all round?
J.: Well, okay, what I have just said ... if I have a belly, if I get fat or like that, that bothers me. But ... no.
I.: Is there never a day when you stand in front of the mirror and think 'Oh, perhaps it would be nice if this or that were different'?
J.: (Pause) Well, yes, I do stand in front of the mirror with a kind of dissatisfaction, but couldn't identify it now; I could just say, well, it's your nose you don't like, or you're not that keen on your mouth. It can't be pinned down to one point which I could name. I don't know, maybe it's a sort of 'Bleah!' at my face in the mirror (...) Yes, maybe, perhaps I could say, I mean in the past I always thought it would be nicer if you had curly hair and not hair like this, that's true, but ...
I.: Yes, that sort of thing, or it could be something really outrageons, something you might wish for sometime but which probably is entirely unrealistic - not really feasible (long pause).
J.: Yes, I still remember, I still think this sometimes, this thing about my hair, that it's just so dead straight. And then I'm rather afraid of, well, losing too much hair. I mean a bald head and so on, and I also know that I have a tendency to it. And that is really, well, stupid.

With about half of the people interviewed, almost no desire for change is apparent; at most, a change of hairstyle and a small change in weight are mentioned. I believe that the question caused a number of men problems related to their feeling of self-esteem. If the basic philosophy 'Accept what is' is adhered to, desires for change threaten stability.

To admit to another person that one's own body should be other than it is seems to be a threatening perception. This contradicts the Mrazek's hypothesis (1984) quoted at the beginning of the chapter that the body does not constitute a part of male identity. It is indeed a part of it, but in a tacit and natural way. Another example will illustrate this. This 22-year-old student expressed many negative self-assessments during the interview, but on the question of change he always said he was content.

I.: ... If you had have the chance to change something about your body, what would you do then?
W.: What?
I.: Well, changes in any respect, realistic or unrealistic.
W.: Hm, well what I've thought sometimes is how it would be if I could see property with both eyes. That would be something, yes, and another thing, it would be nice not to have to shave every morning, but to let a real nice beard grow and just let it bush out. Somehow it's annoying just to let a couple of weeds grow, and they never amount to anything. Apart from that I used to dream about being at least 1.80 m tall, but I've given that up. Otherwise ... Well, for heaven's sake, I've always said, what does it matter, I am as I am, I can't change much simply physically, maybe I could go sunbathing and get a nice suntan (...) but basically these are just minor things. Otherwise, by and large, that's it.
I.: Otherwise you are satisfied with your body?
W.: Yes.
I.: You mean, you don't want to change anything through training or something?
W.: Oh, put it this way, I think it's good, I mean, just some bodybuilding ... that's bullshit ... some things in competitive sports ... basically you ruin your body with that and ... well, OK, I could see myself maybe picking up handball again.
I.: Otherwise you are satisfied?
W.: Most of the time.
I.: When not?

W.: When something is wrong with me ... I was weighed down with this gastritis a rather long time, well you don't exactly want to have this pain, a really 'wonderful' feeling, to feel how the stomach juices were working inside; I wasn't content with that condition at all, naturally.

I.: Everything is OK with the shape of your body?

W.: Well, my God, it was bothered me terribly for a while that some people called me very fat, which was true for a period of time, but then, my God, I accepted it and if somebody says, you look like you have a bun in the oven, then I just think, well, just let him talk. Then I just say, 'Then I won't starve to death right away.' I think it's stupid to strive for ideal beauty, everybody should know for himself what he finds beautiful ... Like I've said, eating is very important for me and if something tastes good, I just eat and don't care, and I don't think about a heart attack or constriction of the blood vessels or whatever. My God, who wants to live forever? And I think one can really mess up one's life with any kind of asceticism. I think, life is dreary enough, why make it worse for oneself?

W. obviously has serious health problems - I think the way he talks about them is typically male: all in all, he is content; naturally he 'didn't want' the gastritis and at this point he becomes ironical. His remarks as to the health consequences of his overweight are even sarcastic: 'Who wants to live forever, life is dreary enough!'

Sarcasm is also typical of other comments by men, when they talk about real health problems: one person who has an allergy commented: 'I have the attitude, "To hell with it, I'll do that, the body will have to put up with it."'

In sarcasm there are obvious auto-aggressive tendencies - obviously the affected men resent their bodies.

The Interviewees and Their Sexuality

A different problem was the relationship of the men interviewed to their sexuality, their sex. Just about one third of the interviewees mentioned their penis in the interviews regarding body-image, two of them to stress that even there they just did not have any sexual sensation. The male sexual organ belongs to the most taboo parts of the body. A 22-year-old student mentioned to the interviewer the following desired change:

X.: ... Well, I wouldn't have anything against that, well, it's only the semen with which I have a difficult relationship. I think, this just isn't necessary.

I.: And how would you like to change that? Just leave it out?

X.: If something like that were possible, then I would just really wish that I could consciously leave it out, that it would just come when I want it ...

In this comment one also can see the desire for a competent sexual technique expressed in front of a woman interviewer, presented even with a certain coquetry. In this I see at least partly a really disturbed relationship to one's own physical sexuality. Why should one be ashamed of one's own semen and one's capacity to procreate? The problem of shame often also appears when the interviewees describe their impact on woman, their sexual aura. Some men dissociate themselves from vanity and ideals of beauty. 'I only look into the mirror for practical reasons ... In puberty I did it more often', 'No, that kind of exaggerated vanity doesn't suit me ...'

Other men admit that they are vain, but then engage in protracted justification exercises.

'I think its good, that I can look into the mirror and not do it furtively, as though somehow it were something not done, that I like to look at myself and take care of myself . . .

I.: Do you feel really bad, because you are 4 kg overweight?
G.: No, no there is no real consequence for my emotional life. It is just real vanity. I guess I could be an athletic type if I worked in that direction, but I don't attach any importance to that . . . Every day I go swimming with somebody. I go because I want to get rid of my extra weight; he goes because he really wants muscles. I think that's overdoing it a bit, really . . . Because I think a belly is just ugly, I think that's a healthy aesthetic feeling - but to build up muscles, I think that's a bit of a cult thing . . .

Men are caught in a contradition: for their sense of self it is important how their body is perceived, but they are not allowed purposely to care for their body and make themselves look handsome.

Some emphasize what an important experience it was to be found attractive: 'My body was weak and so was my identification with myself; since then I have received assurance about my body from people who liked my exterior . . . people who are important to me and who thought that I have value as a person, and I've carried this over to my body.' Self-esteem does not simply develop out of inner values; it is primarily an external social function, the esteem of others perceived as real. Powerful rules forbid a real man to become dependent on something like that - with all the negative consequences for the self-esteem.

In the following interview excerpt a 20-year-old student copes with this conflict by a depreciation of the external ideals.

A. I was never such an ideal type of man, so I can hardly judge, but in principle I'm really glad that I am how I am because somehow I just have the feeling that I am liked not for my looks but because of the rest. So, when I look at others who look more like the dream man - how a female imagines him to be, or how one imagines females' ideas to be - then I see the others as much poorer than I am. Because they always have to put on a show.
I.: How important is your effect on women to you, or what do you think it is? How do you see the effect, how strong is it?
A.: Somehow it will be there I can imagine that well some such effect will be there just how it is and how strong it is, I can't say. Never talked to a woman about that no, I can't say. (Pause)

This reminds one of Jourard's phrases (1971), describing the man as occupant of a tank on enemy territory. One does not reveal oneself. The person interviewed above is glad that he does not have to put on a show, but he also does not know how he appears to women. The armour keeps hurt at bay - and important experiences as well.

This alienated relationship to their own genitals and sexual appeal is also an expression of the complex relationship many men have to women. As in the quotation above, many men are sure that some kind of effect on women does occur, but they have no awareness of what it is in them that works the attraction. They also often lack awareness about their own flirtatious behaviour. This is supported by the strong conviction (ideologically entrenched) that this is the normal way to behave, and it is also a result of a very considerable fear of women. When the sexual attraction of woman becomes a topic, and if there is also physical sensation, for example, in the genital region, in the stomach or in the area of the heart, this is arousing and for many men extraordinarily frightening. The fear of a possible rejection plays an important role in this. A rejection would have a central effect on self-esteem, in order to avoid this, initial feelings will be partly repressed.

In recent years an interesting discussion has developed on the implications of this alienation from body and sex for male sexuality and the male organism (see Norretranders 1983).

Some psychotherapists, with reference to Reich (1969), see in this represssion of feelings and the resultant 'body armour' the cause of many sexual problems.

Summary

The initial superficial positive description of their body-image as expressed by most of the men interviewed did not stand up to an intensive analysis of the dialogue during interview. An indifference, a taking for granted and sometimes even a hostile opposition show up behind the surface.

The ideology of manliness with its numerous demands and an ambivalent attitude to women and sexuality proved to be important influences on male body-image.

The interviews with men averaging 25 years of age, i.e. young men, revealed few indications of new body awareness apart, from the two students who had been in touch with bioenergetic groups.

The consequences of this alienation of the body on health-related and sexual behaviour patterns can only be called alarming.

References

Bongers D (1984) Körperselbstbilder. Research report from the Institute of Psychology, Technical University, Berlin, vol 4, pp 1-33

Bongers D (1985) Männerselbstbilder - Eine explorative Studie über Auffassungen von Männlichkeit im Selbstbild. Ritter, Berlin

Jourard SM (1971) Self-disclosure. An experimental analysis of the transparent self. Wiley, New York

Jourard SM (1974) Some lethal aspects of the male role. In: Pleck JH, Sawyer J (eds) Men and masculinity. Prentice-Hall, Englewood Cliffs

Leontjew AN (1982) Tätigkeit, Bewußtsein, Persönlichkeit. Rugenstein, Cologne

Merton RK, Kendall PL (1979) Das fokussierte Interview. In: Hopf C, Weingarten E (eds) Qualitative Sozialforschung. Klett-Cotta, Stuttgart

Mrazek J (1984) Die Verkörperung des Selbst. Psychologie Heute 2/84: 50-58

Norretranders T (1983) Hingabe - über den Orgasmus des Mannes. Rowohlt, Reinbek

Reich W (1969) Die Funktion des Orgasmus. Kiepenheuer and Witsch, Cologne

Richter HE (1974) Lernziel Solidarität. Rowohlt, Reinbek

Schütze F (1977) Die Technik des narrativen Interviews. Work reports and research material no 1, Faculty of Sociology, University of Bielefeld

Thomae H (1968) Das Individuum und seine Welt. Hogrefe, Göttingen

Fluor Albus: How Doctors and Patients React to a Body Symptom

M. Lohs

If a patient consults the therapist at the very moment the symptoms of a chronic, apparently purely organic disease are fading away, this in itself is unusual enough to be looked into more closely. But if this step is taken to find out whether the disappearance of the physical symptoms is yet another symptom of a hitherto undetected disease, then this case becomes a telling example of the problems arising as soon as the history of an organic disease is conceived of as a mental process. Suddenly one's body turns into a stage where a mental drama with an ever uncertain end takes place. The very fact that the affected person gradually realizes her mental disposition to somatic syndromes causes a feeling of uncertainty - even when the symptoms themselves have disappeared - which was suppressed by the orthodox, purely organic diagnosis, even though treatment on the basis of this had no curative effect. It is this insecurity, evoked if the doctor abandons orientation by somatic interpretation models, that makes the superficially symptom-free patient consult the therapist.

This remarkable constellation was found in the case of one patient, whose case history will now be described.

Mrs K., 41 years old and mother of two, a housewife since the birth of her eldest daughter 17 years ago, came to consult me. She emphasized that she enjoys running the household, especially as the work that needs to be done leaves her enough free time to pursue her own interests. Her husband, very successful in his job and making good money, encourages her to practise her hobbies. After these preliminaries Mrs K. immediately brought up her problem. For about 10 years she had been suffering from recurrent flour albus. During this time she had only been symptom-free for one menstrual cycle at the most. Over the years she had seen various doctors, and eventually she even went to a university hospital, the diagnosis, however, being always the same: *fluor albus* with pathological findings of *candida albicans.* The success of the widely differing drug therapies never lasted longer than to the next menstruation, after which the same symptoms reappeared. Treatment of her partner also had had no lasting effect. The doctors attributed the disease to different causes, but no improvement occurred after these causes were eliminated. Changing contraceptive methods (first different anti-ovulants, then a JUD and finally condoms) had no effect either. Rigorous dieting also gave no relief. She stopped wearing synthetic underpants, always boiled her underwear, used no softening agents, wore no tight slacks, stopped going to public swimming pools or saunas, etc., did not take baths any more - although this was hard for her - did not use ordinary soap but only medical, alkali-free detergents, took all hygienic precautions when she used a public toilet. This list could be continued, but all these changes in her behaviour and habits had just as little effect as the drugs she took according to the doctor's prescription. Psychic causes were ruled out by the doctors who attended her. Thus Mrs K. believed that she just had to put up with the fluor and to learn to live with it.

Three months before Mrs K. consulted me on the recommendation of a woman physician, the fluor had disappeared without any apparent reason. This surprising fact bothered Mrs K. to such an extent that she began to develop ideas which neither she nor her doctors had considered so far. To begin with, she discovered a connection between certain events of her private life and the discharge, which she now regarded to be an indication of some latent problem. This new interpretation immediately gave rise to the fear that her trouble could recur as a consequence of events outside her control. In consulting a therapist she was attempting to get a grip on the bundle of powerful factors that made her feel very insecure. She told me that, about 3 months ago, she had had a violent quarrel with her husband, whom she had married 20 years before. In the early years of her married life, she had very much enjoyed having intercourse with her husband, although their relationship had not been free from sexual problems. After the birth of their second child, her husband had more and more lost interest in her sexually, and increasingly gave her the feeling that she was no longer attractive to him and that he had found himself a mistress - both accusations being strongly repudiated by her husband.

Ten years ago, she had met a man, while playing tennis, with whom she has had an affair since. She met him almost daily and never had any sexual problems with her lover, who was the second man she had sexual intercourse with. This sexual relationship proved very satisfactory for her, and she never had any desire for further relationships. Although she felt guilty towards her husband, she maintained this extramarital affair. When Mrs K. discovered that her husband read magazines for homosexual men and frequented gay bars, she took him to task. Although he denied homosexual interests and preferences, Mrs K. remained suspicious.

About 2 years ago Mrs K.'s husband learnt of her liaison. He showed understanding for his wife and tolerated her affair. Mrs K. now hoped to have become more attractive for her husband, but he showed no renewed interest in her; their quarrels, however, became less frequent. Yet her husband's tolerance made Mrs K. more and more suspicious.

About 3 months ago, she confronted her husband, telling him to his face that she thought he was homosexual. Eventually he conceded that he was more attracted by men than by women and that he had had sexual contacts with several men during his marriage. She was simultaneously shocked and relieved, because hidden fears had now been brought to light. Both agreed to try to save their marriage. She broke with her lover, and from this very moment on the fluor had disappeared.

She now suspected that the disappearance of the fluor was in some way connected with the termination of her affair, especially since she now realized that the chronic fluor had appeared when she had started her extramarital affair. On the one hand she interpreted her sudden freedom from symptoms as a sort of moral reward for her dicision to repair her marriage, but on the other hand she wanted some sort of guarantee for a satisfactory sexual life, which seemed possible with her husband only if he could free himself from his homosexual desires. The aim in seeking therapy was to ensure that, in the case that her husband proves to be incurable, Mrs K. will not again develop the fluor symptom if she resumes her extramarital sexual contacts.

This case history sounds as if it were made up for the sole purpose of having it described in a textbook of psychosomatic medicine for gynaecologists: for years, drug therapy of a recurrent genital mycosis fails to achieve lasting success, whereas the mere talk between the couple, their decision to make an effort to continue and improve their relationship, renders the woman's symptom superfluous and makes her genital mycosis disappear. In my pilot study on fluor albus, however, a high percentage of the women examined ($n=40$) were found to have a similar case history. The therapeutic significance of psychic aspects, so often neglected in the treatment of a body symptom - as, for example, the fluor - was proved here beyond all doubt.

The above case history at the same time illustrates a widespread attitude of physicians as regards their approach to the fluor albus patient: women with recurrent fluor albus are considered difficult patients, often irritating their doctors and making them feel helpless as far as a permanent elimination of the symptom is concerned. The patients repeatedly complain about the same thing, going from one doctor to the next if the therapies prove ineffective. The doctor's own therapeutic efforts hardly ever have any success. Subjectively, the therapists believe that these patients show particularly low compliance with them, that they and, when applicable, their partner do not use the medicaments as prescribed or for too short a times, break off therapy too soon, or do not alter their behaviour and habits.

At the same time, most of the physicians have a vague feeling - as become clear to me in many talks during my pilot study - that the fluor of these patients is more than a mere somatic syndrome or a simple organopathological finding.

The number of patients with recurrent fluor albus with pathological finding is steadily increasing in the physicians' consulting rooms (Effendy and Gieler 1984). At present, approximately every fourth woman who consults a gynaecologist suffers from fluor (Kistner 1979, cited in Shorter 1984); the fluor caused by venereal diseases is not included in this figure. However, since the number of effective medications for the treatment of infectious fluor albus has been increasing on the pharmaceutical market since the mid-1950s, the gynaecologist deals with the main symptom in his practice in the way he was taught and is expected to treat it: he prescribes medicaments. Both doctor and patient concentrate on the physical processes. Psychic causes, the subjective experience of the body symptom, and general psychosocial factors relevant for the development and the chronicity of the symptom are in most cases negated by doctor and patient, if not totally excluded as possible causes and judged to be irrelevant. The personal background of a patient is hardly ever discussed specifically, and equally rare are efforts by the doctor to suggest psychic processes as possible causes for the patient's recurrent fluor.

In order to illustrate the contradictory results to which merely organotherapeutic fluor albus have led, and to clarify what relative importance, within the spectrum of aetiological factors of the fluor, should be attributed to psychic aspects and, above all, women's subjective experience of the symptom, the following points will be discussed in this paper:

1. Fluor albus from the gynaecological point of view
2. Aetiology and therapy of fluor genitalis from the medical historical point of view
3. Latest findings of psychosomatic research on fluor albus
4. A special consideration from the medicopsychological aspect of how the affected women handle and experience chronic fluor: fluor albus as an expression of a woman's attitude to her body.

The Gynaecological Term 'Fluor Albus'

The nuisance number one of many a woman has various names: leucorrhoea, fluor albus, whites, or simply fluor, the latter being in general use as a colloquial term for fluor albus. This list of names has overtones of negative connotations, pointing out how unpleasant this physical phenomenon is for the woman affected. Historically, this is understandable, because effective drugs against vaginal infections of a nonvenereal nature have only been available since about 1930. Yet to this day it remains a symptom that is difficult to treat - as could be seen in the case described at the beginning of this paper - especially if it is recurrent or if laboratory tests produce minimal or no pathological finding.

Since primarily the fundamental psychosomatic and medicopsychological aspects are to be presented here, only a brief organomedical differentiation of fluor albus will be given. In the vagina, a biologically necessary tissue fluid is constantly produced, called a transudate. It is a mucous fluid, produced by the glands of the genital system. Its quantity and quality change with the menstrual cycle. It functions as a chemical biological barrier and serves to maintain the normal condition of the tissue in the vagina. Its production is controlled by the hormones in the ovaries. Because of the differentiation of the female genital system, this normal transudation is susceptible to disturbances caused by manifold anatomical and organic variables. If abnormal hypersecretion occurs in the vagina, this is called fluor albus. In most cases, the fluor itself is not a disease but the symptom of a disease (Bickenbach 1951). There are various diseases that can produce the symptom. Fluor albus is categorized according to its causes, although in practice very often no clear-cut monocausal allocation can be made. Generally, fluor albus is categorized as an exudate if it is an inflammatory vaginal discharge caused by bacteria, (candida albicans) trichomonads or gonococcus entering the female genitalia from outside, or resulting from manifold anatomical and organic disturbances such as an inflammation or teratogenesis of the cervix or the tubae, or chemical irritation due to vaginal douching, etc. Hypersecretion caused by organ insufficiency, e.g. of the ovaries, is called *functional fluor* (for the organic causes see the left-hand and middle in Table 1), whereas hypersecretion caused by vasomotor factors, not brought about by an inflammatory process, is called *psychogenic* or *nervous fluor.* The latter often occurs only intermittently, and is taken to be a consecutive symptom or a concomitant phenomenon of mental stress and disorder (Roemer 1972). This category served as a 'glory-hole' for all those cases in which no organic pathological findings were discovered. Both views of the fluor, as an autonomous psychosomatic disease or as a secondary accompanying symptom, are held among psychosomatically orientated gynaecologists (Perez-Gay 1983).

No organic or anatomical indications can be found as possible causes of the fluor in the case of about 15%-25% of patients suffering from fluor albus; for about 75%-85% of the patients a somatic pathogenesis is diagnosed (G. Karkut, 1984, personal communication). In most cases, the general practitioner contents himself with these objective pathological findings, based upon scientific discoveries and (laboratory) techniques and methods, neglecting the psychic aspects which also play a role in the case of an infectious disease. The organic evidence is believed to explain everything about the aetiology of the fluor, and the psychological state of the patient is left unconsidered. The fluor is treated here solely as a concomitant symptom of a somatic disease (Grützmacher-Sawicka 1982).

Girls can have fluor albus at quite an early age (for the first time often 1-2 years before the menarche) and it can extend far into the menopause. Psychosomatically orientated literature mentions especially that women with superficially neurotic problems or of a so-called nervous constitution are most frequently found among patients with fluor albus, and in psychiatric literature the fluor is mentioned as a frequent concomitant of depression (Faust et al. 1983).

As the descriptions show, medical science allocates the causes of vaginal hypersecretion to three factors: endogenic organic factors, exogenic organic factors and psychogenic factors (see Table 1).

Table 1. Overview of the pathogenesis of fluor genitalis

Exogenous factors	Endogenous factors	Psychosocial factors
- Microbiological causes • Uncleanliness • Excessive hygiene • Uncleanliness of the sexual partner • Frequent change of sexual partner - Vulvitis • Specific: bacteria trichomonads *Candida* parasitic stomatitis • Unspecific: bacterial poly-infections - Mechanical irritation • By foreign substances, e.g. during masturbation • By rubbing, e.g. tampons, tight clothing - Chemical substances • Body and laundry detergents • Vaginal sprays, vaginal douching • Moist and warm environment caused by synthetic under wear and sanitary pads	- Hormonal factors • Hormonal changes immediately before, during, and after puberty • Menstrual cycle and disturbances in it • oral contraceptives • Pregnancy • Breast-feeding • Hormonal changes immediately before, during and after the menopause - Local changes in the abdomen • Injuries • Inflammations (sometimes caused by contraceptive methods, sexual contacts, etc.) • Tumours • Ectopia - General diseases • Diabetes mellitus • Infections • Alcoholism • Vegetative dysfunctions (dystonia, gastric and intestinal disorders) • Cardiac and circulatory disorders - Allergic reactions - Local deficiency of the immunological system - Sequela of certain medicaments - After eating certain kinds of food, e.g. carbohydrates, carminatives	- Unsatisfactory sexuality • Expression of unsatisfied sexual needs and desires ('libido fluor') • Self-punishment after satisfactory sexual experiences ('conscience fluor') • Nonacceptance of one's own sexual desires ('defence fluor') • Sexual experiences unsatisfactory and disappointing ('defence fluor') - Sexual dysfunction e.g. Anorgasmy, vaginism, dyspareunia - Fertility • Frustrated wish for children • Subjective attitude to contraceptives • Sterility in the woman or the man - Neurodystonie in unspecified stress situations e.g. increased perspiration, heart palpitation, migraine - Permanent exhaustion • Permanent tension • Direct damage by environmental factors (profession, life style, etc.) • Weak constitution - Acute psychic strain - General mental disorders of women • Concomitant symptom of depression, general anxiety, compulsiveness (cleanliness), identity or contact disorders, psychoses, etc. - Hypochondriac and phobic reactions to feared diseases of the genital system e.g. carcinomata, venereal diseases, sterility - Compensatory benefits • Control over timing and frequency of sexual contacts • Ascertainment or clarification of the partner's love • Rejection of the partner • Expression of the wish that the partner fulfil one's expectations - Early traumatizing experiences Deprivation, such as lack of attention from one's mother

Fluor Albus in the History of Medicine

Fluor albus is a symptom that women have always regarded as a burden of their sex. Greek and Roman physicians already knew and reported on it. Whether to assess the discharge, formerly called fluor albus as a life-threatening disease or as a normal, even healing, purification process of the female body was controversial for centuries - an important indication of the fact that the fluor was a symptom difficult to define for the physicians and authors of medical treatises, that it was a crux for them, and probably still is.

From Hippocrates to Galen to Mercurialis in the sixteenth century, medical science took the view that fluor is neither a disease nor a symptom of a disease, but rather a purification of the entire body of every woman. Fluor was put on the same level as menstruation, both being considered as normal processes for women of child-bearing age.

In the seventeenth and eighteenth centuries, the assessment of fluor albus underwent a change. It was clearly distinguished from that kind of fluor which is an accompanying symptom of a venereal disease and occurs as a consequence of tumours, etc. When fluor albus became 'too heavy and too strong', it was no longer considered as a normal body secretion of all women. It was supposed to be unhealthy, as soon as it exceeded an unspecified quantity' (Asteruc 1768-1778; Musitanus 1743; Mueller 1790; Stahl 1724). A pathogenic effect as being 'an inner obstacle to marital fertility and love' was attributed to the fluor.

In addition to that, medical literature, manuals, especially marriage guides, and later the encyclopaedias of the time indicate the emotional valuation of the fluor by the women themselves and their husbands. It is called 'annoying' and 'disgraceful', seen as a punishment and distress, and described as a troublesome disease which is considered unclean and' makes a woman unpleasant for 'her husband'. It is understood as a life-threatening disease. The assessment of the physicians changes: the status of a disease is increasingly often attributed to fluor albus, especially if the women complain about pain and if additional symptoms, such as temperature, irregular menstruation, allergies, etc. appear, or if a woman dies 'exhausted by the white flux' (Krüntz 1856; Stahl 1724). Consumption, fatigue, hysteria, and depression are mentioned as frequent side effects of fluor albus. Warnings are given against the fluor albus of women that can end in invalidism and sometimes even proves fatal. The dangerousness and malice of this body secretion is emphasized.

Up to the middle of the sixteenth century, the aetiological explanations were based upon assumptions that the fluor was a sequela or symptom of the following (cf. Krüntz 1856):

1. Women's unhealthy way of living. On the one hand this included such extreme living conditions as the physical over-exertion of women of the lower social strata, the idleness and 'extravagance' of women of the higher social strata, and the reading of 'bad literature', e.g. romances, etc., of women of the upper classes. On the other hand, it referred to so-called sexual hyperactivity and total sexual continence. It is also a late sequela of a woman's breast-feeding her own children and of too little sleep.
2. A woman's unhappy love for a man.
3. The use of certain contraceptives and abortives.
4. Poor nutrition, e.g. if the woman ate and drank too much in general, or if she ate particularly greasy, starchy, and coarse food and drank strong liquor.
5. Insufficient clothing for protection from severely cold and stiflingly hot weather.

6. Lack of or too violent exercise.
7. Lack of, exaggerated, or faulty body hygiene.
8. Certain climatic and ecological conditions to which the woman was exposed; e.g. the fluor was said to have been more widespread in Poland and the Netherlands than elsewhere in Europe.
9. Genetic or constitutional disposition; e.g. the particular fibrous tissue and vascular wall deficiency in some women.
10. Certain personality traits and mental peculiarities; e.g. it was assumed that so-called hysterical and depressed as well as emotionally disturbed women were to a great extent also inconvenienced by fluor.
11. Organic diseases, such as scurvy, herpes, skin diseases, allergies.

Summing up, it can be said that, in the history of medicine, three basic tendencies can be distinguished in the assessment of the body reaction "flour". The recurrent fluor albus

- Was at first (right into the sixteenth century) considered as normal, and thus healthy, up to a certain degree - this degree, however, was not specified any further in the literature.
- Next it was seen as 'becoming increasingly fashionable among the diseases of the female sex in the cities, in high society circles, among the rank and fashion' (Thilenius 1814).
- Eventually a pathological status was attributed to it across the social strata. It was realized that it could develop into a malicious, insidious, and eventually life-threatening disease.

For the therapy of nonvenereal fluor the following recommendations can be found (Thilenius 1814):

1. Diet. The woman should primarily eat food that promotes digestion and is simultaneously light and nutritious.
2. Administration of restoratives, especially preparations rich in iron.
3. Clothing that is appropriate for climate, temperature, and work, and does not restrict the woman's mobility.
4. Plenty of exercise in the open air.
5. Stimulation of body secretion, such as perspiration, e.g. by means of purgatives.
6. The following gynaecological measures are suggested: injections, enemas, hip baths, tinctures, imfusions, and the insertion of sponges soaked with herbal ingredients into the vagina. The recipes for these prescriptions are manifold.
7. Often one finds the advice that married women should abstain from sexual intercourse, whereas 'maidens' are encouraged to get married and bear children.

Current State of Psychosomatic Research on Fluor Albus

Fluor albus may well be the most frequent problem and topic in gynaecological practice and literature. Research concentrates primarily on the functional somatic aspect, on chemical bacteriological studies, on improved and refined technical analyses and interventions, e.g. exact statements concerning the number and quantity of possible strains of bacteria. In contrast to that, only an infinitesmall number of holistic studies has been carried out which, aside from the anatomical, endocrinological, physiological, biochemical, and clinical sides of the problem, address themselves explicitly and in detail to the mental and psychosocial aspects of the fluor, and differentiate and analyze them. Interestingly enough, there is not a single study on women's subjective experience of fluor albus. It is not clear why one woman feels decidedly handicapped by the dampness in her panties, the next woman even considers the fluor as a disease, whereas a third woman experiences it as totally normal, unobtrusive, and healthy, and a fourth woman even enjoys it as a pleasant token of her womanhood, nor is it clear what connection exists between these subjective reactions and the continuation of the sympton.

The fact that the subjective experience of fluor albus is a 'blind spot' in medical and psychological literature, may, among other factors, be explained by methodological difficulties in recording and elucidating these subjective reactions and convert them into objective and thus comparable data. The often emphasized discrepancy between the objective - and that means here medical, pathological - findings and the subjective experience of the women suggests that the perception and assessment of fluor albus depends to a high degree on the individual sensitivity of the woman affected and the importance she herself attaches to the fluor. This subjective sensitivity of a woman, however, is left totally unconsidered in gynaecological literature. It is of course scientifically inadmissible simply to reduce the concept of a disease without further ado to its easily measurable factors, merely because of the methodological problems in collecting reliable data on the subjective experiencing of the symptom. In therapeutic practice this reduction leads to an unfortunate point of view: laboratory findings are used to decide whether the complaints of a patient indeed signal a serious fluor - and that means one of organic origin - or whether there is primarily 'only' a psychogenic fluor albus. In fact, it is often very difficult or virtually impossible to make a differential diagnosis - as in the case history described at the beginning of this article. Both aspects, somatic and mental, should be taken into account by the physician.

Thus, the psychosomatic factors playing a role in the development and chronicity of fluor albus (see right-hand column in Table 1) will be discussed below.

Psychodynamic theories predominate in the explanations of psychosomatic fluor albus. According to these theories, one of the most important causes for the development of the fluor is unsatisfactory or disturbed sexuality (Perez-Gay 1983) of the patient herself. Secondly, fluor is regarded as a woman's reaction to the disturbed sexuality of her partner, e.g. his sexual dysfunction. The classification of the discharge as libido, conscience, or defence fluor (see Table 1) depends on how the woman either denies herself sexual satisfaction or punishes herself for it or how she is denied sexual satisfaction, i.e. depends on her psychodynamic coping pattern.

Additionally, it was noticed that women with sexual dysfunctions or menstrual disorders often develop fluor. Here, on the one hand the fluor seems to be part of a more complex syndrome resulting from various psychodynamic causes - such as negative sexual or menstruation experiences, a negative view of one's sexual identity as a woman, a sexually repressive education, a negative attitude towards one's own sexual needs and desires as well as their satisfaction, lack of sexual experience - but, on the other hand, it could also be a concomitant symptom of a different functional organic disturbance, such as, for example, a regulatory disorder of the autonomic nervous system, or a disorder of the ovarian hormones. Both modes of explanation should be tested in every case. It is also known that a great variety of contraceptives can contribute to an increase of the fluor. In the case of hormonal or mechanical contraceptives, endocrinological, chemical, or mechanical causes ought certainly to be considered. Psychodynamic factors, however, must also be taken into account, such as the 'latent', 'ambivalent', or 'frustrated' wish of the woman, her partner, or both of them, to have a child, as well as the woman's attitude towards the method of contraception practised or her wish and desire to check and reassure herself of her reproductiveness, for the first time or the *n*th. In another area, equally concerning fertility, a woman may react to an organic and/or psychic insufficiency by developing fluor: if either she or her partner is sterile and both desire to have children. The fourth aspect mentioned by the psychodynamic theories consists of early childhood traumatizing experiences, such as, for example, deprivation by one's mother.

Besides the psychodynamic theories outlined here, there are physiological and psychological stress theories which explain the occurrence of fluor albus. Psychosomatic gynaecology employs these theories to trace the appearance of that fluor albus which is a concomitant symptom of other functional disorders. Thus, for example, patients with symptoms of neurodystonia complain about developing fluor in nonspecific stress situations. Moreover, stress factors due to occupational and environmental influences are interpreted as causes of fluor, such as heavy physical and mental strain, lack of competence in stress-producing situations, noxae in food, air and at work, etc.

A third theory tries to establish a connection between specific personality profiles and the occurrence of fluor albus. So far, studies on the personality structure of fluor patients have been reduced to dealing with mental peculiarities and disorders, which were not exactly defined in these papers and therefore rendered no objective data. The results do not allow differentiation, since according to these studies every mental seems to make women complain about fluor. This unsatisfactory result may be a consequence partly of problems in the psychodiagnostic approach and partly of the fact that only very few cases have been specifically studied in this respect. Most of the time it is casual remarks made in passing which are used as a basis for generalizations. No standardized psychological tests have yet been applied in order to collect quantifiable data.

One observation frequently reported is that there is often a striking disproportion between the quantity of the fluor and the patient's assessment of the symptom. Fear of venereal infections, cancer in the genital system, etc., is hidden behind this hypochondriac or phobic attitude of the patient. Sometimes this fear does not originate from the patient herself, but from her partner, who tells the woman to see a doctor, either because he himself has a phobia or because he has a bad conscience after having had 'extramarital' sexual intercourse.

A fourth independent theory for the occurrence of the fluor is the view that this disease holds certain compensatory benefits for the woman. She benefits from the fluor in the sense that she can indirectly influence and determine how often and when she has sexual intercourse with her partner, or she can secretly check if her partner still finds her attractive in spite of her 'disease' or not, etc.

These comments show that the clinical valency of fluor albus can be quite diverse and cannot possibly be determined by a single comprehensive definition. For the psychological study of fluor it is important to remember that fluor can be a phenomenon and a sensation as well as a symptom of physical and/or mental processes; in exceptional cases, however, it can also be a disease (Müller 1972).

Fluor Albus as an Expression of a Woman's Attitude to her Body: A Selected Medicopsychological Aspect of Women's Handling and Experience of Chronic Fluor Albus

The case history outlined at the beginning of this article emphasized the psychic dimension of fluor albus and made it clear that the symptom was rendered 'superfluous' as soon as the relationship with the partner was cleared up. A further aspect of this case is equally striking, and that is the low degree to which Mrs K. was inclined to talk about her personal feelings about the fluor. This example is not arbitrary, insofar as the experiencing of the fluor in the case of the patients who are normally available for research purposes is prejudiced by a double mediation: on the one hand by the diagnoses, aetiological concepts, and therapies of general practitioners, gynaecologists, and/or dermatologists, and, on the other hand, by the theory that partner conflicts in the widest sense are the appropriate interpretation of the body phenomenon of fluor. Although the latter view, used in the psychosomatically oriented or directly psychotherapeutic practice, represents a decisive step towards self-knowledge, it still does not include the concept of the fluor as an expression of one's attitude to one's body, which can have a significance that is independent of the partner situation.

Because of the 'double prejudice', complete investigation of the fluor albus will prove to be fairly complicated. As a consequence of their narrow concepts of the disease, researchers have hitherto also displayed a kind of strategic blindness, so that as a rule even the statements of those of their patients who were spontaneously aware of their reactions to the increased fluor, and mentioned this aspect, were not taken much notice of. I myself became aware of the women's remarks on this subject during my sociopsychological study of female student's potential for orgasm.

The psychosomatic approach, claiming that a woman's attitude towards the fluor reflects her attitude to her body, is certainly correct for all patients with recurrent fluor except one definite group. This group is partly consists of patients whose partners are considered to be the cause of the infection triggering off the fluor, either because of inadequate body hygiene or promiscuous habits together with lack of hygiene, and partly of patients whose fluor is caused by their own practice of inadequate genital hygiene or of having various sexual relationships with partners whose hygiene is inadequate; all this suggesting that the fluor has purely microbiological not psychogenic causes. In their case it would be wrong to assume psychosomatic or medicopsychological causes of the fluor. It is still totally unclear whether the group just mentioned is a tiny minority or rather a majority among the patients with infectious fluor. Opinion is divided, on the one hand because it is difficult to get frank answers to direct questions on this subject, and on the other hand because doctors are influenced by personal impressions of the patient and their own individual concepts of the aetiology of the infectious fluor.

In my pilot study I interviewed and questioned in writing 40 women who consulted their doctor for a medical check-up and then mentioned to him that they were suffering from fluor, as well as women who took part in self-examination classes, female students and women of different ages and professions who had recurrent fluor and took part in the study because they found it interesting. The diagnosis of their doctor as to which kind of fluor - infectious, functional, or nervous - they were suffering from was of secondary interest to the way in which experiencing the fluor. They did not classify the fluor per se as a pathological phenomenon, even if it was caused by an infection or if it evoked strong feelings of irritation and disgust. The following rough classification can be made for women with chronic fluor:

1. Women who experience the fluor as a lustful sensation
2. Women who simply accept the fluor as a given biological fact, even if it is very heavy
3. Women who consider the fluor as a nuisance but irrelevant
4. Women who experienc the fluor as disturbing and disgusting.

It is conceivable that precisely this analysis of how the women in my pilot study experience fluor albus offers another key to an understanding of the condition and a therapy even for those women suffering from chronic fluor albus who so far, due to their 'double predetermination', could neither talk about their subjective reactions to the fluor nor come to terms with them. It is especially important for the group of psychosomatic patients to be made aware of the significance of and the hidden experience structure of their symptom, since it is known from psychotherapy how little these patients are able to talk freely about their sensations and feelings, how much they tend to express their feelings primarily by means of their body symptoms, and how difficult it is for them to engage in any direct dialogue with themselves or their environment.

I would therefore like to discuss some especially striking findings of the pilot study, throwing light upon the complex, partly - prima facie - paradoxical, emotional cathexis fluor albus.

Two contrary attitudes can be found among those women who react positively to their fluor. This attitude can correlate with successful sexual experiences and a stable sexual identity, but also with an extremely low rating of 'womanhood', manifested in a generally low estimation of women as well as in the depreciation of the female genitalia. For example, the vulva is described as ugly, deformed, shrivelled, its smell as pungent, sweetish, putrid, its consistency as amorphous, flabby, and sticky. These women wash their vaginal area frequently (sometines leading the doctors to suspect that here the hypersecretion is a reaction to the disturbance of the vaginal flora by lotions, soaps or sprays, etc.), avoid coitus, and generally have a phobia of germs. Closer investigation reveals that these women consider the fluor itself to be some purification of the essentially detested organ and thus even welcome it. Since single acts of purification are not sufficient, the fluor develops, so to speak, into a chronic 'ablutomania', curbing the women's revulsion from their own genitalia.

But even among the women who violently hate their fluor, there are some who show a seemingly paradoxical pattern of experience. They are disgusted by their surplus of body secretion, while at the same time displaying a positive attitude to 'womanhood', to sexual experiences with their partners and to their own sexual needs. They perform normal or even less than normal vaginal hygiene and are not afraid of germs penetrating their body. A remarkable fact is that these women started to have a sexual relationship with a partner rather late in their life, but from then on led an active sexual life. Various indications (such as, for example, hints of a sexually repressive education) allow the conclusion that in these cases the fluor may be interpreted as the physical expression of an unconscious moral condemnation of their sexual practices. Yet this moral censorship is not strong enough to disturb the woman's 'lust orientation' and to shake her female identity. However, in the form of a feeling of disgust it clings to the fluor, seen as an excess of the secretion stimulated by sexual practices. Here, lust is condemned in an indirect way, with disgust playing the part of one's conscience. Pleasure must be paid for by the disgust at the continuously flowing (independent and nonfunctional) secretion.

Although the concept of paradoxical experience patterns helps to extend the scope of the understanding and treatment of women with recurrent fluor, it must again be emphasized that the transition from a merely organic analysis of the fluor to a psychosomatic view, concentrating on personal experience, does not yield a homogeneous interpretation model but only indicates the complexity of the phenomena connected with the term fluor albus. Thus, identical body symptoms can be experienced in a different way; and even in cases in which these experiences coincide, totally different causes could be at work, as has been illustrated by some examples. How wide the range of such possible causes is will be realized if one reminds oneself that the mere attempt to take particular note of sexual causes - without making any claims to primacy in research strategies - renders such a complex picture.

References

Asteruc J (1768) Theoretisch-praktische Abhandlung von den Frauenzimmerkrankheiten, pp 367 ff. In the Bibliothek Wolfenbüttel

Bickenbach W (1951) Über den Flour genitalis der Frau. Med Klin 43: 1121-1124

Effendy J, Gieler U (1984) Genitalmykosen auf dem Vormarsch. Sexualmedizin 8: 452-457

Faust V, Hole G, von Zerssen D, Wolfersdorf M (1983) Zur Diagnose der Depressionen. In: Faust V (ed) Depressionen. Symptomatik-Ätiopathogenese-Therapie. Compendium Psychiatricum. Hippokrates, Stuttgart, pp 3-11

Grützmacher-Sawicka I (1982) Der psychogene Fluor - Von der Selbstreflexion zum ordnenden Prinzip Eros. Sexualmedizin 11: 471-474

Krüntz JG (1856) Ökonomisch-technologische Enzyklopädie, pp 12-37. In the Bibliothek Wolfenbüttel

Mueller (1790) Medicinisches practisches Handbuch der Frauenzimmerkrankheiten, zum Gebrauche der Ärzte und verehelichten Damen, pp 176-196. In the Bibliothek Wolfenbüttel

Müller H (1972) Fluor genitalis. In: Käser (ed) Gynäkologie und Geburtshilfe, Vol 3. Thieme, Stuttgart, pp 81-109

Musitanus C (1743) Weiberkrankheiten, pp 303-337. In the Bibliothek Wolfenbüttel
Perez-Gay B (1983) Fluor vaginalis et cervicis aus psychosomatischer Sicht. In: Prill (ed) Der psychosomatische Weg zur gynäkologischen Praxis. Schattauer, Stuttgart, pp 186-191
Roemer H (1972) Psychogener Fluor. In: Käser (ed) Gynäkologie und Geburtshilfe Vol 1. Zyklusabhängige psychogene Störungen. Thieme, Stuttgart, pp 528-530
Shorter E (1984) Der weibliche Körper als Schicksal - zur Sozialgeschichte der Frau. Piper, Munich
Stahl GE (1724) Ausführliche Abhandlung von den Zufällen und Krankheiten des Frauenzimmers, pp 172-184. In the Bibliothek Wolfenbüttel
Thilenius MG (1814) Medicinische und Chirurgische Bemerkungen, part 2, pp 177-191. In the Bibliothek Wolfenbüttel

The Role of Body Experience in Women's Desire for Children and During Pregnancy, Birth and the Time after Delivery

M. Jarka

Plenty of medical, psychological and sociological literature already exists on the topics of pregnancy, birth lying-in and breastfeeding. While in medicine it is the elimination of or coping with risks during pregnancy and birth that is of primary interest (which actually makes it possible in the first place to pay more attention to psychological aspects in practice; cf. Hillemanns et al. 1983), psychology and psychoanalysis deal with endo-psychic and interpersonal conflicts concerning generativity (Deutsch 1954; Benedek 1960; Molinski 1972; Lukesch and Lukesch 1976) or regard this period as a crisis in life (Bibring 1961). The sociological problems of the mother's role have also been described in detail (Beauvoir 1968). However, the effect of body experience during this period has hardly been considered a central theme in scientific literature, which is rather surprising as one can assume that, for most women (mothers), pregnancy, birth, lying-in and breast-feeding are connected with an intense experience of the body, in both a sensual and a nonsensual way. Descriptions of body experience during this time have usually been confined to 'pseudoscientific' literature and empirical reports.

The perspective of this article differs from that of medical discourses on bodily processes in that here the main interest is focused on the perception and subjective experience of physical changes or the condition of the body. Feldmann, who studied body experience during pregnancy, defined it as the experiential representation of the body as perceived directly, though barely consciously; his definition includes the act of emotionally taking possession of the body, evaluating statements, and physical experiences of obstacles such as work and stress. The awareness that 'I, as a body, also exist for others and in the consciousness of others' (Feldmann 1977) plays another important role. Women allegedly define themselves through their bodies to a far greater extent than men (Hardach-Pinke 1982).

We must assume that there is a special connection between psychological condition and body experience during pregnancy, birth and the time after delivery. Three questions may be asked here:

1. What role does body experience play in the desire for children and in the course of pregnancy, birth and lying-in?
2. How does body experience change during pregnancy, birth, lying-in and breast-feeding?
3. What significance do experiences during pregnancy and birth have for a woman's subsequent perception of her own body and personal sexual identity?

When these questions are asked it becomes obvious that hardly any satisfactory answers are possible, and that they serve rather to open up new areas for research (Hardach-Pinke 1982).

This paper will try to collect arguments for the significance of body experience from the medical, psychological and psychosomatic literature on pregnancy, birth and lying-in, in order to give a provisional survey; it will include empirical studies and reports of special cases as well as theoretical concepts. The background to this is the recent discussion about research into the desire for children (Sichtermann 1983; Jagenow and Mittag 1984; Gambaroff 1984). In addition changes regarding the role of women - and thus changes in female body experience, with a tendency towards repossession of the body and ending the estrangement between 'head and belly' - have to be considered. The widespread debate in the feminist movement about changing views on pregnancy and birth shows that emancipation should enable women to realize both, their mental and physical abilities; the prerequisite for this is an end to fixed social roles.

In dealing with this topic one runs the risk of supporting a new ideology of motherhood (Beckmann 1984) and therefore should bear in mind that body experience can be only one aspect of the complex psychosomatic processes during pregnancy, birth and lying-in: an aspect that is closely connected with physiological and psychosocial processes, in which the importance of pregnancy ranks high for the woman concerned. Under fascism, however, women were reduced to the biological function of motherhood and were actually considered 'birth machines' for the production of human beings, as defined by the system (Davies-Osterkamp and Beckmann 1982). This may explain the reluctance of the social sciences to look into the physical aspects of maternity.

Body Experience and women's Desire for Children

Circumstances favourable to a potentially sensual aspect of motherhood (despite the stress of having children) have developed recently, as a result of women's increased freedom of choice in the realization of their own fertility, sometines after years of planned childlessness:

- Since the advent of the pill 20 years ago, it has been possible to plan the number of children and time their births with reasonable accuracy, and only during this period has the desire for children become a subject to cause conflict.
- The availability of contraceptives facilitates the separation of sexuality from procreation; against a background of centuries of moral hostility towards sensuality, this is actually to be seen as a liberation (sexuality only for the purpose of reproduction: 'the curse of procreation').
- Consequently - with the advent of family planning and birth control - children were wanted only when all consumer needs (house, career, etc.) were satisfied and when well-organized circumstances prevailed: the child became an acquisition.
- The resultant drop in the birth rate and newly developing endopsychic and interpersonal conflicts about the desire for children (because planning is possible)

have led to a situation where this desire has become the object of psychological and sociological research (Berninghausen 1980; Mittag and Jagenow 1984).

By means of questionnaires, numerous motives and motive categories have been ascertained (which cannot here be discussed in detail), in the course of which it has finally been confirmed that (a) the desire for children is always more or less ambivalent, according to the personal and social situation of the persons interviewed; (b) this changes in the course of the individual life cycle and (c) there are more rational arguments *against* than *for* having children (Heinkelmann 1978; Berninghausen 1980; Jarka 1981; Mittag and Jagenow 1984). If, despite this, people still have children, the arguments given for doing so are rather general and emotional, or diffuse expectations of happiness (Berninghausen 1980), which give rise to the assumption that there are physical and psychological possibilities inherent in the relationship with a child which are not to be found in a partner relationship alone. Thus psychological and sociological research into the desire for children provides important findings, but some questions still remain beyond rational explanation.

Whether the possibility of sensually experiencing the generative processes indicates a 'desire for fertility' (during coitus), as Jagenow and Mittag (1984) suggest, or whether the wish for procreation is already integrated in the female sex drive, as Sichtermann (1983) assumes, are interesting questions, which, however, in my opinion, cannot be answered with certainty. This discussion will remain a 'tightrope walk' (Jagenow and Mittag 1984). The biological fact(or)s of reproduction, however, have in any case to be distinguished from the psychological experience of sensual pleasure or aversion as otherwise we shall descend into a new biological determinism of the woman as mother.

The desire for children remains a complex system of motives. We observe (only) for the aspect from the point of view, of body experience that, first of all, a woman's desire for her *own* children coincides with the wish to realize female physical potential at some time during her life, and thus includes a desire for widened physical experience. There is also the wish to be able to continue to live through the physical product of oneself and the loved partner, which in a way represents a synthesis of the two. Another important factor is the desire for intensive physical contact with a baby and a growing child.

This body-oriented lust is always interwoven with psychosocial motives, as human beings are social beings and thus not biologically determined. Only real freedom to decide for or against children, and an end to the exploitation of women's child-bearing ability as a justification for stereotyped social roles (Mitchell (1976), allow us to examine the significance of these physical possibilities for the development of female sexuality and identity without supporting a new 'mother cult'.

Body Experience, the Desire for Children, and Psychoanalysis

Freud explained the origin of the desire for children by means of the oedipal theory based on a physical fact, namely the female lack of penis:

> The wish, with which the little girl turns to her father is originally the wish for the penis which her mother has denied her and which she now expects from her father. Womanhood, however, is

reached only when the wish for a penis is replaced by the wish for a baby, when the child, according to ancient symbolical equivalence, takes the place of the penis. (Freud 1932, p. 137)

Other psychoanalytically oriented authors such as Mack-Brunswick (1940) and Mitscherlich-Nielsen (1978) place the origin of the desire for children earlier, at the stage of pre-oedipal identification with the mother. Menne and Moersch (1980) connect the pre-oedipal and oedipal theories and come to the conclusion that the desire for children, because of the specific psychosexual development of the girl, is already integrated in the female sexual identity at an early stage (see also Chasseguet-Smirgel 1979).

On the subject of Freud's oedipal approach, Schmiedbauer-Schleibner writes that the term 'penis envy' is to be understood symbolically and that it refers to the 'social castration' of the woman and her striving for equality: 'Man and child are required to fill the body, which is felt to be damaged, and serve as substitutes for the lacking ego' (Schmiedbauer-Schleibner 1979, p. 353). Hagemann-White (1979) argues that the present reality of motherhood often does not fulfil the longing for sexual identity hidden in the unconscious penis envy and the conscious wish for a baby. Thus Freud is interpreted to the effect that he explained the desire for children as a reaction to the supposed social discrimination against women. Both his original theory and the interpretation are probably justified.

However, proceeding on the assumptions that the inferiority of women an ideological fallacy (Mitchell 1976), even if social reality at the moment, and that the sexes are biologically different but of equal value and functionally related in a complementary way, one could also understand Freud's theses with the following model:

Male sexual identity is already expressed in the externally visible and tangible existence of the penis and can therefore be physically experienced at any time. Physical experience of the hidden female genitalia is indeed possible through coitus, masturbation and sensory stimulation (of the breasts, for example), but in its diversity it is only fully exhausted with the realization of fecundity through pregnancy, birth and the child. Thus, in female sexuality, perception is focused on the interior of the body and the processes that are possible there: women's sexuality does not necessarily end with coitus but can go further, as shown by Jagenow and Mittag (1984).

The Freudian equation namely that the wish for a baby equals the wish for a penis, also applies on the social level: penis and child are phallic symbols representing power and potency. Consequently, a child per se need not be a substitute serving as compensation for insults to a woman's ego (Gugel 1976). This may be true sociologically but is not supported by biology. The psychoanalytical theory according to Freud covers and explains both aspects of the female desire for a child: that of body experience, arising from actual anatomical differences between the sexes, and the psychological aspect, or identification with the mother as a result of the oedipal conflict situation.

The extent to which a woman actually needs the realization of her physical potential to confirm her whole female identity is a different question and obviously depends on what other (intellectual and social) sources for finding her identity are available. However, the experiences of intellectual women who had their children late in life (Gambaroff 1984; Chessler 1980) show that the realization of this physical possibility can bring about an expansion of identity. In exceptional cases, of course, neurotic motives can dominate the desire for children: if a woman has doubts about her femininity because of parental insults to her ego, a problematic relationship with her mother or a boyish or masculine appearance, then pregnancy (the realization of fecundity) may be a welcome chance to heal the wounds to fill the depressive void and thus to prove her femininity. For depressive women in particular, pregnancy can be an opportunity to feel alive inside and to experience their own productivity. These factors perhaps explain why so many unintended pregnancies come about (Menne and Moersch 1980).

As to the timing of a woman's pregnancy, one matter of importance could be when the act of experiencing her physical reproductive capacity seems advantageous to the development of her identity, or when she wants and is able to get involved in the regression connected with motherhood. This might be the case at 20 or not until the age of 40, when the fear of missing the chance is a problem for many women. Erikson (1976) offers an appropriate model in his book Identity and Life Cycle.

Descriptions of known bodyoriented motives for and against the desire for offspring follow in support of these theoretical observations. The above-mentioned ambivalence in the desire for children is also expressed in the area of (anticipated) body experience.

In surveys, the wish to become a full, mature, satisfied woman has been given as an argument in favour of having children (Berninghausen 1980; Heinkelmann 1978), which calls to mind archaic representations of women as receptacles (Macy and Falkner 1980). The child is seen by women (and men) as a personal product and as proof of sexual potency, which from the physical point of view it is. The child also represents a 'narcissistic extension' (Friday 1979), which in the physical sense is again applicable here: the expression 'our own flesh and blood' is vividly metaphorical. Precisely because these body-oriented motives are beyond any rational explanation, people easily succunb to an ideological approach: under fascism the child was in fact propagandized as 'your own flesh and blood' (Beckmann 1984).

Contrasting with the above, the body-oriented fear of (and defence against) the child shows the ambivalence in attitudes towards procreation. Molinski writes that excessively intellectual women are afraid of the temporary regression in their own state of awareness which is necessary when dealing with a young child (and during the process of birth - author's note). 'Related to this is the fear of being a mere tool of nature' (Molinski 1978, p. 103). The fact that, having once got involved in it, one cannot consciously direct the course of pregnancy and birth causes fear in some women: the biological process is equivalent to a total loss of control over one's own body. This state of affairs must psychologically affect any woman forced to carry a child through an unwanted pregnancy. Expressions like 'breeding machine' and 'milk cow' make the rejection clear. In some cases the baby is feared to be a physical parasite (Mühlenau 1984); indeed, this is biologically true. Hertz and Molinski state that sometimes, together with a serious disturbance of the ego and of a woman's perception of her own body, the fear can be detected that 'the child could become as unattractive as I am myself' (Hertz and Molinski 1981, p. 76).

Other body-oriented arguments against pregnancy include the fear of losing physical and sexual attractiveness (Heinkelmann 1978), as the common ideal of female beauty is hardly compatible with gravidity. (The contradictory roles of the woman as Madonna and whore come to light here; see Hays and Hoffmann 1978). Additionally, there is the fear of injuries and damage resulting from the birth itself (Heinkelmann 1978), which possibly stems from deeply rooted infantile fantasies of the exploding belly (Moeller-Gambaroff 1981) or the imagination of a discrepancy between the size of the baby's head and the narrow vagina, namely the fear of being torn apart during the birth. These apprehensions are increased by dramatic descriptions of birth supplied by other women, the exaggeration of medical risks and real traumatic experiences recalled from earlier deliveries.

In conclusion: the decision to carry a child to full term requires confidence in one's own adaptability and capabilities. Possibly, explanations for psychogenic infertility (see Brähler, this volume) or psychogenically determined habitual abortions are to be found in a disturbance of body experience.

Body Experience During Pregnancy

Many women become aware of being pregnant at a very early stage, when the nidation of the fertilized egg in the uterus causes tension in the breasts about 6–10 days after inpregnation. This tension is more marked than premenstrual tension but can be confused with the latter, especially if there is hope that pregnancy might not have occurred: the motive influences the attribution. Sensitive body experience can therefore signal pregnancy before it is confirmed by biochemical tests or gynaecological examinations.

Morning sickness, *nausea gravidarum*, which starts from about the 6th week, and its intensification towards vomiting are physiologically due to increased gastric secretion. It is astonishing that such symptoms have been observed neither in other cultures (Macy and Falkner 1980) nor in other mammals; we may therefore assume that psychological factors also have an influence here, possibly on the degree of physical symptoms. From the psychoanalytical point of view, ambivalence towards the fetus is expressed in the alternation between ingestion and vomiting: retention versus expulsion. Molinski (1972) looks into the psychosomatic background of hyperemesis (pathological excessive vomiting in later pregnancy) and comes to the conclusion that the experience of one's own orality or oral inhibitions and the image of femininity currently held by the woman (the author distinguishes between different stages of maturity) play a role in psychosomatic symptoms during pregnancy. The significance of orality is also evident in the various cravings experienced by pregnant women.

Women who are in a serious decision conflict (whether to have the child or to have an abortion) can develop the idea that in an abortion the inside of the body is scraped and sucked out. They feel the fetus to be a part of their body; whereas in a totally unwanted pregnancy it is considered rather as a foreign substance. This would affect the way in which an abortion is coped with psychologically.

From about the 6th month the belly becomes tangibly and visibly bigger. The woman has to adjust her body scheme to the new physical limitations, for example in her choice clothes, or behaviour among crowds of people. Feldmann, who questioned 50 women on experienced body experience during pregnancy, concludes that the early swelling is at first connected with feelings of embarrassment, as the woman has the impression of getting bigger. The belly is still perceived as such and not as child: 'The baby is still too deep inside' (Feldmann 1977). With advancing pregnancy the body experience changes, tending to separate the belly and the child from the rest of the body and finally even from the ego. The author distinguishes the following levels of separation:

1. 'I am not getting bigger, it is the child.'
2. 'I no longer feel my belly as belly, but rather as child.'
3. 'This belly is the child, not me.'
4. 'The child is not growing within me any longer, it is growing out forwards.'
5. 'I am behind the child.'
6. Unexpected bumping into obstacles with the belly.
7. The limit of the body image is no longer experienced at the periphery of the belly but more proximally, even behind the child. (Fig. 1).

The separation of the child is seen as a predominantly active achievement on the part of the pregnant woman. In this research distinct separation was found in only some of the pregnant women, while others achieved a partial separation or none at all. Hence we are faced with the question as to whether pregnant women who do not experience any separation at all have difficulty in giving up the narcissistic identification with the child that is fully incorporated in the self, and in accepting the child's own existence and identity (Feldmann 1977). The author further sug-

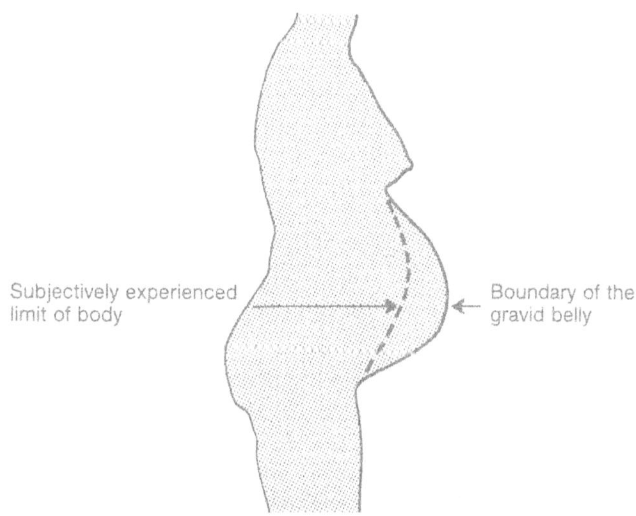

Fig. 1. Restriction of the body as experienced in relation to the actual extension of the gravid belly (in cases where the tendency to separate the belly and the child from the rest of the body is strong)

gests that the separation of the child from the rest of the body is connected with the importance of the pregnancy and the attitude towards the child.

At this point, mention may be made of rare disorders such as denied pregnancy, which, in extreme cases is recognized only shortly before the birth, and phantom pregnancy, in which physical changes including vomiting and expanding girth of the belly occur although no pregnancy exists. This shows that psychic factors probably have an influence on body experience.

The physical expansion of the belly can have a narcissistic effect and be regarded as an expansion of the ego, or be a source of pride and a feeling of potency ('pregnancy is power'). In other women, however, feelings of shame (the belly is skilfully concealed behind clothes), withdrawal from the public (mainly from swimmingpools and saunas; cf. Voigt-Hägerbäumer 1977) and lethargy are observed, according to the woman's own body image and ego as well as the significance of the child. Advertising slogans such as 'pregnant but still beautiful' highlight the contradictions. The attitude of men towards the pregnant woman is rather different, too: possibly men perceive her primarily as a mother (with associations to their own mother) and less as a lover, which may explain the increased sexual desire for other women on the part of some partners.

Concerning inner body experience, doctors usually emphasize that fetal movements are significant for the attitude towards the fetus: women who had an ambivalent attitude in the early stages of pregnancy now tend to identify with it.

> That 'something is growing and living in one's body' is obviously experienced particularly intensely. Initially the fetal movements can be felt like a pounding, 'like a body function, the pulsating of one's own heart', that express the symbiosis of mother and fetus. Later the fetal movements are experienced as an expression of an 'independent being', stronger fetal movements ('kicking') even as 'the child's own energetic initiative'. (Feldmann 1977, p. 315)

Thus an abortion in the second trimester (genetic or medical indications) is often experienced as a traumatic intervention both physically and psychologically, a fact which, among other things, has prompted the development of new methods of prenatal diagnosis (Kessler 1984).

I should be mentioned that, in general, fewer psychological disturbances occur during pregnancy than at other times (Krüger 1964, 1965). According to Hertz and Molinski,

> biologically, considerable somatic changes occur. The genitals are loosened up and, in conjunction with an increased blood supply, restructured. The different hormonal condition has an effect on every cell of the body: water is intercalated; the belly grows larger; the breasts change. All these changes lead to copious physical sensations and to a different perception of the body, although pregnancy biologically makes many women feel particularly well. (Hertz and Molinski 1981, p. 91)

One reason for this feeling of wellbeing could also be that pregnant women can now actually live out their narcissism without any feelings of guilt, for example, with intensive body care, good food and relaxation, because everything is done 'for the child'. Deutsch (1954) writes that for some women pregnancy means something like a 'vacation from the ego', as they can escape demands from others and are now the focus of attention, a state of affairs which ends after the birth.

Sexual desire may change during pregnancy and is probably influenced by factors of attitude (Macy and Falkner 1980, Haeberle 1983).

Towards the end of the pregnancy, before delivery, some women experience themselves primarily as an enormous body or 'mother animal'. Owing to their immobility and the limitations connected with it, most women long for the birth, which will bring physical relief. Hertz and Molinski (1981) state that, with the onset of the birth, the consiousness is dimmed and the functions of the ego are reduced: a regression in preparation for the intense bodily processes of labour.

Birthing Experience is Body Experience

Modern obstetrics are concerned with optimizing the safety of mother and child and reducing pain without depriving the mother of positive birthing experiences (Hillemanns et al. 1983). Davies-Osterkamp and Beckmann (1982) are of the opinion that 'natural' birth (without obstetrics - author's note) will remain an abstract concept, as obstetric practices of one kind or another exist in all cultures (Kitzinger 1980). Assistance during parturition, whether medical help or self-help through certain breathing techniques and co-ordination of the tensing and relaxing rhythm with the labour activity, should generally support the natural somatic functions when the cervix opens and the baby is expelled ('out of paradise').

Psychoprophylactic methods of birth preparation start from exactly this point. In spite of considerable differences between the theoretical approaches of Read (1950) and Lamaze (Ewy and Ewy 1981) (Read bases his ideas on the triad 'fear - tension - pain'), in practice similar elements are employed, such as explanation, relaxation techniques, breathing exercises and body perception exercises (e.g. for tensing and relaxing the pelvis). For some years now, methods of increasing body sensibility and body experience have also been used to support biological processes during birth. Thus, in our society 'natural' birth is to be understood as a coordination between the various kinds of assistance and the natural body functions. On birthing experience in artificially induced births Davies-Osterkamp and Beckmann (1982) report that about 80% of the women in a survey who had an induced birth did not want to experience this kind of assistance again. The routine scheduled birth, a method that fortunately has fewer supporters nowadays, can be assessed as for as body experience are concerned as a disregard of female childbearing functions and ability.

That technical aid is necessary in especially complicated cases goes without saying. Schreiber (1981) looks into the effects on birthing experience of routine technology in the delivery room. Preparation for parturition today often resembles the preparations for an operation: the pubic hair is shaved off and an enema is administered. In general, painkillers are given during labour (barbiturates, epidural anaesthesia or pudendal block) which result in a partial loss of physical sensitivity, so that the mother loses direct, active experience and physical realization of the birth.

Macy and Falkner (1980) observe that the physical reactions of the female body during contractions and delivery are very similar to the reactions during sexual orgasm (Kitzinger 1981: 'Birth is basically a sexual act'): some women even have an orgasm in the course of it. In both birth and orgasm, breathing becomes deep and heavy or the breath is held. During orgasm, the woman groans and gasps and her face sometimes takes on a strongly painful expression which can be mistakenly interpreted as a sign of suffering. At this point the proximity of pain and lust becomes obvious:

> The belly contracts at regular intervals; the mucous plug in the cervix loosens; the whole body can fall into rhythmic movement, stronger than ever before. In both cases sensitivity and alertness are at first increased and then turn into almost complete unconsciousness when the climax is near. A sudden return to full consciousness follows, accompanied by dizziness and happiness. The same hormone, oxytocin, plays an important role in both occurrences. (Macy and Falkner 1980, p. 78)

Davies-Osterkamp and Beckmann (1982) state that, during the perception of birth pangs, a number of psychological factors are involved. About 5%–7% of all women have painless births, some women report sexual experiences during the birth, but the majority describe the contractions as painful to unbearable. Others claim that they experience labour pains as 'physical, heavy work without actually suffering from pain' (Davies-Osterkamp and Beckmann 1982; see also Gambaroff 1984. Subjective accounts of birth pangs are not necessarily correlated to the medical course of the labour (Nettelbladt et al. 1976). According to Martling (1979), for instance, women who had delivered at home without any analgesics recalled the delivery as less painful than did a comparable group who had given birth in a clinic. This shows that psychological factors such as attitudes and fears are significant.

Davies-Osterkamp and Beckmann (1982) report that women, doctors and midwives can come to divergent accounts of the painfulness of the same birth. The high pitch of excitement of the woman in labour can prompt administration of an analgesic, although the woman is actually only experiencing the birth very actively. This is not to preach a total ban on analgesics (which would be tantamount to torture), but rather to advocate, as far as possible, that the parturient should participate in deciding when and how much should be given. Molinski (1972) says that the course of labour can certainly be hindered by rigidity of the cervical os, but this can also be caused by psychosomatic processes.

Nowadays in most deliveries a perineotomy is carried out prophylactically in order to facilitate expulsion of the baby's head and to prevent slow-healing *tears*. Although extremely few women actually feel the cut because no pain sensation is possible in a tense perineum at the climax of a contraction, the suture is often experienced as very unpleasant or painful (Gafka-Fehse and Schuhl 1979). Tocophobia is possibly in many cases a fear of the technical interventions described earlier, such as shaving off the pubic hair, enema, being attached to drip apparatus, and perineotomy. Hence Gambaroff (1984) suggests that the perineotomy, in particular evokes castration anxieties (see also Laing 1981).

All in all, the attitude towards pregnancy and birth has changed in recent years (ultimately owing to the commitment of many women). Hence, we may assume a change in body experience: while formerly the father of the child was habitually spared the unaesthetic view of a woman in labour, nowadays men in the delivery room are quite the norm. Thirty years ago delivery in a clinic was welcomed by women not least 'in order not to have the mess at home anymore' (personal communication). In this respect, the loosening of religious mores, 'In sorrow thou shalt bring forth children', plays a role, as do the significant approaches of Read (1950), Lamaze (Ewy and Ewy 1981), Leboyer (1974) and others.

Body Experience After Delivery

After delivery, the body experience can be very varied and changeable (an ambivalence is also apparent here). This is reflected on the one hand in the unpleasurable crises and depressions of lying-in (Jarka 1981) and on the other hand in a rather sensual description of the early relationship between mother and child (cf. Sichtermann 1981).

Crises and Depressive Reactions

The psychological and physical problems of women after delivery have been rather neglected in the literature. When using the term 'puerperal depression' one must distinguish between 'maternal blues' (the onset of crying on about the 3rd-5th day after delivery), crises and depressive reactions within the first months, and puerperal psychoses (Oakley 1979; Gödtel 1979; Jarka 1981)

In the case of the 'maternal blues', a drastic drop in the progesterone level within a few hours after delivery creates a psycho-autonomic state of emergency: decreased stability combined with simultaneous sensibility (which will be elaborated upon later), entailing unusual reactions including crying as a result of stress and trouble. Thus hormonal factors seem to play a role in the heightened level of agitation. The quality of the sensation feelings of extreme happiness versus deep sadness) is conditioned rather by psychical stimuli:

'On the third day I was just crying: I thought everything was terrible ...' '... Around lunch time the mood swings started. During the visiting hours in the evening I finally couldn't suppress my tears any longer'. (Gafka-Fehse and Schuhl 1979, p. 76-77).

'I kept looking at her and crying. I knew absolutely that these were sentimental tears, but after all these fears the relief was so immense ... that I simply had to go on crying all the time'. (Barber and Skaggs 1980, p. 25)

In explanation of the considerably rarer puerperal psychoses, nonhormonal physical factors are mentioned, together with difficult operative deliveries or endogenic predisposition. Premorbid personality disorders are also said to have an effect (Gödtel 1979; Krüger 1964, 1965; Pauleikhoff 1964; Molinski 1972).

Psychoanalytically, these depressive reactions are explained as a mourning of the separation from the baby (the loss of prenatal unity through delivery), conflict between self-interest and the reproductive function, disappointment caused by the child (e.g. the 'wrong' sex), reactivated conflict with one's own mother (Payne 1936; Deutsch 1954; Benedek 1960) and increased aggression (caused for example, by a screaming baby) combined with a simultaneous prohibition of aggression imposed by clichés of the happy mother (Jarka 1981). For women with an ego-weak personality, with oral and aggressive inhibitions, these conflicts can be the trigger for psychic disturbances (Molinski 1972). Sociologically, social stress and reorientation in fundamental spheres of life (partnership, profession, leisure activities, isolation) are seen as promoting crises (Dyer 1976). Thus the crises and depressive reactions after delivery are overdetermined (Deutsch 1954), the body experience being one aspect which will here be described in more detail. To promote better understanding, the physiology of lyingin will be briefly outlined, because this is not generally well known.

Towards the end of the pregnancy, production of female sex hormones reaches its climax, in order to set off parturition when optimal growth of the uterus and size of the baby in relation to the placenta have been reached. The hormone progesterone then prepares the ground for co-ordinated contractions, which are additionally caused by the release of the hormone prostaglandin. At the end of the pregnancy the progesterone level is at its maximum, and it rapidly drops within a few hours of the birth. This hormone is supposed to have a physiologically and psychologically relaxing effect, which is allegedly intensified during pragnancy as a result of the rise in the progesterone level. The latter also prevents the occurrence of premature effective contractions and possibly acts as a causal factor in the subjective wellbeing of the pregnant woman despite the physical strains associated with her condition (Bardwick 1972, p. 34). After the birth, production of this 'natural tranquillizer' ceases, which is seen as a possible cause for sudden changes of mood.

The concentration of estrogens as well as of a number of other hormones also rapidly decreases after delivery or changes during the lying-in period. The natural contraction of the uterus after delivery is sometimes furthered by the administration of ergot preparations. The healing of internal injuries to the walls of the uterus, such as the insertion of the placenta, is lengthy and complicated. Injuries to the birth organs, such as a perineal tear, a perineotomy or lacerations of the vagina take about 3-4 weeks to heal completely. Blood and tissue are expelled from the uterus with the lochial secretion, which is susceptible to the effects of different medicaments as well as to psychological and physical stress. It lasts for about 6 weeks, in the course of which the bloody afterbirth turns into a yellowish discharge. Breast-feeding accelerates the process of involution. Menstruation recommences at different times: for women who are not breast-feeding, 6 weeks after delivery at the earliest.

Extragenital organs are also affected by the birth: the small and large intestines, stomach and gallbladder can re-expand after delivery and the diaphragm is more intensely involved in respiration. Changes such as striae and pigmentations become less conspicuous or disappear; proteo- and lipometabolism, blood volume, blood pressure and pulse rate become normal. The loss of weight through the delivery amounts to approximately 10 kg (baby, placenta, blood and mobilization of, oedema fluid).

On about the 3rd day the 'milk comes in' which can cause painful tension in the breasts. The milk-giving reflex is set off by indirect nervous excitation of the nipples (sucking), which brings about a release of prolactin, regulated by the hypophysis. Gödtel (1979) states that the process of breast-feeding - and, more significantly, any disturbance in this process - has a physical and mental influence on the mother. For instance, lactation can be negatively affected by complicated operative delivery, illness, painful sucking by the baby, sore nipples or psychological factors.

Because of severe physical weakening and the resultant increased susceptibility to illness (such as thrombophilia), the puerpera should avoid overexertion, even towards the end of the lying-in period.

It seems likely that the experience of such drastic physical changes within a very short time at least contributes to emotional reactions after delivery, although at the same time the significance of social factors and of existentially experiencing the birth is not to be underestimated. Somatic influences on the psychological condition during lying-in can work in different ways: through hormonal changes, through nonhormonal factors, including physical stress and medical complications, and through subjective body experience, which is described below.

In her multidimensional study, Heitler (1976) was able to confirm correlations between physical difficulties and depressive reactions within the first 6 weeks after delivery. Gafka-Fehse and Schuhl (1979) interviewed women after delivery and came to the conclusion that in the last days of pregnancy most women long for their original body shape, their physical powers, their mobility and former looks. Some women, however, have unexpected difficulties with their body during lying-in. One of the most frequent causes for complaint is the perineal suture: women often cannot walk or sit in the first days after delivery and some suffer from painful defaecation and urination for a prolonged period. In rarer cases it happens that, because of careless treatment, the suture tears open again. Even the fear of later, possibly painful, sexual intercourse can be psychologically oppressive. Because of psychological factors, routine perineotomy has been disputed among doctors for some time:

'The perineal suture was very painful; this actually was the worst of all; I had difficulty sitting and walking.'

'I found the scar really bad: I needed half an hour to squat down on the toilet and get up again ... I really found that impossible ... All this afterwards with the cut and everything, that's actually worse than the delivery itself ...'

'After both deliveries the perineotomy hurt quite a lot. After the first delivery "proud flesh", a little proliferation, had grown at the rim of the vagina.' (Gafka-Fehse and Schuhl 1979, p. 71-93)

The lochia is experienced as unpleasant by some women:

'The discharge gave me a lot of trouble. It lasted so long. I suffered from it for nearly 6 weeks and it was disgusting; I was finished with my body from the breasts down, there was just nothing any more.' (Gafka-Fehse and Schuhl 1979, p. 74)

A lot of puerperae also suffer from haemorrhoids caused by bearing down on the baby:

'I'd got awful haemorrhoids from all the pressing, so I couldn't sit properly and couldn't even go to the toilet.' (Gafka-Fehse and Schuhl 1979, p. 72)

After delivery some women suffer from muscular weakness caused by decompression of the abdominal organs:

'A friend of mine, she couldn't even walk, she just kept wetting her pants, because there was such muscular weakness. This was the same for me at the beginning; I always felt as if urine was permanently dripping. It took quite a while ... but definitely several weeks, and I found that really unpleasant.' (Gafka-Fehse and Schuhl 1979, p. 72)

Heavy sweating and circulatory insufficiency are also quite frequent during lying-in. Several women reported incontinence: a 'leaking of liquids out of the body'. Describing the case of a 20-year-old patient with tocomania (puerperal psychosis). Gödtel (1979) writes:

'She had the feeling that water was running through her body by the litre ... She developed an obsession for washing and insisted on cleaning herself with *Sagrotan* ...' (Gödtel 1979, p. 43)

These are illusions which could have reference to incontinence.

The harmonious, tender breast-feeding relationship presented in most illustrations fairly frequently starts with unexpected difficulties. Some women feel the milk-flow as a painful tension. Sensitive nipples can become inflamed because the baby is sucking too strongly or even biting. In some cases feverish mastitis causes problems for further breast-feeding. An imbalance between the baby's appetite and the milk secretion is also unusual necessitating pumping off of the milk (which is time-consuming and physically awkward) or supplementary feeding. Problems with breast-feeding can result from the timetable of hospital routine or from the social pressure, nowadays widespread, concerning breast-feeding.

For many women, recovery from this overall state of physical weakness takes about 6 months. One reason for depression arising from these bodily problems is that women have little opportunity to talk about such difficulties because excretory and sexual processes are taboo. Many women feel hardly any desire for sexual contact with their partner for a long time (Gafka-Fehse and Schuhl 1979). This may be connected on the one hand with physical problems and on the other with the fact that, through intense bodily contact with the baby, the mother can feel already 'occupied'.

Early Maternal Love

Even if depressive reactions can occur in many cases, the early relationship between mother and child can also be experienced as very pleasurable. The psychoanalyst Winnicott (1960) describes an unusual state of extreme sensitivity towards the end of the pregnancy and in the first weeks after delivery, a state which he calls 'primary maternal preoccupation'. The author compares this empathy for the child, combined with simultaneous disorientation, to a schizoid condition in which a single aspect of the personality temporarily becomes dominant. This state of heightened sensitivity, which Winnicott likens to an 'normal illness', susceptible of rational understanding, enables the mother sympathetically and judiciously to adjust to the baby's needs. Schmiedbauer-Schleibner writes that this state, according to her experience and observations, may be biologically conditioned, which seens reasonable as the new-born infant is dependent on extreme sympathy from the person who looks after it (Schmiedbauer-Schleibner 1979). This author adds that social influences certainly contribute to determine and overlap with this state.

If we assume that the extreme sensitivity of Winnicott's (1960) 'primary maternal preoccupation' and the heightened sensitivity of the 'maternal blues' (which occur within the same period) are equally biologically conditioned, i.e. by hormonal influences, then we could regard these states as two psychological sides of the same physiological process, a hypothesis that would have to be examined. External factors such as the clinic, family conditions and intra- and interpersonal situations may be important in determining whether a woman experiences the state of 'primary motherliness' or rather reacts depressively.

In this respect Leboyer's (1974) recommendation of intense bodily contact between mother and child directly after delivery (allow the umbilical cord gradually to stop pulsating, lay the baby on top of the belly and prepare for nursing) is justified and necessary. Even the introduction of 'rooming-in' in clinics has been long overdue.

Schmiedbauer-Schleibner remarks that the state of 'primary motherliness' is psychophysiologically comparable to that of being in love in its extreme. This hypothesis is supported by Sichtermann (1981) with her descriptions of the pleasurable aspects of the early relationship between mother and child, especially breast-feeding:

> The child sucking on the breast and the mother enjoying suckling: both, with closed eyes, go back to the time 'before the great separation' ... It may be essential for any being, even for the human, to dive back from time to time into the 'ocean' of prenatal life, of amniotic fluid, of weightlessness, without any tension. Sleep benefits from it, and so does sexuality, in which breast-feeding, however, is not actually included - how the women and babies are defrauded! Trying to attribute an intervention to nature, one could say that nature protects the reproduction of the species by giving pleasure on top of procreation, and we can add that she protects the survival of the new-born by allowing mother and child to find pleasure in breast-feeding ... 'Breast-feeding is a part of female sexuality as well as the first intense sexual experience of the new-born child.' (Sichtermann 1981, p. 76)

This author continues that, if the aspect of high-quality nutrition in breast-feeding is one-sidedly emphasized, a sexual process is reduced to its usefulness and the woman is defined by her renunciatory role: 'Doesn't the child give her [the mother] close contact, warmth, rhythm and lust, too?' (Sichtermann 1981). On the similarity of breast-feeding to the heterosexual act, the author states that in both situations the nipple, a highly, sensitive organ, becomes erect, although the 'lust curve' runs in a flat rather than a steep arc of excitation. However, to what extent a mother experiences the breast-feeding relationship as pleasure or burden must be partly determined by her ability to cope with the endopsychic and interpersonal conflicts that arise during this period (Jarka 1981).

Despite everything, early motherly love is physical love and exists through breast-feeding, caressing, changing nappies and caring for the child. This physical love in conjunction with slowly increasing physical separation may precede the psychological relationship with the child. Unfortunately, the abstract concept of motherly love has become a cliché which makes women expect certain feelings and realize with fear that there is not (yet) any abstract psychic relationship with the child (Sichtermann 1981). Possibly this cliché is another cause for the feeling of being a bad mother, and resultant depressive reactions.

Looking at human evolution we notice that increased physical sensitivity plays a role both in the earlier stages of evolution and in the early relationship between mother and child (Spitz 1976; Renggli 1976; Hassenstein and Morath 1983).

The extent to which the child is actually wanted and what problems it causes by its mere existence are certainly significant for the expression of this early love. Badinter's theories (1981) on the social and historical 'nature' of motherly love are therefore by no means contrary to the experiences mentioned, as his historical analyses refer to periods when women were left to the 'curse of procreation', so that pleasurable motherly love could hardly develop (Aries 1975; Gambaroff 1984). Even today this can be the case in unfavourable psychosocial conditions.

Prospects for the Future

In summary one can say that the desire for children, and pregnancy, birth, lying-in and breast-feeding are spheres of female sexuality. The immediate experience of these somatic processes is reduced by cultural and ideological influences ('In sorrow thou shalt bring forth children').

The status of the physical experience of the generative processes is made clear in cases of infertility, in renewed hopes for fertility, in miscarriage and stillbirth, i.e. when the complete body experience is denied (Meyer 1984; Borg and Lasker 1983). The idea of a new-born child being given away for adoption causes a feeling of uneasiness, as the continuous physical relationship is abruptly broken off. It is Possible that the physical relationship with the child precedes the psychological relationship.

At a time when human reproduction can be achieved by medical technology (Silber 1985), it seems especially necessary to look closer into the role of body experience and sexuality in women and men during the origination and development of human life, to feel one's way carefully forward into unknown and unconscious spheres of the body-soul relationship and to learn to stand the fear of contact with biological theories.

References

Aries P (1975) Geschichte der Kindheit. Hauser, Munich

Badinter E (1981) Die Mutterliebe - Geschichte eines Gefühls vom 17. Jahrhundert bis heute. Piper. Munich

Barber V, Skaggs MM (1980) Die Mutter. Rowohlt, Reinbek

Bardwick JM (1972) Psychology of women. Harper and Row, New York

Beauvoir S de (1968) Das andere Geschlecht. Rowohlt, Reinbek

Beckmann D (1984) Mutterideologie. In: Becker H et al. (eds) Psychosozial 21. Rowohlt, Reinbek

Benedek T (1960) Elternschaft als Entwicklungsphase. In: Dräges K et al. (eds) Jahrbuch der Psychoanalyse, vol 1. Westdeutscher Verlag, Cologne

Berninghausen J (1980) Der Traum vom Kind - Geburt eines Klischees. Ullstein, Frankfurt

Bibring L (1961) A study of the psychological processes in pregnancy and of the earliest mother-child relationship. Psychosom Study Child 16: 9-72

Borg S, Lasker J (1983) Glücklose Schwangerschaft. Tomus, Munich

Boston Women's Health Book Collection (ed) (1971) Our bodies, our selves. Simon and Schuster, New York

Chasseguet-Smirgel J (ed) (1979) Psychoanalyse der weiblichen Sexualität. Suhrkamp, Frankfurt

Chessler P (1980) Mutter werden - Die Geschichte einer Verwandlung. Rowohlt, Reinbek

Davies-Osterkamp S, Beckmann D (1982) Psychosoziale Aspekte von Schwangerschaft und Geburt. In: Beckmann D, Davies-Osterkamp S, Scheer (eds) Medizinische Psychologie. Springer, Berlin Heidelberg New York

Deutsch H (1954) Psychologie der Frau, vol 2. Huber, Bern

Dyer ED (1976) Parenthood as crisis - A re-study. In: Moos RH (ed) Human adaptation. Lexington, Massachusetts, pp 177-187

Erikson EH (1976) Identität und Lebenszyklus. Suhrkamp, Frankfurt

Ewy D, Ewy R (1981) Die Lamaze-Methode. Goldmann, Munich

Feldmann H (1977) Untersuchungen zum Körperleben in der Schwangerschaft. Psychosom Med Psychosanal 23: 310-328

Freud S (1932) Neue Folge der Vorlesungen zur Einführung in die Psychoanalyse: Die Weiblichkeit. In: Gesammelte Werke, vol 15 (1949). Imago, London, pp 119-145

Friday N (1979) Wie meine Mutter - My mother my self. Fischer, Frankfurt
Gafka-Fehse A, Schuhl A (1979) Vom Widerspruch zwischen der Ideologie vom Mutterglück und der Wirklichkeit von Müttern - Probleme nach der Entbindung. Thesis, Pädagogische Hochschule, West Berlin
Gambaroff M (1984) Utopie der Treue. Rowohlt, Reinbek
Gödtel R (1979) Seelische Störungen im Wochenbett. Fischer, Stuttgart
Gordon RE, Karpartins EE, Gordon KK (1967) Factors in postpartum emotional adjustment. Obstet Gynaecol 25: 158-166
Gugel E (1976) Sexualität und Identität der Frau. Focus, Giessen
Haeberle EJ (1983) Die Sexualität des Menschen - Handbuch und Atlas. De Gruyter, Berlin
Hagemann-White C (1979) Frauenbewegung und Psychoanalyse. Stroemfeld/Roter Stern, Basle
Hardach-Pinke I (1982) Schwangerschaft und Identität. In: Kamper D, Wulf C (eds) Die Wiederkehr des Körpers. Suhrkamp, Frankfurt
Hassenstein B, Morath M (1983) Fragen zur Betreuung von Neugeborenen aus der Sicht der Verhaltensbiologie. In: Hillemanns H-G, Steiner H, Richter D (eds) Die humane, familienorientierte und sichere Geburt. Thieme, Stuttgart
Hays R, Hoffman R (1978) Mythos Frau - Das gefährliche Geschlecht. Fischer, Frankfurt
Heinkelmann E (1978) Einstellungsfaktoren und Risikoverhalten in der Empfängnisverhütung. Thesis, University of Marburg
Heitler SK (1976) Postpartum depression - A multidimensional study. New York University 1975. Dissertation Abstracts International, May 1976, 36: (11-B) 5792-5793
Hertz DG, Molinski H (1981) Psychosomatik der Frau. Springer, Berlin Heidelberg New York
Hillemanns H-G, Steiner H, Richter D (eds) (1983) Die humane, familienorientierte und sichere Geburt. Thieme, Stuttgart
Jagenow A, Mittag O (1984) Weiblicher Kinderwunsch und Sexualität. In: Becker H, Beckmann D (eds) Psychosozial 21. Rowohlt, Reinbek
Jarka M (1981) Krisen und depressive Reaktionen nach der Entbindung. Thesis, University of Marburg
Kessler J (ed) (1984) Psychologische Aspekte der genetischen Beratung. Enke, Stuttgart
Kitzinger S (1980) Frauen als Mütter - Mutterschaft in verschiedenen Kulturen. Kösel, Munich
Kitzinger S (1981) Die Geburt ist im wesentlichen ein Geschlechtsakt. In: Schreiber M (ed) Die schöne Geburt. Rowohlt, Reinbek
Krüger H (1964) Die Wochenbettpsychosen im Wandel der Anschauungen. Nervenarzt 35: 448-458
Krüger H (1965) Zur Psychodynamik der Gestationspsychosen. Z Psychother Med Psychol 15: 230-252
Laing RD (1981) Die technologische Geburt ähnelt einer weiblichen Kastration. In: Schreiber M (ed) Die schöne Geburt. Rowohlt, Reinbek
Leboyer F (1974) Pour une naissance sans violence. Seuil, Paris. (Der sanfte Weg ins Leben. Kösel, Munich, 1984)
Lukesch H, Lukesch M (1976) Konstruktion und Validierung eines Fragebogens über die Einstellung zur Schwangerschaft und Sexualität. Z Entwicklungspsychol 8: 142-144
Lukesch H, Rottmann G (1976) Die Bedeutung soziofamilialer Faktoren für die Einstellung von Müttern zur Schwangerschaft. Psychol Prax 20: 4-18
Mack-Brunswick R (1940) Die präödipale Phase in der libidinösen Entwicklung. In: Chasseguet-Smirgel J (ed) Psychoanalyse der weiblichen Sexualität. Suhrkamp, Frankfurt
Macy C, Falkner F (1979) Pregnancy and birth: pleasures and problems, Multimedia, Willemstad, Curacao
Martling A-E (1979) Einfluß der Entbindungsart auf das Geburtserleben am Beispiel von Haus- und Kliniksgeburt. Thesis, Technical University of West Berlin
Menne K, Moersch E (1980) Psychoanalytische Erfahrungen aus der Supervision von Schwangerschaftskonfliktberatungen. Psyche (Stuttg) 2: 121-151
Meyer A (1984) Das Mutterglück wiedergegeben. In: Becker H, Beckmann D (eds) Psychosozial 21. Rowohlt, Reibek
Mitchell J (1976) Psychoanalysis and feminism. Freud, Reich, Laing and women. Pantheon, New York
Mitscherlich-Nielsen M (1978) Psychoanalyse der Weiblichkeit. Psyche (Stuttg) 8: 669-694

Mittag O, Jagenow A (1984) Motive zur Schwangerschaft, Geburt und Elternschaft. Ergebnisse einer empirischen Untersuchung an verhütungswilligen Frauen. Psychother Med Psychol 34: 20-24

Moeller-Gambaroff M (1981) Wenn der Bauch explodiert, komm'n die Kinder rausmarschiert - Über den Einfluß der Lebensgeschichte auf die Geburt. In: Schreiber M (ed) Die schöne Geburt. Rowohlt, Reinbek, pp 43-60

Moeller-Gambaroff M (1984) Schwangerschaftsphantasien. In: Kursbuch 76. Kursbuch-Verlag, West Berlin

Molinski H (1972) Die unbewußte Angst vor dem Kind. Kindler, Munich

Molinski H (1978) Schwangerschaft als Konflikt. In: Koschorke M, Sandberger JG (eds) Schwangerschaftskonfliktberatung. Vandenhoek and Ruprecht, Göttingen, pp 97-104

Mühlenau M (1984) Mutterliebe. In: Kursbuch 76. Kursbuch-Verlag, West Berlin

Nettelbladt P, Fagerström CF, Uppenberg N (1976) The significance of reported childbirth pain. J Psychosom Res 20: 215-221

Nott PN, Franklin M, Armitage C, Gelder MG (1976) Hormonal changes and mood in the puerperium. Br J Psychiatry 128: 379-383

Oakley A (1979) The baby blues. New Society, 5 April, p 11

Pauleikhoff B (1964) Seelische Störungen in der Schwangerschaft und nach der Geburt. Enke, Stuttgart

Payne S (1936) Zur Auffassung der Weiblichkeit. Int Z Psychoanal 22: 19-39

Read GD (1950) Mutter werden ohne Schmerz. Hoffmann and Campe, Hamburg

Renggli F (1976) Angst und Geborgenheit - Soziokulturelle Folgen der Mutter-Kind-Beziehung im ersten Lebensjahr. Rowohlt, Reinbek

Schmiedbauer-Schleibner U (1979) Mutterschaft und Psychoanalyse. In: Verein 3. Sommeruniversität für Frauen 1978 e.V. (ed) Frauen und Mütter - Beiträge zur 3. Sommeruniversität von und für Frauen. Basis, Berlin, pp 351-378

Schreiber M (1981) Unendliches Vergnügen, unendlicher Schmerz - Protest gegen die Technik im Kreisssaal. In: Schreiber M (ed) Die schöne Geburt. Rowohlt, Reinbek, pp 11-42

Sichtermann B (1981) Leben mit einem Neugeborenen. Fischer, Frankfurt

Sichtermann B (1983) Weiblichkeit - Zur Politik des Privaten. Wagenbach, West Berlin

Silber SJ (1985) Endlich schwanger. Rowohlt, Reinbek

Spitz RA (1976) Vom Säugling zum Kleinkind. Klett, Stuttgart

Stark EM (1976) Geboren werden und Gebären. Frauenoffensive, Munich

Voigt-Hägerbäumer B (1977) Schwangerschaft ist eine Erfahrung, die die Frau, den Mann und die Gesellschaft angeht. Rowohlt, Reinbek

Winnicott DW (1960) Primäre Mütterlichkeit. Psyche (Stuttg) 7: 393-399

Infertility: Injury and Challenge

C. Brähler

It is estimated that about 20% of marriages in West Gemany today are involuntarily childless. At the beginning of the 1970s the percentage was assumed to be lower (10%-15%), but it is not clear whether the number of cases of infertility has actually increased or whether, as a result of recent advances in medicine and the apparently unlimited treatment possibilities, more childless couples are consulting their doctors sooner than they used to.

Human fertility is determined by so many factors that for the majority of couples it is not possible to arrive at a definite statement as to the exact causes of their infertility. Only in very few cases are irreversible disorders in the husband and/or wife, such as chromosome aberrations or deformities, found to be the sole cause. Psychological conflicts and ambivalence can influence fertility too. Opinions as to their significance are very divided; between 6% and 50% of all infertile couples are estimated to be affected by functional sterility.

However, in practice it is hardly possible to draw such distinctions between physical and psychological processes in the area of human fertility. This becomes particularly evident during the course of a couple's treatment. Quite apart from questions of aetiology, the very knowledge that they suffer from a fertility disorder has to be coped with by every couple on a psychological level.

Treatment Perspectives and Sexual Ethics

The enormous developments in medical technology in recent years have opened up perspectives for treating infertility which potentially have such a radical influence on marriage and the family structure that discussions on questions of sexual ethics in this connection are in progress even outside medical circles. Emotional controversies flare up especially when traditional conceptions of marriage and the family unit are upset by the introduction of donor semen, donor eggs or surrogate mothers to help a childless couple to parenthood. Ethical questions are particularly apparent here. Less spectacular forms of therapy, e.g. with hormones or artificial insemination using the husband's sperm (AIH), impinge on our ideas about marriage and sexuality.

We can begin to get an idea of the full significance of fertility and parenthood through the reactions of couples who have agreed to treatment. This they experience as such a hurtful invasion of their most intimate sphere that they are usually extremely anxious to hide both the fact of their infertility and of the treatment from other people. These couples' shame has its roots in their sense of personal failure and their awareness of involuntarily deviating from the norm.

The ethics of marriage and sexuality are based on fundamental beliefs about the purpose and value of people living together. These basic assumptions are closely related to social structures and norms and have changed repeatedly in the course of history. Awareness of the connection between coitus and conception was an important factor in the development of social attitudes towards sexuality. In our culture this knowledge was used by the Church as a means of moral control, in that reproduction was declared to be the only legitimate justification for sexuality. The strong influence of social changes on moral concepts is clearly exemplified in the period of transition from feudal to capitalist economy. The new economic system with its demands for organized labour also altered peoples' way of life and attitudes. Self-discipline, self-control, efficiency and productivity became the guiding norms not only in the sphere of production but also in personal life. The human body was expected to function in as precise and controlled a manner as a machine. Spontaneity and pleasure stood in contradiction to this system of functionality and were supressed as being subversive. The value of sexuality lay solely in its productive function, i.e. in reproduction. Economic and religious demands supplemented one another here (cf. also Haeberle 1983). Later, in the course of the industrial revolution, the woman's role became more and more modelled on the ideal of the loving, providing housewife and mother, whose productivity lay in her reproductivity (Berninghausen 1980).

The ideals of self-discipline and efficiency are still influential today, but the enormous advances in science and technology and our greatly increased contact with other cultures have led to an increase of knowledge that has broken through rigid moral standards and brought forth a multitude of new values. However, looser expectations with regard to roles mean not only greater freedom of decision for the individual, but also greater personal insecurity. Deep-rooted traditional morals and values maintain their influence in the individual's psyche for a long time, impeding free decisions. This conservative tendency comes out in the shame of infertile couples. The attitude which demands that reproduction be the ultimate justification for sex still wields its influence.

In our culture, a change has come about in the past few decades, in the direction of earlier puberty and a longer life-expectancy. That means an extension of the period of life during which an individual can be sexually active outside the phase of reproductivity. It therefore seems desirable to loosen the moral connection between sexuality and reproduction (Haeberle 1983). Contraception and treatment for infertility are medical methods which clash with obsolete moral concepts and so give rise to inner contradictions and emotional insecurity.

The Dynamics of Treatment for Infertility

The starting-point for treatment of infertility is external and internal pressure on the couple. The questions of friends, colleagues and relatives, often in the form of joking allusions and hints about the baby which is failing to materialize, strike at deep-rooted inner expectations about procreation and potency in the couples concerned.

The couples' own ambivalence usually remains hidden. Their very failure on this head makes them see fertility unreservedly as the source of all meaning and happiness in life. Shadows and doubts have no place in these dreams of ultimate fulfilment. Particularly when treatment continues over a long period of 2 or more years, there often develops a bitter struggle to try, with the help of modern medicine, to extort one's happiness, come what may.

The treatment itself usually amounts to a compromise solution between contradictory tendencies. If unconscious anxieties and defences prevent parenthood being achieved, the conscious wish for a child can be lived out to the full in the endless new efforts that are made to conceive one. The permanent preoccupation with this conflict-ridden wish helps reduce tension. The battle with one's own body, which is experienced like a defective machine, is an aid in the deeper struggle to overcome the huge narcissistic injury.

This intrapsychic significance which the treatment takes on for the individuals concerned lends it an addictive quality. Couples who for years have been trying everything possible to acquire the longed-for child find it hard to give up the fight. In spite of their resignation and desperation over the daily restrictions it demands of them, they dare not give up treatment because it might just have succeeded in the very next menstrual cycle.

These couples hope for an authoratitive word from the doctor, who will make the decision for them to break off treatment. The couple themselves do not want to take responsibility for such a step, but then neither does the doctor in many cases.

The infertile couple try to cope with their helpless anger at their own failure by forcing the body into submission. Complete control and regimentation of the body take the place of sexual desire. Sexuality becomes a means to an end - to conception - which, however, often remains out of their reach.

Example of One Couple's Treatment

The couple whose treatment will be outlined below are approaching 30 years of age. They married 5 years ago and planned a child right from the start. They have been in treatment for infertility for 4 years. First of all the wife went for a gynaecological examination and has been keeping temperature charts ever since. Apart from slight irregularities in her menstrual cycle there were no pathological findings.

Then the husband had an andrological investigation. Several specimens of semen were tested, which had sperm counts fluctuating between 20000 and 70000 per ml. In addition, slight gynaecomastia was diagnosed. To improve sperm production the man was treated with hormones which, however, brought about no significant change. The spermiogram fluctuated as before.

The next step was a postcoital test of the wife's cervical mucus to check its permeability for her husband's sperm. This involves the wife going to the gynaecologist's directly after intercourse. This arrangement she found particularly upsetting.

The appointment for the test was made in advance, so that even during intercourse she had visions of how all the staff at the clinic would be thinking of what she was doing at this moment and would look at her in a funny way when she appeared for her appointment. This postcoital test was carried out twice, with no notable results.

For the past year the gynaecologist has been trying artificial insemination with the husband's sperm (AIH) to bring about conception. The course of treatment carried out every month involves the following stages: The wife takes her temperature every morning to find the time of ovulation. To encourage follicle ripening and to control ovulation she takes a hormone preparation from the 3rd to the 7th day of her cycle. The exact date of ovulation is then checked again in an ultrasonic examination. In the proliferative phase, the artificial insemination is carried out in the gynaecologist's practice or hospital out-patients' departement. Five days of sexual abstinence beforehand is recommended to guarantee optimal quality of the husband's semen.

The seminal fluid obtained from the husband by means of masturbation is tested immediately for its sperm count, then sucked up into a syringe and - because the wife's cervical mucus has been made viscous by the hormone treatment - injected directly into her womb.

Each time the couple is as nervous as if they were taking an examination. Is there an egg ripe enough? How will the sperm quality be this time?

The insemination technique itself is painful for the wife. The doctor advises her to relax and relieve her pain by coughing as he penetrates the neck of the womb. But she refuses; she does not want to distract herself but would rather feel the pain.

After 4 years of treatment the wife in particular is getting desperate and is psychologically in a bad state. Nevertheless, it is impossible for her to break off treatment. She also rejects the offer of a more pleasant method of insemination, whereby the doctor fits a cap over the neck of the womb so that she can inject the seminal fluid into it herself at home. Both find the insemination process at the doctor's practice painful and embarassing, but do not feel able to do it alone themselves. All responsibility is delegated to the doctor. The couple expects him either to bring about conception or to make the decision to terminate treatment. In the psychotherapeutic councilling sessions which they then attend, they also remain passive for a long time and wait to be told what to do next.

Both of them know all about their bodily processes in minute detail, but this knowledge gives them no security. Both experience their body as a badly functioning mechanism which, even with all possible medical assistance, they are still not able to master. Seen in this light it is understandable why the wife rejects all offers to alleviate the treatment and wants to experience the painful manipulations of her (bad) body to the full. Their pleasure in sex is of course also impaired, since coitus always reminds them of their deficiency. Their partnership in the marriage is by now defined purely through their common struggle to have a child.

Let me stress once again that, from the medical point of view, there is no explanation for this couple's infertility. In the majority of couples undergoing long drawn-out courses of treatment like the one described above we find slight irregularities in the wife's menstrual cycle or fluctuations in the husband's sperm count but no serious organic disorders. The doctors responsible feel challenged and try endless new strategies which in fact have the effect of increasing the couple's unconscious anxiety and resistence.

The treatment involves a whole series of restrictions with which many couples willingly comply; for example, they organize their entire sex life according to the calendar, give up smoking, reduce their alcohol consumption and withdraw from social life around the date of ovulation - all for the sake of creating the best possible conditions for conception. This sort of regimentation leads to the paradoxical result that on the date calculated they have no desire at all to sleep together. Many of the women report that when they find out from their temperature chart in the morning that the optimal period for conception is beginning, the rest of the day is spoilt for them. Full of aversion, all thay can think of is their self-inflicted duty to have intercourse that night.

All of these restrictions have a clearly punishing quality. If only for this reason, all resistance against becoming pregnant has to remain unconscious because it contradicts the ego-ideal and is to be condemned. The punishing aspect of treatment applies to these unacceptable tendencies (on treatment methods, see also Silber 1985).

Parallels with the Clinical Picture of Anorexia Nervosa

The dominant symptoms in anorexia nervosa are eating disorders, including both refusal to take food and bouts of bulimia and vomiting, resulting in extreme and often dangerous loss of weight. A secondary symptom in women is amenorrhoea, which is frequently interpreted as a defence against accepting the woman's role. This points to areas of conflict similar to those observed in cases of functional sterility. But the overriding theme in both symptoms is the need for body control as a flight from an oppressive and apparently unalterable situation.

Common to both groups of patients is their inner conviction of their own inadequacy and helplessness. They feel unable to lead their lives in the way they would like and so seek at least to retain control over their own bodies, which are experienced as seperate entities. Their deep insecurity makes them see this extreme control over their bodies as a special achievement (see also Bruch 1980).

Although every fertility disorder necessarily arises in the context of a relationship between two people and both partners share the self-controlling rituals involved in treatment, it is nevertheless the women who carry on this power struggle with their bodies with far greater intensity than the men. This may partly be because the treatment involves them to a greater extent than their husbands and that the evidence of the success or failure of their attempts to have a child is registered in their bodily processes. However, the driving force behind these couples' efforts lies ultimately in the special significance that pregnancy and birth hold for the women.

The great physical changes, the experience of having another person growing inside oneself, the creativity but also dependency inherent in the development of the child - all of these processes in pregnancy are so closely interwoven with a woman's identity that a far greater ambivalence in the women than the men is to be expected. What both partners have in common is their insecurity about their sexual identity, which is expressed in - and perpetuated by - their infertility. Goldschmidt and De Boor (1976) claim that this ambivalent attitude towards fertility would already have been a decisive factor in the choice of a partner, which was bound up with the unconscious goal 'to have a special sort of relationship, in which childlessness played a certain positive role'. This positive role lies in the prevention of a situation which may be consciously sought after but whose realization, it is feared, would bring about an intolerable role conflict. Particularly 'oral-providing' or 'hysterical-rivalry' collusions between partners can be identified in this connection (Willi 1975).

The symptom of anorexia nervosa is also ambiguous and can be understood either as a hysterical symptom or as a defence against oral aggression (Loch 1983), However, whilst the female anorexic patient shows off her emaciated body, infertile couples try to remain as inconspicuous as possible. Their infertility is hidden from the outside world like a stigma. Thus, each individual couple is only aware of its own difficulties, and they feel like outcasts in a fertile environment.

The special status which makes the anorexic patient dream of having supernatural powers is for the infertile couple yet another injury and a further reason for redoubling their efforts yet again. In this way the women, especially, move further and further away from the posture of openness and receptivity which belongs to conception. On the conscious level, reproduction becomes a highly technical affair, stripped of its mythological associations, whose special and fearsome significance works on in the unconscious, where it cannot be worked through in a realistic way. For these couples, their treatment for infertility represents an attempted compromise between conscious and unconscious motives.

References

Berninghausen J (1980) Der Traum vom Kind - Geburt eines Klischees. Mutterschaft: Ideologie, Wunsch und Wirklichkeit. Ullstein, Frankfurt

Bruch H (1980) Der goldene Käfig. Das Rätsel der Magersucht. Fischer, Frankfurt

Goldschmidt O, De Boor C (1976) Psychoanalytische Untersuchung funktionell steriler Ehepaare. Psyche (Stuttg) 30: 899-923

Haeberle EJ (1983) Die Sexualität des Menschen. Handbuch und Atlas. de Gruyter, Berlin

Loch W (1983) Die Krankheitslehre der Psychoanalyse. Hirzel, Stuttgart

Silber SJ (1985) Endlich schwanger. Informationen für Paare mit Kinderwunsch. Rowohlt, Reinbek

Willi J (1975) Die Zweierbeziehung. Rowohlt, Reinbek

Body Complaints Among Recovered Genital Cancer Patients and Their Partners

P. Möhring and E. Brähler

One way of experiencing one's own body is through physical complaints. These are perceived with varying degrees of clarity, depending on how a particular part of the body is represented in consciousness, i.e. the intensity with which a complaint is felt does not have to be directly related to the extent of an organic lesion but is rather a measure of one's relations with one's own body.

A malignant disease shatters an individual's relationship with his or her body. Even if treatment is successful, the initial threat to life will inevitably give place to a life-long uncertainty as to the the final outcome of the illness. Being the centre of events, the body, in particular the organ or organ system affected, remains the focus of all uncertainties. If the genitals are affected, a person's whole sexual identity can be upset and, since the sexual encounter with another person is focused on these organs, their relations with a partner as well. How one pair coped with just such a malignant disease is shown in the following example.

Six years after her operation, Mrs. S. remembers the situation well: she and her husband had longed for a child which, after years of trying, still failed to materialize. So they sought medical advice. During the gynaecological examination, an ovarian tumour was discovered. She was advised to have an operation immediately and the tumour, which proved to be malignant, was removed. Soon after the operation, Mrs. S. and her husband were informed of the diagnosis by the doctor. Before the operation she had already had fears in the direction of cancer, but when she heard the news she was seized with paralyzing horror; for a whole day she contemplated suicide. She recovered from the operation without complications and tolerated the after-treatment well. She made it clear to her husband that the best way in which he could help her was by distracting her from her condition. This he did for all his worth: he took her on outings and accompanied her to the theatre, museums and to visit friends. At home they talked about every possible topic, just not about her cancer and the anxieties connected with it. This helped the patient to get over the crisis. As she had longed so very much for a child in the years preceding, it was especially bitter for her to hear that she would now never be able to have one, particularly since she was only 25 years old at the time.

In the initial interview briefly outlined below, the interviewer found her to be a delicate, defenceless, childish creature. Her husband had driven her to the interview but did not stay.

She tells the interviewer that although they spend all their free time together

her illness is never mentioned between them. Their marriage is very harmonious. Asked about how the illness has affected their sex-life, a momentary look of pain passes over her features before she recovers her usual conventional and somewhat formal facial expression and way of speaking. She then says that she has fortunately reached an agreement with her husband that they should have no further sexual intercourse. After a few attempts following the operation she had realized that she simply could not tolerate it any more. She cannot say why, as there is no anatomical reason for this reaction of hers. She just sensed that the act of intercourse was something she could no longer tolerate. Perhaps psychological, she surmises, with a questioning look.

This subject clearly bothers her. She says that intercourse had begun to upset her; it left her tense and nervous afterwards. It gave her no pleasure and she has no desire for sex any more. The interview turns to the subject of her husband, whom she praises with enthusiastic admiration for his self-sacrificing willingness to renounce sex for her sake. She is very glad that she has him: he is the great stabilizing factor in her life, her parents living hundreds of miles away so that she does not see them often.

Distraction and work are clearly the coping mechanisms she chose from the start to get over the shock of the dreadful news. The whole sphere of illness and being ill has been banned from consciousness, for which the husband's supportive attitude is largely responsible. Nevertheless, she could not prevent these unpleasant feelings - in the form of a diffuse sense of strain at first, then an inner tension rising to the pitch of trembling and shaking - from occurring whenever she was forced to become conscious of her genitals again through sexual contact with her husband. In trying to deal with the severe illness through repression and disavowal she had attempted to ban the corresponding body representative from consciousness in the same way. This defence mechanism was successful, too, as long as it was not endangered by her husband's sexual approaches. The moment it was, the entire defence threatened to collapse, giving rise to anxiety and physical tension. The mutual regression of this couple onto a childish, almost symbiotic level of interaction succeeded in stabilizing the relationship, so long as neither tendencies towards loosening the bond nor sexual impulses were permitted to endanger the common defence against the past trauma. A decisive factor in the success of this strategy was the husband's behaving in symmetry to his wife. If he had continued to press her sexually, she would have been forced to resort to a more difficult sort of intrapsychic defence, such as the repression of her own genital sensations or perhaps a form of hysterical symptom-formation, which would surely have been a greater stress for her.

In this example, one can observe how the body has become more than just the scene of the patient's struggle for survival; it has also become cathected with a psychic function as a part of her effort to master the double trauma of the immediate threat to life and the loss of her hopes of motherhood. As long as the patient's genital sphere was not activated or stimulated in any way, the desired result - coping with anxiety, mourning, disappointment etc. - could be maintained, albeit at the price of a discontinued sex life and a reduced emotional life. The fact that it was possible in the case in question to involve the husband in such a defence system had a positive influence on the patient's psychic economy, for only his willingness to share her regressive stance of self-denial and self-protectiveness guaranteed the stability of the marital relationship.

In the case outlined above, the patient's body and bodily sensations were directly involved in her psychological strategy for coping with the illness. From the literature on other patients' reactions to malignant diseases affecting the genitals, it is well known that in a high proportion of such cases the women subsequently complain of disturbances in the sexual sphere or give up sexual activity altogether. Abitbol and Davenport (1974), for example, report that 75% of women complained of sexual dysfunctions following radiological treatment of genital carcinomas. Similarly, in a study on patients who had had an operation for cervical carcinoma, Beck and Nikorovicz (1980) found that in 61% both the desire for sex and the capacity for sexual enjoyment had decreased or they had lost interest altogether. In men who had had a partial testectomy because of a malignant scrotal tumour, a third suffered from sexual disturbances as a result, which in part took the form of compensatory sexual overactivity in an attempt to master their fears of potency loss (Janssen and Weissbach 1978).

Thus, the way in which individuals experience their own body is unquestionably a relevant dimension in considering how they cope with malignant disease. The fact that aspects of body experience can be important even years after the illness itself was illustrated in the example quoted above. Since illness in general, and malignant disease in particular, is frequently experienced as a threat to or failure of the body, and since this deficiency is still felt years later in the form of recurrent anxiety states, it is important to investigate body experience after an illness by obtaining a complete picture of all the ex-patient's physical complaints. The example demonstrated further how much a person's attitude to their body is also dependent on their partner's behaviour. Thus, in asking about bodily complaints, it can be helpful to include the patient's partner in the inquiry to obtain additional information on relevant aspects of the couple's interaction.

The fact that the body is an important, albeit often neglected, dimension of identity is discussed at length in this volume. We would like to report here on a study involving two samples of male and female genital carcinoma survivors. The ex-patients and their partners were asked to report on their body experience insofar as it was expressed through physical complaints. Included in the whole inquiry were 103 married couples who were questioned 5-10 years after the illness of one of the partners. In study 1 ($n = 46$), the women had had a carcinoma of the corpus uteri, ovarian or collum uteri in stages I-III, usually I and II. The average age of this group was 53.4 years (SD = 6.1). In study 2 ($n = 57$), it was the men who had been ill. They had had a seminoma, teratoma or embryonic cell carcinoma or, in 15% of cases, some other malignant testicular tumour; the stages here were unknown. This sample had an average age of 40.6 years (SD = 13.1). The age difference corresponds to the differing age of manifestation of the various tumours. Each subject, i.e. 206 individuals, answered questions about the nature and frequency of his or her own physical complaints, as well as on what they knew of their partner's complaints and complaint frequency. In this way we obtained four subjective descriptions for each couple:

The husband's self-report

The wife's report on her husband's complaints

The husband's report on his wife's complaints
The wife's self-report

The details about the complaints were gathered by means of the Giessen Subjective Complaints List (GSCL; cf. Brähler and Scheer 1983; Brähler and Möhring, this volume). This is a questionnaire on the degree of distress caused by physical symptoms, i.e. it asks for subjective impressions - bodily distress as a psychological dimension. It contains 57 items, 24 of which are grouped into the four scales 'exhaustion', 'gastric complaints', 'pains in limbs' and 'cardiac complaints', the sum of these making up the fifth scale, 'overall distress'. The scales will be interpreted below, along with selected items.

First of all, the results of both studies will be presented, starting with study 2.

Table 1 shows the profile of the scale means over the four questionnaires that were filled out by the male genital cancer survivors and their wives. In comparison with the standard sample, the wives show no significant deviations from the norm. Their husbands, who had been ill, have significantly raised scores on the scales 'exhaustion', 'pains in limbs' and 'overall distress'. Looking at the self-reports on item level, the women as a group again show no unusual deviations from the standard sample. The ex-patients, on the other hand, have significantly elevated scores on 22 items, especially the following:

29 Exhaustability
42 Weariness
37 Numb extremities
53 Abdominal pain
41 Tired legs
14 Difficulties in walking
20 Lump in the throat
12 Excessive sweating
24 Oversensitivity to cold
9 Pains in limbs

Items 29 and 42 belong to the scale 'exhaustion', items 41 and 9 to the scale 'pains in limbs' and item 12 to the scale 'cardiac complaints'.

Reviewing the results on the husbands' and wives' reports about each other's complaints in Table 1, we find that each has given a fairly accurate picture of the

Table 1. Profile of GSCL scale means for men after genital carcinoma and their wives ($n = 57$)

Scale	Husband's self-report		Wife's report on husband		Husband's report on wife		Wife's self-report	
	Mean	SD	Mean	SD	Mean	SD	Mean	SD
Exhaustion	5.68[a]	4.95	5.88	5.46	5.47	4.71	5.46	4.87
Gastric complaints	3.37	3.71	4.37[c]	4.90	2.21[c]	2.94	3.30	3.01
Pains in limbs	5.70[a]	5.12	5.77	5.45	6.28[b]	5.00	7.14	5.18
Cardiac complaints	2.88	4.12	2.65	4.42	3.30	3.81	3.77	3.56
Overall distress	17.63[a]	14.43	18.67	16.97	17.26	13.37	19.67	13.82

[a] $p < 0.05$ compared with standard sample (men 18-60 years)
[b] $p < 0.05$, [c] $p < 0.01$ } self-report as compared with partner's report

other on the scales 'exhaustion' and 'cardiac complaints'. The wives tend to overestimate their husbands' 'gastric complaints' as compared with their husbands' own self-reports, whereas the husbands have the opposite tendency to underestimate their wives' complaints on the same scale. The husbands also understimate the intensity of their wives' 'pains in limbs'.

In Table 2, the self-reports and partners' impressions are compared and presented as correlations over the whole sample. The self-reports of both partners correlate positively throughout, with highly significant correlations on the scales 'pains in limbs', 'cardiac complaints' and 'overall distress'. The correlation between the husbands' self-reports and their wives' impressions of them is very high, higher than the test-retest correlations for the questionnaire and in some cases even exceeding the internal consistency of the scales (see Brähler and Scheer 1983). This means that the wives can give an accurate description of their husbands' complaints.

If one takes the wife's impressions of her husband's subjective physical condition as being made up partly of her true perceptions of his complaints (as compared with his self-report), and partly of her projections (as compared with her own self-report), then one finds that her impressions of her husband are indeed based almost entirely on correct perception of his complaints and contain practically no elements of projection.

The correlation between the husbands' impressions of their wives' complaints and the wives' own self-reports is also very high on the scale 'pains in limbs', is somewhat less on the scales 'exhaustion', 'cardiac complaints' and 'overall distress' and reaches only 0.59 for 'gastric complaints'. If, as above, one views the men's reports on their wives as a linear combination of 'true perceptions' (measured by comparison with the wives' self-reports) and projections of the men's own subjective conditions, the scales 'pains in limbs' and 'overall distress' can be seen to contain certain projective elements, which are, however, less dominant than the accurate perceptions.

Table 3 presents the correlations between the self-reports and the partners' impressions for the three selected items which relate directly to the affected organs: low sexual excitability, high sexual excitability and abdominal pain. The correlations between both self-reports are significantly positive for the item 'low sexual excitability', but very low for the other two items. Whereas on all three items the men's self-reports are strongly confirmed by their wives' impressions of them,

Table 2. Congruence between self-report and partner's report for men after genital carcinoma and their wives ($n = 57$)

Scale	Husband's/wife's self-reports	Husband's self-report/ Wife's report on husband	Wife's self-report/ Husband's report on wife
Exhaustion	0.21	0.84	0.69
Gastric complaints	0.16	0.85	0.59
Pains in limbs	0.40	0.81	0.83
Cardiac complaints	0.44	0.85	0.73
Overall distress	0.46	0.89	0.73

Table 3. Congruence between self-report and partner's report on selected items

Item	Husband's/wife's self-reports	Husband's self-report/wife's report on husband	Wife's self-report/husband's report on wife
Low sexual excitability	0.32	0.73	0.47
High sexual excitability	0.10	0.66	0.19
Abdominal pain	0.06	0.80	0.38

there is far less congruence between the partners when it comes to the question of the wives' position with respect to these three items. Especially low is the agreement on the wives' 'high sexual excitability'.

Taking the partners' impressions once again as a combination of both self-reports, one arrives at the interpretation that the women's impressions of their husbands are largely influenced by accurate perceptions of their husbands' self-impressions and contain hardly any elements of projection. This is also the case with the men's impressions of their wives on the item 'low sexual excitability', but when it comes to the items 'high sexual excitability' and 'abdominal pain' we find that the men's impressions of their wives are very strongly influenced by their own self-images, i.e. they contain strong elements of projection.

And now to study 1. Table 4 shows the profile of scale means over the four reports by the women who had had a genital carcinoma and their husbands. The women's self-reports here had significantly raised scores on the scales 'exhaustion', 'pains in limbs' and 'overall distress'. Their husbands were also troubled to a significant extent by 'pains in limbs'. Taking the self-reports on item level the women who had been ill had significantly higher scores than the standard sample (women, 35-60 years) for 30 complaints, most of all on the following:

8 Low sexual excitability
43 Diarrhoea
12 Excessive sweating
21 Frequent urination
29 Exhaustability
38 Constipation
40 Hot flushes
41 Tired legs
42 Weariness
30 Insomnia

In this group the husbands, too, had significantly elevated scores on 25 items, particularly for the complaints:

9 Pains in limbs
11 Backache
13 Pains in neck and shoulders
41 Tired legs
56 Bouts of heart trouble
14 Difficulties in walking

16 Visual disturbances
49 Cold feet
21 Frequent urination.

The four items with the highest scores all belong to the scale 'pains in limbs'.

Looking at Table 4, if one compares the scales means for the self-reports with those for the partners' reports, one can see that the complaints reported by the men themselves and their wives' impressions of their complaints have roughly the same frequencies. On the other hand, the men regularly underestimate the extent of their wives' complaints on the scales 'exhaustion', 'pains in limbs' and 'overall distress'. Table 5 shows the correlations between the self-reports and the partners' impressions. On all scales there is a very high rate of correspondence between the self-reports of both partners, particularly for 'gastric complaints', 'cardiac complaints' and 'overall distress'. The agreement between self-reports and partners, impressions is good throughout, with coefficients on a level with those reflecting the internal consistency of the scales.

In the husbands' impressions of their wives' complaints there is an element of projection which, however, is not as influential as the correct perceptions. Accurate perceptions are dominant in all the other partners' reports.

Table 6 presents the correlations between the self-reports and the partners' impressions for the selected items 'low sexual excitability', 'high sexual excitability' and 'abdominal pain'.

The correlations between the self-reports are positive and significant. The agreement between husband and wife on the husband's 'low sexual excitability' is very high, but on his 'abdominal pain' relatively low. In their judgements of the wife's 'abdominal pain' they show a particularly high rate of agreement.

If one sees the partners' impressions as linear combinations of the individual self-reports, no projective elements are to be found in the husbands' impressions of their wives. In the wives' impressions of their husbands there are clearly strongly projective elements in the items 'high sexual excitability' and 'abdominal pain'. On the item 'abdominal pain', the wives' judgement of their husbands are even more strongly influenced by projective aspects than by their actual perceptions.

Table 4. Profile of GSCL scale means for women after genital carcinoma and their husbands ($n = 46$)

Scale	Husband's self-report		Wife's report on husband		Husband's report on wife		Wife's self-report	
	Mean	SD	Mean	SD	Mean	SD	Mean	SD
Exhaustion	4.59	4.66	4.96	4.82	6.98[c]	4.73	8.00[b]	5.10
Gastric complaints	3.15	3.67	3.24	3.48	3.39[c]	3.65	4.11[a]	4.03
Pains in limbs	7.93[b]	4.97	8.33	5.38	9.24	5.88	10.04[a]	6.00
Cardiac complaints	3.61	4.29	3.91	4.29	5.07	4.33	5.28	4.15
Overall distress	19.28	13.72	20.43	13.93	24.67[d]	14.99	27.43[b]	15.61

[a] $p<0.05$, [b] $p<0.01$ } compared with standard sample (men/women 41-60 years)
[c] $p<0.05$, [d] $p<0.01$ } self-report as compared with partner's report

Table 5. Congruence between self-report and partner's report for women after genital carcinoma and their husbands ($n = 46$)

Scale	Husband's/wife's self-reports	Husband's self-report/wife's report on husband	Wife's self-report/ husband's report on wife
Exhaustion	0.31	0.89	0.75
Gastric complaints	0.53	0.89	0.85
Pains in limbs	0.40	0.93	0.89
Cardiac complaints	0.59	0.89	0.92
Overall distress	0.60	0.91	0.90

Table 6. Congruence between self-report and partner's report on selected items

Item	Husband's/wife's self-reports	Husband's self-report/ wife's report on husband	Wife's self-report/ husband's report on wife
Low sexual excitability	0.25	0.87	0.72
High sexual excitability	0.44	0.63	0.72
Abdominal pain	0.54	0.51	0.92

Interpretation

In interpreting the results, deviations from the standard sample as well as similarities and differences arising between the two groups will be discussed.

In study 1 (where the wives had been ill), the high scores of both partners are striking; at item level this applies to 30 items for the women and 25 for their husbands. The women suffer particularly from complaints in the areas of temperature regulation, exhaustion and abdominal troubles. The men's highest scores are on items belonging to the scale 'pains in limbs', to the extent that the whole scale deviates significantly from the norm. The fact that the women complain of abdominal pain may be an indication that they watch this part of their bodies with special attentiveness, or the complaints may be consequences of past treatment. The relationships between self-report and partner's report at the scale level in this group demonstrate a high degree of congruence and very good mutual perceptions. There is a tendency among the men to underestimate their wives' exhaustion, gastric complaints and overall distress, perhaps because the women do not communicate the full extent of their complaints to their husbands, but basically the men's impressions correspond to their wives' self-reports. Mutual identification and empathy are features characteristic of this group. The partners have moved closer together with respect to their self-perceptions and show that they know each other well. Their capacity for body perception has increased, perhaps as a reaction to the wife's illness having begun unnoticed, so that both now watch their bodies more carefully.

After a genital tumour, the area of sexuality is of particular interest. Here we do in fact find one important difference between these items and the judgements on the other scales. Dividing the partners' reports in this group into a perceived and a projected part, one arrives at the conclusion that the wives' impressions of their husbands with respect to high sexual excitability and abdominal pains are to a considerable extent projections; these even make up the dominant part of their reports on his 'abdominal pain'. In other words, in this area, the wives' judgements of their husbands' complaints are based more on their own self-perceptions than on the way the husbands see themselves. This suggests the further interpretation that the women's own attitude to the part of their bodies which has proved to be unreliable and vulnerable has subsequently coloured their judgements of their husbands.

In study 2, the men who had been ill had significantly elevated scores on 22 items, including - along with those complaints belonging to the scales - the item 'abdominal pain', which again is related to their past illness. The region of the abdomen has been ill and still demands continued attention years afterwards. In this group, it is striking that the wives report no increase in their own complaints. Their whole attention is focused on their husbands' troubles, so that these are even overestimated on one scale, whilst the wives' complaints are underestimated by their husbands on two scales. An increase in complaint level common to both partners, as in the group where the women had been ill, does not occur here. The complaints remain specific to the partner who had the illness and are not shared, as with the other group. But here, too, the partners' judgements of each others' complaints correspond closely to the self-reports; empathy is still there. On the scales, the elements of projection are minimal.

Here, too, the responses to the items on sexuality were examined separately. In this group, the women perceive their husbands' level of sexual excitability and abdominal pains almost entirely without projection. Not so the men. Their judgements of their wives' abdominal pains and high sexual excitability are strongly influenced by projections, which is further evidence of the fact that an individual's relationship to a certain part of their body distorts their view of a partner's true situation.

In psychopathology, the conflict model of symptom formation shows how the areas of one's own conflicts distort one's perceptions of others in those areas. For this reason, projections and transference phenomena are a constituent part of every neurosis. Here we can see that the same mechanisms are applied in coping with a physical trauma occurring in adulthood.

A person who has had cancer has been betrayed by their body. In the cases in question, the affected partner was struck on a part of the body which is inseparably bound up with reproduction and sexual identity, i.e. an area which is essential to one's sense of one's own value. Furthermore, the genitals are the parts of the body where the most intimate encounter between man and woman takes place, where they not only metaphorically but also literally become united and fused with one another, so that an illness here can bring about a disturbance in their sexual communication. At this point, at the latest, it must become clear why any consideration of the problem of coping with the illness must involve the patient's partner. In both studies, processes of mutual identification and assimilation have taken place between the partners to an unusual degree. The studies differ in that the men whose wives had been ill have increased their own complaint level, which has no equivalent in the other group.

Increased exhaustion, pains in limbs and overall distress all suggest that the husbands of the women who had been ill are overburdened. Where the husband was the ill partner, the wives show no correspondingly detrimental responses. In this group the mutual assimilation is also less. The fact that here the suffering is shared less may be an expression of the mens' stronger orientation towards autonomy. On the whole, then, the pattern of complaints among the men who had been ill and their wives shows less deviation from the norm and the general complaint level is lower.

We interpret this process of assimilation between partners, which can be observed in marriages threatened by a malignant disease, as a common response to this very deep threat. It is an identificatory defence process which, even if it has the advantage that the partners discover more things that they have in common, inevitably means also that each individual has to partially renounce or at least reduce his or her claim to a separate identity, i.e. a change in self-perception is necessarily involved as well. Although the observed increase in mutual empathy is clearly an indication of improved perceptions and intensive and close communication within these marriages - of an enrichment in the relationship, in fact - the similarity of the self-reports leaves one with a divided impression. It may be that the remaining conflict potential is now less and the personal sense of security in an insecure situation greater, but it is also a fact that renouncing differences in a marriage at the same time has the effect of reducing the opportunities to come to grips with conflicts fully. Anyone who clings to a partner out of anxiety gives up a degree of independent identity. That may be a price which these couples are willing to pay when confronted with a threat to life. Working out remaining anxieties in a psychotherapeutic context could give them courage for further development, although these people hardly belong to the psychotherapist's usual clientele. In the case quoted at the beginning, both partners were left with considerable restrictions, even if they appeared to have come to terms with their situation. But giving up all claims to a sex-life is a heavy demand on a young married couple, even if in this case it was the solution which enabled their life together to continue without the assistance of a psychotherapist.

Acknowledgement. This work was supported by the Robert-Bosch-Stiftung.

References

Abitbol MM, Davenport J (1974) Sexual dysfunction after therapy of cervical carcinoma. Am J Obstet Gynecol 119: 181

Beck A, Nikorovicz F (1980) Das Sexualleben nach Radikaloperationen des Zervixkarzinoms. Onkologie 3: 26

Brähler E, Scheer JW (1983) Der Giessener Beschwerdebogen (GBB) - Testhandbuch. Huber, Bern

Janssen PL, Weissbach L (1978) Zur Psychosomatik behandelter Hodentumor-Patienten. Psychosom Psychoanal 24: 70

D. Measuring Body Experience and Body Complaints

Psychological Research into Body Experience: Models and Methods

P. M. Wiedemann

Introduction

Research into body experience was a nearly forgotten topic in psychology but has recently attracted more interest. Social and clinical psychologists are attempting to explore dimensions and types of body experiences for different groups under various conditions (Jodelet 1984; Pervin 1976: Wiedemann et al. 1984). A further topic is the relationship between body experience and emotion (Fehr and Russel 1984; Shields and Stern 1979). Researchers in the fields of medical psychology and psychosomatics focus on perception of symptoms and pain (Pennebaker 1982) and on body experience in relation to various illnesses. For psychotherapists, body experience is interesting as a tool for change, especially in the Reichian approach and in gestalt therapy (Lowen 1981; Perls 1978).

The results and conceptions of psychological body research are divergent: there are numerous approaches and models and it is often hard to detect any connections between them. To give an example, it is nearly impossible to connect Pennebaker's (1982) model of symptom perception, Leventhal's (1982) conception of illness representation, Fisher's (1970) body feeling guidance system and his conception of body boundaries, and Gendlin's (1978) 'felt sense' approach in psychotherapy. The same is true for the various diagnostic instruments in this field (Miller et al. 1981; Paulus 1982; Strauss and Appelt 1983). These divergences are caused by different conceptions but also by the different methods used in the investigation of body experience: each method creates a different perspective on the body. This interaction between method and emergence of data is the topic of this article. The questions are:

- Which techniques produce which kind of data?
- Which aspects of body experience are highlighted and which are hidden by different methods?

The Problem: How to Gather Data on Body Experience

The most important precondition for gathering data on body experience is the subjects' ability to verbalize their body feelings. This sounds trivial but is in fact a very restrictive condition, since without verbalization there are no data and, furthermore, in the process of verbalization people interpret their feelings, and thereby construct the meaning of their body experience.

This corresponds to findings in cognitive psychology (Neisser 1979): Perception is not a passive but an active process of interpreting stimuli, and it is not only the subject who interprets her or his bodily feelings in the process of communicating them, but also the researcher or investigator, who elicits these data by the use of diagnostic methods, which constrain and structure the data in a specific way.

The choice of a diagnostic instrument influences the communication between subject and researcher and thus determines which kind of data we get. Data can differ in respect to type, response format and verbalization scheme.

Type of data refers to the difference between quantitative and verbal data. Data are quantitative if they are numerical; verbal data can vary in scope, i.e. they can reach from associations to reports and narrations. *Response formats* differ in the degree of freedom the subject has to express her or his experience. Closed response formats constrain the subject to given categories, whereas open formats leave more room for subjective and meaningful responses. The choice of closed response formats will often lead to misinterpretations, especially for subtle phenomena such as body experiences, and special characteristics could be neglected. Open response formats, on the other hand, enable self-presentation and direct expression of feelings. *Verbalization scheme* refers to the type and extent of verbalization. The simplest case is a description of body experiences as a list of associated concepts (verbs as well as adjectives or nouns). The subject can also be asked to provide a detailed account of events related to a certain body experience or feeling. These accounts may have the form of descriptions, reports or narrations, and each of these verbalization schemes has certain psychological characteristics and implications for data analysis and interpretation.

We can now summarize the perspective on psychological body research developed so far:

1. Body experience interacts with cognitive structures and forms part of more comprehensive representations of experience. It is related to situations, emotions, and behaviour.
2. The detection of these relationships depends on the choice of data-gathering techniques and data analysis. Open response formats are hereby preferable to closed ones, since the former allow the elicitation of data from the subject's point of view.
3. Data given in open response format pose a problem: it is difficult to analyse them in an objective way. In the remainder of this article I shall propose different ways of collecting and analysing verbal data. The focus will be on the development of a classification scheme of body experience along two dimensions: relevance structure and time perspective. This classification scheme can be used as a guideline for data gathering and analysis.

Relevance Structure of Body Experience

The term 'relevance' goes back to Schütz and Luckmann (1973) and is used to describe the system which controls attention, perception and interpretation. Schütz and Luckmann differentiate between three kinds of relevance structures:

1. Thematic relevance
2. Interpretational relevance
3. Motivational relevance

Thematic relevance is introduced to answer the question 'How does it come about that precisely this object, whatever it may be, draws attention to itself? Why has it become the focus of attention?' The most important condition is unfamiliarity, i.e. a departure from the normal course of events or general routine expectations. This type of thematic relevance is called forced attentiveness or imposed thematic relevance, since the new theme intrudes or imposes itself. Schütz and Luckmann define a second type, the voluntary advertence or 'motivated' thematic relevance, which is a conscious and motivated focusing of attention by the subject.

Once a theme has been adverted to, i.e. has become thematically relevant, it is brought into congruence with relevant elements of knowledge. This is what Schütz and Luckmann call *interpretational relevance* which can also be imposed or motivated. Imposed interpretational relevance refers to a more or less automatic interpretation of a given theme. Things are routinely understood. Motivated interpretational relevance comes into play when the theme is problematic, i.e. when the automatically activated knowledge structures are not sufficient for the explication of the phenomenon. In this case an active step by step search is initiated to match the problematic theme and the stock of knowledge at hand.

The first type of *motivational relevance* is 'motivation in the "in-order-to" context', which is a goal-directed projection of acts for coping with the problematic theme. The second type, which is of less importance here, is 'motivation in the "because" context' and refers to the causal explanation of actions.

In the context of body experience these relevance structures prove to be very useful. The core of a more narrowly defined body experience is the perception of physical processes and states. Usually attention is not focused on the body; the body becomes thematically relevant under specific circumstances only.

This thematic relevance of the body is not abstract, it is not the knee or the stomach which are thematically relevant, but a throbbing sensation in the knee, or indigestion. The thematic relevance always alludes to bodily sensations. With Schütz and Luckmann we can distinguish between imposed and motivated body attention. Thorbecke's (1979) concept of 'unsuccessful acts' (mißglückte Handlungssituationen) are prototypical for imposed thematic relevance of the body, e.g. when I get out of breath by climbing stairs. Motivated thematic relevance, on the other hand, refers to situations in which the subject consciously guides her or his attention towards the body, for example in a psychotherapeutic setting.

Interpretational relevance concerning the body means the emotional and cognitive framing of body sensations. These translations from sensations into body experiences can range from simple positional interpretations such as stressful/relaxing, comfortable/uncomfortable to associations or analogical or metaphorical descriptions (e.g. 'it feels like a stone in my stomach; it feels like needles ...').

Interpretational relevances can be conceptualized as schemata (Leventhal 1982; Mason 1959); schemata enable the interpretation of thematically relevant body sensations in a consistent way. Mason, for instance, found strong regularities in the interpretations of body sensations; body feelings are connected to specific physical processes or states. Another example is Fisher's 'landmark model': 'The kind of circuit envisioned in this model involves focus upon a body area because of its coded meaning which is congruent with a learned attitude or set; feedback from the resulting perceptually highlighted locale which reinforces the original set; consequent intensified drive to continue focusing upon that body locale which in turn might increase its degree of physiological activations ...' (Fisher 1970, p. 580).

The framing of bodily sensations is not only of emotional nature; Leventhal (1982) shows how physical states are organized in complex cognitive units such as schemata or frames. According to Leventhal the conceptualization of physical sensations depends on four interpretative dimensions:

1. Identity, i.e. the availability of a label such as a specific illness for the bodily sensations
2. Perceived causes, i.e. the perceived conditions for the occurrence of the sensations or symptoms
3. Expected consequences of the bodily state
4. Expectations concerning the time-line of the present body condition

Leventhal's model is of special importance for coping with illness. The first step - the identification of symptoms with a diagnostic label - is crucial, since it focuses attention towards monitoring bodily states and interpreting them in terms of symptoms. This process is useful and will lead to adequate coping strategies if the matching of sensations and diagnostic label is correct. But it can also be misleading: sensations might be wrongly interpreted as symptoms for the illness, which results in inefficient illness behaviour.

Simonton et al. (1978) provide another example for the importance of cognitive framing of body sensations. They develop a therapeutic technique for cancer patients based on cognitive reframing of symptoms. The core of this technique is a guided imagination process: patients are advised to visualize the cancer cells as enemies attacked by their own white blood cells. This metaphor changes patients' attitude towards their illness. They experience themselves as more active, able to influence the illness, which results in a more positive emotional state.

Motivational relevance of body experiences refers to the acts or behaviours which result from the interpreted body sensations. Fisher (1970) calls this linkage between experience and behaviour 'body feeling guidance system', which according to Fisher is of special importance in critical situations.

It should be noted that the interpretational as well as the motivational relevances consist of very complex inference processes; they reach from the perception of a body sensation to the inferring of possible causes and the generation of coping strategies. Contextual information, the specific situational features are also incorporated. Such complex interpretational and motivational structures can be described by the scipt concept developed in the field of cognitive psychology (cf. Abelson 1981). Scripts are more or less stereotypical act-event sequences which reduce complexity and guide action.

Time Perspectives in the Analysis of Body Experience

The data relevant for the analysis of body experience can be given in different time perspectives, i.e. as scenes, episodes and biographical accounts. These units differ in scope and details; the largest unit is the biographical account or the body biography, the smallest but most detailed units are body scene, while body episodes have a medium scope and a medium degree of particularization. Each of these units provides specific possibilities and limitations for analysis.

Body episodes are the prototypical unit for the organization of body experiences. They share the following structural parts:

1. A Description of a situational context
2. A course of events, characterized by
3. A peak or complication and
4. An outcome

This corresponds to the story schema as analyzed by Labov (1972) and the drama conception by Politzer (1974). Description of a situational context provides an orientation: where, under what circumstances and when did it happen, who was involved. The course of events refers to the acts, behaviours and interactions, i.e. the occurrences which constitute the episode. The peak or complication is the kernel of the drama; it is defined as a break with the expected normal course of events. Something startling, new or unexpected happens which attracts attention. Usually the subject describes her or his motives and strategies to cope with the unexpected. It has been shown that episodes are the preferred natural unit of subjective representation of experience (cf Wiedemann and Becker 1986). Episodes have some important advantages: they are highly salient and available in memory, and thus easily accessible. People asked about body experiences will usually report them as episodes, e.g. they give stories about the onset of an illness, an accident or a stressful situation and describe the related bodily sensations. It is difficult to remember specific temporarily encountered body feelings unless they are connected with a drama. Thus the experience of the body is always combined with characteristics of the situational context, emotions, cognition and behaviour.

Body biographies refer to biographical relevant events and conflicts which formed the attitudes to, the perception of and the way a person treats her or his body. They are highly idiosyncratic and can include episodes about accidents, diseases, sports, operations, etc. There are also critical life periods for body experience, such as adolescence and aging. Furthermore, there are various contexts which can be relevant for biographical body episodes, for instance sexuality, illness, physical education. Body biographies consist of such peak experiences - in the form of episodes - and a number of general evaluation aspects connected to the self:

- Basic competencies of body perception, i.e. the sensitivity to physical states
- Basic dispositions, i.e. bodily shape and attractiveness
- Basic relations to the body, i.e. attitudes to the body and styles of body treatment
- Basic strategies of coping with the body, i.e. routine strategies and strategies in critical situations

To give a biographical account means selection and chronological and thematic ordering of body episodes combined with the general self-evaluation aspects listed above. The following questions can be asked in exploring a body biography:

- Which parts are of thematic relevance? Has the thematic relevance structure changed over time?
- Are there contexts which are typical for several episodes in a body biography?
- What interpretation schemes for body experience are generated and how have they changed?
- What are the typical aspects of self-evaluation in different life phases?

Body scenes are the smallest but most differentiated unit of body experience. An example of the significance of body scenes is Gendlin's (1978) focusing technique. He works with the felt sense, i.e. the bodily experience of a problem. The client has to focus on this felt sense and symbolize it in pictures, analogies, metaphors until she or he has found the adequate conceptualization. The criterion for the adequacy is again a bodily one: the noticeable change of the felt sense which Gendlin calls 'body shift'. A more precise analysis of body scenes is provided by the techniques of neurolinguistic programing (NLP) developed by Bandler and Grinder (1981). The NLP model treats subjective experiences as being coded in four different representation systems (Bandler and Grinder 1981; Gordon 1978; Dilts et al. 1980): the visual, the auditive, the kinaesthetic and the olfactory. A complex stimulus can be coded in all four systems: for instance the word 'fire' may trigger a body sensation (warmth), an 'inner' picture (flames, and an auditive representation such as the crackling of the fire. Bandler and Grinder assume that each experience can be traced as activities in the four representation systems. The sequence of these activities is called a strategy.

The NLP technique provides some advantages for the analysis of body scenes. The most important advantage is that microprocesses of body experience can be considered in detail. The subject is asked to describe precisely the development of her or his experiences, e.g. an asthma patient gives a detailed account of bodily sensations and the connected inner pictures (visual representation) as well as the accompanying inner speech (verbal/auditive representation). Thus, body experiences can be analyzed in their interrelations with other forms of experience, i.e. with activities in the other representation systems.

The model presented here consists of two dimensions, structure of relevance and time perspective. It will be used for the derivation of criteria for the evaluation and selection of methods in psychological body research.

Criteria for the Evaluation of Research Methods

Methods for gathering and analysing data can be classified according to four criteria:

1. Methodological orientation
2. Focus of data
3. Time perspective of data
4. Relevance structure

Methodological orientation refers to the differentiation between objective and subjective approaches. An objective approach determines the structure of the data as well as the content; questions, scales and response categories are defined and standardized a priori. Subjective approaches, on the other hand, do not impose structure or content but attempt to represent content and structure as given by the subject. Methodological orientation is correlated with the research objectives. For the field of body experience objectives could be: screening for a previously defined distinctive feature of body experience, its exploration in a single case study or its exploration in a therapeutical context. For a screening test it is sufficient to search for specific characteristics using standardized techniques with closed response formats such as questionnaires (Strauss and Appelt 1983), attitude scales (Miller et al. 1981) or a semantic differential (Feldman 1975). Methods with open response formats such as the repertory grid technique (Kelly 1955) or open interviews are preferable for single case studies and especially so in therapeutic contexts.

Focus of data means diachronic or synchronic organization of the data, i. e. do the data describe processes (diachronic focus) or states (synchronic focus). States can be beliefs, goals, or aspects of self-identity; such states are explored in most studies aiming at attitudes to the body such as risk orientation (Feldmann 1975), physical attractiveness and health (Paulus 1982). Diachronic data refer to sequential data describing the development of a body experience. They are different from longitudinal data: the latter consist of a series of measurements over time, whereas diachronic data usually refer to one measurement and the time aspect is given in the data themselves. Diachronic data can be collected by the use of open interviews. They require special qualitative techniques for analysis (Wiedemann and Becker 1986) since most quantitative methods do not adequately handle diachronic data (Everitt 1980; Jones 1983; Shoben 1983).

Synchronic as well as diachronic data can be valid for different time spans, i. e. they can refer to unique scenes, to episodes such as an illness, or they can be valid for certain biographical periods, e. g. childhood, adolescence, etc. This is meant by the third criterion, the *time perspective of data.*

Collecting data on body scenes is relevant for the exploration of microprocesses, e. g. for therapeutic intervention. When the research aims at investigating the living conditions or life history which determined the individual characteristic of body experience, the focus should be on body biography. Body episodes are in between these two levels or time perspectives. They consist of data of a medium time range and medium degree of particularization which can be further detailed into scenes as well as related to the biographical context. The ideal starting-point for the exploration of body experience is body episodes. They provide a framework for the analysis of body scenes and, furthermore, they allow tracing of the genesis of general attitudes towards the body relevant in a biographical context.

The fourth criterion refers to the different *relevance structures* mentioned above: thematic, interpretational and motivational relevance of body experience to focus on thematic relevance means, for instance, to ask what symptoms a patient monitors for evaluating the course of her or his disease or how and when an anorexic feels that she or he is overweight. The interpretational relevance of body experience can be analyzed in two directions: first, one can ask what bodily sensations are interpreted, e.g. what sensations in what situations a patient suffering from bulimia interprets as hunger. Second, one can investigate what patterns of interpretation a person uses to make sense of a body sensation - here, for example, the researcher might be interested in exploring the pattern of interpretation a person applies to her or his heart attack. Motivational relevance concerns the behaviours and acts motivated by body experience. One research topic in this field is connected to the psychomaintenance of chronic illness: what coping behaviour is evoked by the perception and interpretation of the symptoms?

The four criteria summarized in Table 1 are useful for the evaluation and modification of methods in psychological body research. This will be illustrated by the Body Focus Questionnaire (Fisher 1970), which focuses on the thematic relevance of body sensations. Interviewees are asked to compare parts of their body. They have to decide which part is more salient in their experience at that moment (e.g. mouth versus eyes). The Body Focus Questionnaire is an objective approach since the body areas and the comparisons are prescribed by the method. The specific features of individually structured body zones which might be larger or narrower is ignored. Furthermore, data gathered through the Body Focus Questionnaire are synchronic; changes in body experiences over time are neglected. The concentration of the current body experiences corresponds to focusing on body scenes. But Fisher (1970) assumes that his questionnaire provides data which are biographically valid.

The above-mentioned criteria allow construction of variations on the Body Focus Questionnaire. One variation might concern a change in the focus of data: from synchronic to diachronic data. This might be useful for the analysis of the development of an asthma attack. Here, the researcher could explore the sequence of body sensations preceding the spasm of the bronchial system. An further variation could be accomplished by a change in the time perspective. Leithäuser et al. (1980) give an example of how the thematic relevance of the body can be analysed in the biographical time perspective. They asked the subjects to draw the parts of their body strained by the specific conditions of their jobs. These thematic body relevance structures, elicited by the drawings, were verbalized in follow-up interviews. With this procedure it was possible to get data on the thematically relevant body zones in the biographical context of labour.

Table 1. Classification scheme for data-gathering techniques

Dimension	Feature		
Methodological orientation	Objective	Subjective	
Focus of data	Diachronic	Synchronic	
Time perspective of data	Biography	Episode	Scene
Relevance structure of data	Thematic relevance	Interpretational relevance	Motivational relevance

A Synopsis of Methods in Psychological Body Research

In the final part of this article I shall discuss the power of three different classes of methods in body research. These classes are derived from the criterion of methodological orientation introduced above. A shown in Table 2, the distinction between objective and subjective approach can be made regarding content and structure. Content refers to the data focused upon, whereas structure means the principle of data organization. In both domains an objective or a subjective approach is possible. In the content field an objective approach is realized by the choice of a closed response format, a subjective by an open response format. In the objective approach data organization is determined by the characteristics of the method or the statistical technique, whereas in the subjective approach the subjects themselves organize the data.

Purely subjective methods (subjective content and structure) are basically interview methods which give interviewees the freedom to express themselves without or with only minimal constraints. Which type of interview should be used depends on the preferred time perspective: the elicitation of body biographies demands the use of the biographical method (Thomae 1968), body episodes can be elicited by the narrative interview (Schütze 1976; Wiedemann and Becker 1986), and body scenes by an interview focusing on associations. This class of methods should be preferred in single case studies and for diagnostic tasks in therapy. It should also be mentioned that the analysis of data gathered with purely subjective methods requires special knowledge; for details see Wiedemann and Becker (1986).

Purely objective methods are the most frequently used in psychological body research, although they have the most restrictions. The prototypical objective approach is the standardized questionnaire (cf. Feldmann 1975; Paulus 1982; Strauss and Appelt 1983). The content is determined by the selection of the items (with closed response format) and the structure is determined by the methods used in constructing the questionnaire. Very often factor analytic methods are used for developing scales which are considered as basic dimensions of body experience. It is supposed that these dimensions have universal validity and that each case can be subsumed under them. The underlying assumption is that the body experience of different persons has identical content and structure and that interindividual differences show in the different scores on the dimensions. Individual differences in body experiences are assumed to be of pure quantitative nature, qualitative differences are excluded. Thus, the application of purely objective methods should be limited to screening tests aiming at global attitudes to the body or at symptoms and complaints.

Table 2. Methodological orientation

		Content	
		Subjective	Objective
Structure	Subjective	Purely subjective methods	
	Objective	Mixed methods	Purely objective methods

Methods where the structure is objective and the content subjective: The prototypical example here is the Repertory Grid Test by Kelly (1955). The Rep Grid only imposes the structure, but not the content, since there are no a priori defined items or questions. Thus the Rep Grid aims at the elicitation of 'subjective' constructs, and it covers a whole range of techniques for data collection (Fransella and Bannister 1977). The elements for the elicitation of personal constructs can be body parts (Feldman 1975), body sensations, emotions or body episodes (Wiedemann et al. 1984).

The method used for data analysis imposes a structure on the data: principal component analysis, cluster analysis, multidimensional scaling techniques - all imply a certain model structuring body experiences. Principal component analysis represents body experiences as independent factors, cluster analysis defines a categorical order, and the multidimensional scaling techniques imply a dimensional model of body experiences. This class of methods is useful for the diagnosis or evaluation of changes, for example in the therapeutic process.

References

Abelson RP (1981) Psychological status of the script concept. Am Psychol 36: 715-729

Bandler R, Grinder J (1981) Die Struktur der Magie, vol 1/2. Junfermann, Paderborn

Coxan APM (1982) The user's guide to multidimensional scaling. Heinemann, London

Dilts R, Grinder J, Bandler R, Bandler LC, deLozier J (1980) Neuro-linguistic programming. The study of the structure of subjective experience. Meta, Cuperlin

Everitt B (1980) Cluster analysis. Halsted, New York

Fehr B, Russell JA (1984) Concept of emotion viewed from a prototype perspective. J Exp Psychol 113/3: 464-486

Feldman MM (1975) The body image and object relations: Exploration of a method utilizing grid techniques. Br J Med Psychol 48: 317-332

Feldmann H (1975) Hypochondrie. Springer, Berlin Heidelberg New York

Fisher S (1970) Body experience in fantasy and behavior. Appleton-Century-Crofts, New York

Fisher S, Cleveland SE (1958) Body image and personality. Dover, New York

Fransella F, Bannister D (1977) A manual for repertory grid technique. Academic, London

Gendlin E (1978) Focusing. Everest, New York

Gordon D (1978) Therapeutic metaphors. Meta, Cuperin

Haug F (ed) (1983) Sexualisierung der Körper. Argument special edn 90, Frauenforum 2. Argument-Verlag, Berlin

Helm J (1954) Über den Einfluss affektiver Spannungen auf das Denkhandeln. Psychol 154 (1-2): 23-105

Hogarth RM (1980) Judgement and choice. The psychology of decision. Wiley, Chichester

Jäger AO (1967) Dimensionen der Intelligenz. Hogrefe, Göttingen

Jodelet D (1984) The representation of the body and its transformation. In: Farr RM, Moscovici S (eds) Social representation. Cambridge University Press, Cambridge, pp 211-238

Jones EJ (1983) Multidimensional models of social perception, cognition and behavior. Appl Psychol Measure 7 (4): 451-472

Kelley H (1983) Epiloque: Perceived causal structures. In: Jaspars J, Fincham F, Hewstone M (eds) Attribution theory and research: Conceptual, developmental and social dimensions. Academic, London, pp 388-415

Kelly G (1955) The psychology of personal constructs, vol 1. Norton, New York

Kohli M (1978) Offenes und geschlossenes Interview: Neue Argumente für eine alte Kontroverse. Soz Welt 78 (1): 1-25

Labov W (1972) Language in the inner city: Studies on black English vernacular. University of Pennsylvania Press, Philadelphia

Leithäuser T, Senghaas-Knobloch E, Volmberg B (1980) Arbeitserfahrung und Bewußtseinsbildung. Eine sozialpsychologische Untersuchung über die subjektive Bedeutung der Arbeit in sozialen Problemsituationen. Research report, University of Bremen

Leventhal H (1982) Illness cognition and the perceptual-motor theory of cognition. In: Clark MS, Fiske ST (eds) Affect and cognition. Lawrence, Hillsdale

Leventhal H, Meyer H, Nerenz D (1980) The common sense representation of illness danger. In: Rachman S (ed) Medical psychology, vol 2. Pergamon, New York, pp 7-30

Lowen A (1979) Bioenergetik. Rowohlt, Reinbek

Lowen A (1981) Körperausdruck und Persönlichkeit, Kösel, Munich

Mason RE (1959) Three studies relating internal sensory experiences to feeling reactions. J Gen Psychol 60: 211-228

Miller L, Murphy R, Buss A (1981) Consciousness of body: Private and public. J Pers Soc Psychol 41 (2): 397-406

Neisser M (1979) Kognition und Wirklichkeit. Klett-Cotta, Stuttgart

Paulus P (1982) Zur Erfahrung des eigenen Körpers. Beltz, Weinheim

Pennebaker JW (1982) The psychology of physical symptoms. Springer, Berlin Heidelberg New York

Perls F (1978) Gestalt-Therapie in Aktion. Klett-Cotta, Stuttgart

Pervin LA (1976) A free-response description approach to the analysis of person-situation interaction. J Pers Soc Psychol 34 (3): 465-474

Politzer G (1974) Kritik der klassischen Psychologie. Europäische Verlagsanstalt, Cologne

Rathod P (1981) Methods for the analysis of repgrid-data. In: Bonarius H, Holland R, Rosenberg S (eds) Personal construct psychology: Recent advances in theory and practices. Macmillan, London, pp 117-146

Schank RC (1982) Dynamic memory. A theory of reminding and learning in computers and people. Cambridge University Press, Cambridge

Schank RC, Abelson RP (1977) Scripts, plans, goals and understanding. Erlbaum, Hillsdale

Schütz A (1982) Das Problem der Relevanz. Suhrkamp, Frankfurt

Schütz A, Luckmann T (1973) The structures of life-world. North-Western University Press, Evanston

Schütze F (1976) Zur Hervorlockung und Analyse von Erzählungen thematisch relevanter Geschichten im Rahmen der soziologischen Feldforschung. In: Arbeitsgruppe Bielefelder Soziologen (eds) Kommunikative Sozialforschung. Fink, Munich, pp 159-260

Shields SA, Stern RM (1979) Emotion: The perception of bodily change. In: Pliner P, Blankenstein KR, Spigel M (eds) Emotion in self and others. Plenum, New York, pp 83-117

Shoben EJ (1983) Application of multidimensional scaling in cognitive psychology. Appl Psychol Measure 7 (4): 473-490

Shontz FC (1969) Perceptual and cognitive aspects of body experience. Academic, New York

Shontz FC (1974) Body image and its disorders. Int J Psychiatry Med 5: 461-472

Simonton OC, Matthews-Simonton S, Creighton JL (1978) Getting well again. Bantam, New York

Strauss B, Appelt H (1983) Ein Fragebogen zur Beurteilung des eigenen Körpers. Diagnostica 24: 145-164

Thomae H (1968) Das Individuum und seine Welt. Hogrefe, Göttingen

Thorbecke R (1979) Missglückte Handlungs- versus Krankheitssituationen. In: Sigrist J (ed) Wege zum Arzt. Urban and Schwarzenberg, Munich, pp 56-80

Wiedemann PM (1985) Deutungsmusteranalyse. In: Jüttemann G (ed) Qualitative Forschung in der Psychologie. Beltz, Weinheim (in Vorber.)

Wiedemann PM, Becker U (1986) The use of narrative data in social research. A contribution to methodology, conduct and analysis of qualitative interviews. Research report 82-2 from the Institute of Psychology, Technical University, Berlin

Wiedemann PM, Breckner R, Fliegener B, Janofske F, Tasche KG (1984) Zwischenbericht zum Forschungsbericht "Körpererleben in Tonräumen". Technical University, Berlin

Results Obtained with a Body Experience Questionnaire

B. Strauss and H. Appelt

Introduction

The Body Experience Questionnaire (BEQ, Strauss and Appelt, 1983a) was originally developed to test some specific hypotheses within a psychoendocrinological study of women suffering from hirsutism. Women suffering from this hormonal dysfunction (the chief symptom of which is the occurrence of masculine-type body hair growth) seemed to show some peculiarities in their body experience. This hypothesis is based upon two observations. One of these originated from some earlier studies of hirsutism (Meyer, 1963a), which revealed that the symptoms of body hair growth are experienced by the patients as extremely stressful. Meyer (1963a) showed that the distress may have far-reaching negative consequences for the patient's self esteem and even may lead to an avoidance of any social activity. Meyer called this phenomenon a 'complex of acceptance', referring to the fact that the perception of the body hair growth as a blemish restricts the acceptance of the person as a whole.

Another observation of importance originates from some physicians treating patients with hirsutism. According to these reports, the patients' description of the symptoms often differs from that given by the doctors, in that they tend to describe their symptoms as more pronounced than their doctors do (Strauss and Appelt 1984).

These observations raised the question of whether patients with hirsutism generally experience their body in a different way to other women, for instance in relation to their attractiveness, their identification with their body, and whether this special type of body experience might determine the patients' estimation of their symptoms as well as the effects the symptoms have on their self-esteem. Many authors have speculated about the peculiarities in the body experience of hirsute women; however, attempts to empirically test these hypotheses so far have been rare (see, e.g., Meyer 1963b; Ross et al. 1965).

Suitable methods for testing these hypotheses have been lacking. In the psychological literature, one can find different concepts related to the theory of body experience which are sometimes very imprecisely defined. Table 1 gives a systematic overview of these concepts and shows that two basic approaches can be differentiated. The construct of *body schema* is connected with a theory of perceptual psychology and describes the representation of the parts of the body and the body as a whole as perceived by the individual. The aim of empirical studies related to

Table 1. Theoretical concepts of body experience

A. Body schema	Perceptual theory Representation of the body and its parts in an individual's perception
B. Body image	Personality theory
a) Body awareness	Conscious, verbal representation of single body characteristics
b) Body boundary	Experience of the boundaries of the body
c) Body cathexis	Degree of satisfaction with the body and its parts
d) Body experience	Conscious experience of the body and attitude towards the body as a whole

this approach is mainly the objectification of the subjective body perception (examples of these studies concern the body schema of patients with eating disorders such as obesity or anorexia nervosa that are reviewed by Meermann and Fichter, 1982). One of the methods used to measure body schema is described by Askevold (1975).

Personality theories of body experience are mainly linked with the construct of *body image* (see Kiener 1973). The concepts of body awareness, body boundary, body cathexis and body experience belong in this category.

According to Fisher (1970), the term *body awareness* describes the conscious verbal representation of single body characteristics. Fisher developed different methods to assess this construct, such as the 'body prominence score' or the 'body focus questionnaire' (Fisher 1970).

The concept of *body boundary* has been extensively described by Fisher and Cleveland (1958). This concept is part of a comprehensive theory of personality development and describes the extent to which an individual feels distinct from his or her environment. As a method to assess body boundary, Fisher and Cleveland suggested a projective test such as the Rorschach or the Holtzman Inkblot Technique. Based upon the answers to these tests, scores are calculated describing the degree to which a person is 'sealed off' vs. 'permeable' in relation to his or her body.

The term *body cathexis* was introduced by Secord and Jourard (1953). It describes the degree of satisfaction with the body and with single parts of the body. Secord and Jourard developed a questionnaire providing a systematic assessment of the degree of satisfaction felt in association with different body parts.

The last of the personality theory constructs is that of *body experience* in its narrowest sense, which describes the conscious experience of the body and a person's attitude towards their own body as a whole. An attempt to assess this concept empirically is described by Paulus (1982). The concept seemed to be most relevant for the questions formulated above and of special significance for the study of the importance of body image in psychosomatic patients.

The Body Experience Questionnaire

The development of the present form of the BEQ is described in detail by Strauss and Appelt (1983a). A sample of 527 women and men filled out an earlier version of the questionnaire, developed by Cormann and Holtschoppen (1978). The present version comprises 52 items, forming three factorially derived subscales (Table 2).

The first subscale, *'Insecurity/discomfort'*, is defined by 19 items. It covers mainly negative aspects of body experience, such as the expression of a lack of sensitivity (mainly with respect to sexuality), insecurity and a rejection of one's own physical appearance and of the reactions of one's body.

The second subscale, *'Attractiveness/self-confidence'*, comprises 13 items relating to a more positive evaluation of the body, including expressions of satisfaction with the body, the identification with one's own physical appearance, body shape and different individual body characteristics. They further comprise statements related to confidence in the body and its reactions.

Finally, the third subscale defined by 20 items, is called *'Accentuation of the body/sensitivity'*, and deals with the importance of the exterior of the body and of body care. The body's effect on others, sensitivity to physical appearance and body reactions, and personal health care are all expressed in these items.

Analyses of the scales provided satisfactory psychometric characteristics (Strauss and Appelt, 1983a). Results obtained with the BEQ concerning the correlations of single scales with other variables, and the use of the questionnaire in studies with different clinical and nonclinical groups of subjects, are summarized below.

Table 2. Marker items of the three subscales of the BEQ (+/− coding of the items)

Subscale: Insecurity/Discomfort	
29. There often seems to be a sort of blockage in my sexual feelings	+
52. I am perfectly content with my sexual responses	−
3. I can rely on my body	−
40. I often wish I could feel more	+
38. I often imagine I'm going to hurt myself	+
Subscale: Attractivenes/self-confidence	
27. I am content with my figure	+
48. I am proud of my body	+
34. It is hard for me to believe that others find me attractive	−
31. I am attractive	+
Subscale: Accentuation of the body/sensitivity	
16. I often look in the mirror	+
30. When I'm not looking good, I don't feel right	+
21. I enjoy looking at myself and often do so	+
47. I have often been hurt by remarks about my body	+
6. If something is troubling me, it has a marked effect on my body	+

Results

Correlations with Other Variables

The following results are based upon studies with four different subgroups and relate to several correlations of the subscales of the BEQ with other characteristics.

Sixty-four men and women filled out the BEQ and rated their psychological wellbeing using an adjective checklist (*Eigenschaftswörterliste,* Janke and Debus 1978). They also answered in a questionnaire related to their 'present body experience' (*momentanes Körpererleben,* Baumann and Rathje, unpublished work; Table 3). The latter serves to assess situation-dependent judgements of the body experience, especially related to sensations of different body parts. The questionnaire comprises the subscales 'faintness', 'liveliness', 'activation' and 'tension' with items such as 'My knees tremble', 'I can feel all my bones', or 'My head is very clear.' The original purpose of this questionnaire was the differentiation of body experience in specific situations. In the present context the questionnaire was presented with a general instruction: 'Please indicate how you experience your body generally.'

Table 3. Correlations of the subscales of the BEQ with other variables

Insecurity/discomfort
+ Bodily complaints (GBB)
Tension (MK)
Irritability (EWL)
Nervousness (FPI)
− Self-assertiveness (Rathus)
Liveliness (MK)
Self-assertiveness (EWL)
(Males) masculinity (FPI)
Nonconformity with sex role (SAQ)
Attractiveness/self-confidence
+ Liveliness (MK)
Extraversion (FPI)
Nonconformity with sex role (SAQ)
− Tension (MK)
Accentuation of the body/sensitivity
+ Bodily complaints (GBB)
Irritability (EWL)
Nervousness (FPI)
Depression (FPI)
Arousability (FPI)
Neuroticism (FPI)
− Self-assertiveness (EWL)
(Males) masculinity (FPI)

GBB, Giessen subjective complaints list; MK, questionnaire on present body experience; FPI, Freiburg personality inventory; Rathus, Self-assertiveness scale; SAQ, sexual attitude questionnaire

\+ Significant positive correlation
− Significant negative correlation

In another study, 85 men and women answered the BEQ and the large version of the Freiburg Personality Inventory (FPI, Fahrenberg et al. 1978). A small group of 29 men and women filled out the BEQ together with the German version of the Rathus self-assertiveness scale (Rathus 1973) and the Giessen Subjective Complaints List (Giessener Beschwerdenbogen, Brähler and Scheer 1983). Finally, the BEQ was used in a study serving to reconstruct and validate the Menstrual Attitude Questionnaire (MAQ, Brooks-Gunn and Ruble 1979), in a sample of 220 women (Strauss et al. 1987). In this study correlations were calculated between the subscales of the BEQ, the five German scales of the MAQ, the GBB (see above) and a sexual attitude questionnaire developed by Arentewicz et al. (1975).

The German version of the MAQ comprises the scales 'menstruation as handicap', 'positive view of menstruation', 'denial of any effect of menstruation', 'menstruation as an impairment of sexuality' and 'menstruation as an impairment of wellbeing.' The sexual attitude questionnaire consists of the subscales 'permissiveness', 'nonconformity to sex role', and 'romanticism'.

The direction of the significant correlations of the three BEQ scales with the other variables are summarized in Table 3. As the table shows, there were significant associations of the body experience scales with most of the other variables. An exception was the MAQ. There were some significant correlations, but with a very small proportion of common variance. Further relations between body experience and specific experiences of menstruation are extensively described by Strauss et al. (1987); Lange (1985).

Studies of Different Subgroups

Nonclinical groups

One important finding in the development of the questionnaire was a significant difference between the response of men and women in the subscales 'Accentuation of the body sensitivity' and 'Insecurity/Discomfort'. Women generally expressed more insecurity in their body experience as well as more emphasis on their appearance and they described themselves as more sensitive than men. No sex differences in the estimation of the attractiveness and satisfaction with the body were revealed.

On the basis of this result, care was taken in the studies reported below to match groups according to their sex, and also according to age and socio-economic status, variables that have also been shown to influence evaluation of body experience (Strauss and Appelt 1983 a).

In the meantime, results of different subgroups of healthy subjects were obtained with the BEQ. In a first investigation, women were studied who used different methods of contraception (155 using the diaphragm, 78 taking the pill, and 33 using the intrauterine device; cf. Appelt et al. 1984; Appelt and Strauss 1985; Table 4). In a further study, psychological intolerance of the contraceptive pill was investigated in 106 students using hormonal contraception as compared to a matched group of students who had stopped taking the pill at least 6 months previously ($n = 85$; for details see Ulrich et al. 1987). In all these studies, the hypothesis tested was if women who decided to use 'natural' contraceptives showed a more conscious body experience than those taking hormonal contraceptives. The

Table 4. Overview of different groups investigated with the questionnaire

'Nonclinical' groups		
Women using various contraceptives		
diaphragm	$n = 155$	
pill	$n = 78$	
IUD	$n = 33$	
'Pill-takers' vs. 'pill-stoppers' (students)		
pill-takers	$n = 105$	
pill-stoppers	$n = 85$	
Participants in yoga and fitnessgroups		
yoga	$n = 20$	
fitness	$n = 20$	
controls	$n = 20$	
'Clinical' groups	Women	Men
Hirsutism (50 treated, 50 untreated)	$n = 100$	
Anorexia nervosa	$n = 27$	
Obesity	$n = 15$	
Sexual dysfunctions	$n = 23$	$n = 20$
Alcoholism	$n = 50$	

Table 5. Mean values of scales for several clinical and nonclinical subgroups

Groups	*n*	Insecurity/ discomfort Mean (SD)	Attractiveness/ Self-confidence Mean (SD)	Accentuation of the body/ sensitivity Mean (SD)
Initial sample				
Total	527	5.32 (4.09)	8.91 (2.91)	11.11 (3.77)
Women	364	5.76 (4.09)	8.95 (2.97)	11.83 (3.62)
Men	163	4.36 (3.70)	8.80 (2.79)	9.54 (3.62)
Nonclinical groups				
Diaphragm	155	5.20 (3.17)	9.81 (2.69)	13.20 (3.14)
Pill	78	5.17 (3.95)	9.34 (3.21)	12.44 (3.35)
IUD	33	5.08 (3.17)	9.05 (2.77)	12.41 (3.05)
'Pill-takers'	85	4.33 (2.98)	9.55 (2.94)	12.46 (3.17)
'Pill-stoppers'	105	4.81 (3.24)	9.47 (2.83)	11.94 (3.35)
Yoga group	20	4.10 (2.63)	8.65 (3.01)	11.60 (2.76)
Fitness group	20	5.15 (3.23)	8.55 (3.41)	11.95 (3.22)
(MC)	20	5.55 (3.47)	9.63 (2.14)	11.60 (3.24)
Clinical groups				
Hirsutes, treated	50	7.02 (4.07)	6.50 (3.22)	11.57 (2.61)
Hirsutes, untreated	50	8.17 (5.10)	5.70 (3.98)	12.33 (3.49)
(MC)	50	4.86 (3.20)	9.04 (3.79)	13.28 (3.12)
Anorectics	27	8.86 (3.57)	5.04 (2.49)	11.88 (3.11)
(MC)	27	4.36 (2.88)	9.92 (3.01)	12.23 (3.24)
Obese women	15	6.85 (2.98)	3.58 (3.01)	12.67 (3.68)
(MC)	15	5.70 (3.14)	7.50 (2.33)	11.05 (3.41)
Sexual dysfunctions				
Women	23	9.13 (3.75)	8.19 (3.09)	12.18 (3.68)
Men	20	5.26 (3.19)	9.35 (2.76)	9.65 (3.80)
Alcoholic women	50	7.70 (4.50)	6.02 (3.64)	13.72 (2.68)
(MC)	50	5.82 (3.99)	8.53 (3.34)	11.78 (3.33)

MC, matched controls

results (Table 5) contradicted this hypothesis; no differences between the groups were obtained.

A further hypothesis was tested in groups of men and women participating in yoga ($n=20$) and fitnessgroups ($n=20$). Both groups were compared with a matched control group. It was suggested that persons who are specially concerned with their bodies in their leisure time should have a more positive body experience than the controls. This assumption too proved untenable (see Table 5). In none of the three subscales significant differences revealed. All the results indicate that the BEQ seems to be of limited value for discrimination between groups of healthy subjects.

Clinical groups

The most important results concerning different clinical groups are summarized in Table 5 and Fig. 3.

Women Suffering from Hirsutism. Two groups of hirsute women, each comprising 50 Patients, were investigated with the BEQ. One group was being treated with anti-androgens at the time of the study; the second group was not receiving any medication at that time (Strauss and Appelt, 1983b). Both groups were compared with matched controls recruited from gynaecological out-patient clinics. The results indicate that both patient groups differed significantly from the controls in the subscales 'Insecurity/discomfort' (showing higher values than the controls) and 'Attractiveness/self-confidence' (showing lower values than the controls). Patients treated with anti-androgens also showed significantly lower values in the

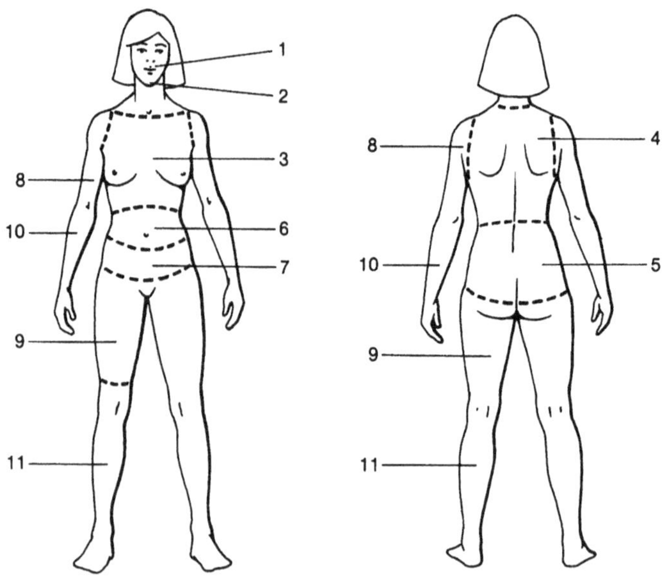

Fig. 1. Chart for the assessment of body hair growth (Ferriman and Gallwey 1961). For each of the eleven parts of the body, the degree of hair growth has to be rated on a 7-point scale. Patients are also asked to judge the distress caused by the symptoms on the individual body parts

third subscale (Accentuation of the body/sensitivity) as compared to the control group without hirsutism.

In the study of hirsutism, relations between the patients' body experience and their estimation of the symptoms, i.e. the degree of body hair growth, were of special interest. The symptom ratings were performed using a modified form of the chart developed by Ferriman and Gallwey (1961; Fig. 1). For 11 separate parts of the body, patients were asked to judge their symptoms as well as the distress caused by the symptoms on 7-point scales. The correlation of the symptom ratings and the ratings of the distress (averaged for 11 body parts) and the scores in the subscale 'Attractivenes/self-confidence' was negative ($r = -0.36$ for the symptom ratings; $r = -0.38$ for the distress ratings; $p < 0.05$). A significant positive correlation of both aspects was found with the subscale 'Accentuation of the body/sensitivity' ($r = 0.42$ for the symptom ratings; $r = 0.37$ for the distress ratings; $p = < 0.05$). This result, together with those of the group comparisons, indicates that the hypothesis of some peculiarities in the body experience of hirsute women may be seen as confirmed (see Strauss and Appelt 1984).

Women with Anorexia Nervosa and Obesity. The results related to different groups of patients with eating disorders are described in detail by Strauss and Appelt (1983a). Twenty-seven patients with anorexia nervosa who were investigated with the BEQ differed significantly from a matched control group in the aspects 'Insecurity/discomfort' (considerably higher values) and 'Attractiveness/self-confidence' (considerably lower values). A group of obese women ($n = 15$) treated in group therapy differed from matched controls only in the subscale 'Attractiveness/self-confidence'. The obese women rated their attractiveness significantly lower.

Males and Females with Sexual Dysfunctions. Groups of women ($n = 23$) and men ($n = 20$) with various sexual dysfunctions were also investigated with the questionnaire. The results reveal that men as well as women showed more insecurity and discomfort than a control group, but were not different in the other two subscales. In this group a study of changes in body experience during a psychotherapy was performed separately. 10 couples who participated in couples therapy according to Arentewicz and Schmidt (1980) for 3 weeks (massed therapy) filled out the questionnaire at the beginning and at the end of the treatment. In each couple one partner was declared as having the symptom. The other did not reveal any sexual disturbance. Pre/post comparisons (t Tests) of the scale values of these two groups showed that, during the course of therapy, the persons with the symptom drew closer to their partners' values in the subscales 'Insecurity/discomfort' and 'Attractiveness/self-confidence', thus showing significant changes in these aspects (Fig. 2). In the third scale no significant pre/post differences were obtained. It might be of interest that the partners without symptoms did not show any changes in their body experience during the 3 weeks of treatment.

Alcoholic Women. In a further study, investigating the sexual history and sexual life of women alcoholics (Scherotzki-Hanninger et al. 1986), the BEQ was also included. Comparisons with a control group of women (gynaecological patients

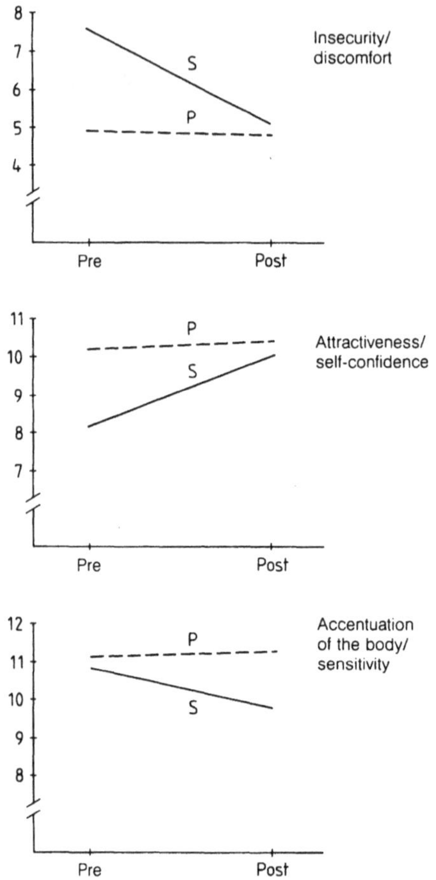

Fig. 2. Body experience measured at the beginning and end of a 3-week couple therapy. S, partner presenting the sexual symptom; P, Partner without sexual dysfunction. Pre/post differences were statistically significant for the partners with symptoms in the first two subscales ($p < 0.05$)

matched according to age and socio-economic status) revealed that alcoholics showed slightly higher values in the subscale ‚Insecurity/discomfort' and slightly lower values for 'Attractiveness/self-confidence'. These differences did not reach statistical significance. The only significant difference was found in the third scale (accentuation of the body/sensitivity), where the alcoholics showed higher values than the controls.

Discussion and prospects

The results reported indicate that the BEQ could be suitable for differentiating between clinical groups and normal controls (Fig. 3). The content of the subscale 'Insecurity/discomfort' seems to be of special importance for psychosomatic patients and for women suffering from hirsutism, whereas the subscale 'Attractiveness/self-confidence' mainly differentiates out those groups who have visible symptoms (such as hirsute women and anorectics and obese patients).

Based upon their scores in the subscale 'Accentuation of the body/sensitivity', only hirsute women and female alcoholics differed from matched controls. It should be noted that this subscale is the most heterogeneous one.

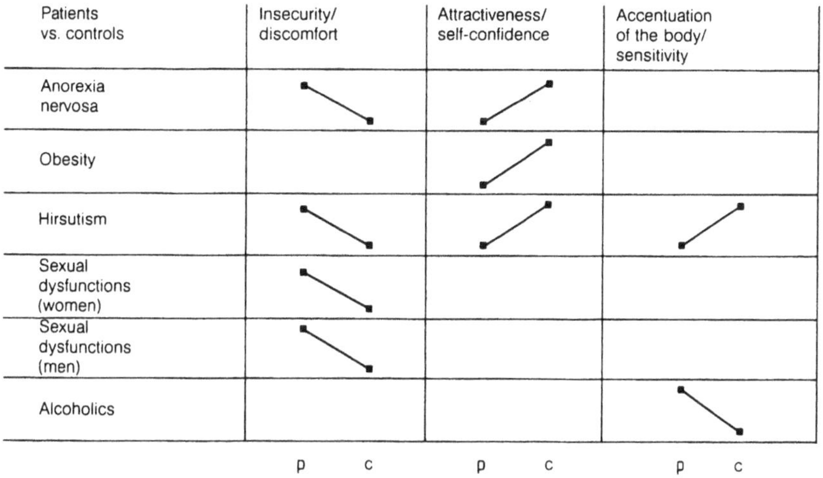

Fig. 3. Summary of several comparisons of clinical groups (p) and matched controls (c) for each subscale of the BEQ. The figure shows the directions of significant group differences ($p < 0.05$; *t* Tests)

In summary, it can be concluded that the questionnaire obviously covers some aspects of body experience that are of clinical relevance. These aspects are possibly sensitive for psychotherapeutic interventions, as the pre/post comparisons of the patients with sexual dysfunctions showed. Discussion of the single aspects covered by the items of the BEQ has been shown to be useful in therapies with groups of patients suffering from eating disorders. Group comparisons of single items of the questionnaire might also be fruitful (see Strauss and Appelt 1984). The further use of the BEQ in studies aiming to characterize psychosomatic and psychiatric patients and their treatment might be most promising for the future.

Acknowledgement. This work was supported by the Deutsche Forschungsgemeinschaft, SFB 115, Project C 24.

References

Appelt H, Strauss B (1985) Die Verhütungskarriere von Frauen, die Pille, Spirale oder Diaphragma als Kontrazeptionsmethode benutzen. In: Bericht über den 34. Kongress der Deutschen Gesellschaft für Psychologie in Wien 1984. Hogrefe, Göttingen

Appelt H, Strauss B, Iendra A, Schneider D (1984) Erfahrungen mit dem Diaphragma. Sexualpad Familienplanung 12: 6-26

Arentewicz G, Schmidt G (1980) Sexuell gestörte Beziehungen, Springer, Berlin Heidelberg New York

Arentewicz G, Bulla R, Schoof-Tams U, Schorsch E (1975) Verhaltenstherapie sexueller Funktionsstörungen. In: Schorsch E, Schmidt G (eds) Ergebnisse zur Sexualforschung. Kiepenheuer und Witsch, Cologne

Askevold F (1975) Measuring body image. Psychother Psychosom 26: 71-77

Brähler E, Scheer J (1983) Der Giessener Beschwerdebogen (GBB). Huber, Bern

Brooks-Gunn J, Ruble D (1979) The menstrual attitude questionnaire. Psychosom Med 42: 503-512

Cormann G, Holtschoppen U (1978) Dimensionen des subjektiven Körpererlebens. Thesis, Marburg University

Fahrenberg J, Selg H, Hampel R (1978) Das Freiburger Persönlichkeitsinventar, 3rd edn. Hogrefe, Göttingen

Ferriman D, Gallwey JD (1961) Clinical assessment of body hair growth in women. J Clin Endocrinol 21: 1440-1447

Fisher S (1970) Body experience in fantasy and behaviour. Appleton-Century-Croft, New York

Fisher S, Cleveland SE (1958) Body image and personality. Van Nostrand, Princetown

Janke W, Debus G (1978) Die Eigenschaftswörterliste. Hogrefe, Göttingen

Kanfer FH, Goldstein AP (1977) Möglichkeiten der Verhaltensänderung. Urban und Schwarzenberg, Munich

Kiener F (1973) Untersuchungen zum Körperbild. Z Klin Psychol Psychother 21: 335-351

Lange C (1985) Validierung eines Fragebogens 'Einstellung zur Menstruation'. Thesis, Hamburg University

Meermann R, Fichter MM (1982) Störungen des Körperschemas (Body Image) bei psychischen Krankheiten - Methodik und experimentelle Ergebnisse bei Anorexia nervosa. Psychother Med Psychosom 32: 162-169

Meyer AE (1963 a) Zur Endokrinologie und Psychologie intersexueller Frauen. Enke, Stuttgart

Meyer AE (1963 b) Körperstörungen und Sexualität, dargestellt am Beispiel des genuinen Hirsutismus. Prax Psychother 8: 1-7

Paulus P (1982) Zur Erfahrung des eigenen Körpers. Beltz, Weinheim

Rathus SA (1973) A 30-item schedule for assessing assertive behaviour. Behav Ther 4: 398-406

Ross JR, Mastrodanato RA, Cassell WA et al. (1965) Psychological problems associated with hirsutism. Int Psychiatr Clin 2: 625-640

Scherotzki-Hanninger F, Appelt H, Strauss B (1986) Sexuelle Erfahrungen alkoholabhängiger Frauen. Suchtgef 32: 386-399

Secord PF, Jourard SM (1953) The appraisal of body cathexis and the self. J Consult Psychol 17: 343-347

Strauss B, Appelt H (1983 a) Ein Fragebogen zur Beurteilung des eigenen Körpers. Diagnostica 29: 145-164

Strauss B, Appelt H (1983 b) Antiandrogene in der Gynäkologie. Sexualmedizin 12: 515-518

Strauss B, Appelt H (1984) Psychologische Einflüsse auf die Beurteilung körperlicher Symptome am Beispiel des Hirsutismus. Psychother Med Psychol 34: 179-185

Strauss B, Appelt H, Lange C (1987) Deutsche Neukonstruktion und Validierung des 'Menstrual attitude questionnaire'. Psychother Med Psychol 37: 175-182

Ulrich D, Appelt H, Strauss B (1987) Eine empirische Untersuchung zum Phänomen der Pillenmüdigkeit. Psychother Med Psychol 37: 322-333

The Body and Its Complaints: A Review of Findings Using the Giessen Subjective Complaints List

E. Brähler and P. Möhring

Introduction

Even when expressing itself throug complaints, our body remains our own personal body, but in a special way. As self-reflective beings we can recognize the double function it has for us: we are a body and we have one. We can feel ourselves in our bodies; if we have complaints, we feel unwell. In the early stages of childhood, with growing maturity, we achieve the degree of distance to our bodies necessary for the development of symbolization and speech. With increasing alienation, we long for sensations and perceptions that help keep alive our awareness of our physical being. But somatic complaints are troublesome. They may reassure us that our bodies are still there, but they have a way of imposing themselves. Ailments are experienced at uncomfortably close quarters and are a clear expression of the fact that something is wrong, Psychotherapists have an ear for their patients' complaints – they try to understand their significance for the individual. They are used to seeing more than an organic dysfunction or lesion behind each ailment. They are familiar with the many ways in which problems in peoples' lives find expression through their bodies. Thus, a person's description of their health troubles takes on a psychological dimension: in the manner in which it is presented as a complaint, as an articulation of body-centredness, it tells us something about each individual's special relationship with his or her body. It is a subjective statement which does not necessarily correspond to an objective finding. Whilst traditional medicine generally defines health and disease through the presence or absence of objective organic findings, as far as the patient is concerned these things are necessarily linked up with the complaints that he or she experiences subjectively (see Brähler and Scheer 1984).

In recent years, numerous questionnaires for recording physical complaints have been developed and in some cases empirically tested (see, e.g., the reviews in Brähler and Scheer 1983, Fahrenberg 1983). Some of these have similar origins and certain features in common, whilst others are extremely heterogeneous with respect to their administration and objectives. Some have only been used a few times and others have become quite popular, e.g., in Germany, the *B-L-Liste* by von Zerssen (1971, 1976), the *Freiburger Beschwerdenliste* (known as the FBL) by Fahrenberg (1975) and the *Beschwerdefragebogen* (Höck and Hess 1975). For the FBL, group comparisons and other validity studies have been published (Hampel and Fahrenberg 1982).

This chapter offers a review of the results obtained so far with an instrument which has become very widespread in German-speaking countries and is now available in English translation as the 'Giessen Subjective Complaints List', or GSCL (in German, *Giessener Beschwerdebogen* or GBB, formerly BSB). It takes the form of a checklist, which was developed out of an early form of another German questionnaire, the *HHM-Liste* (Kerekjarto et al. 1972; Zenz 1971). It contains 57 items covering the areas of general physical wellbeing, functional complaints, pains and emotionality. The subject is asked to estimate the degree of discomfort caused by each of the 57 complaints listed (in columns headed 'not at all', 'slightly', 'somewhat', 'considerably' and 'very much'). The data from a sample of 4076 patients seen in the Clinic for Psychosomatics in Giessen, Federal Republic of Germany, between 1968 and 1975 and from a representative sample of 1601 other West Germans was evaluated using factor and item analysis, which produced 4 scales containing 6 items each and an overall score made up of the sum of these 24 items.

The scales are:

(E) - Exhaustion
(G) - Gastric complaints
(L) - Pains in limbs
(C) - Cardiac complaints
(D) - Overall distress

The first 4 scales have a range of possible scores extending from a minimum of 0 to a maximum of 24, whilst the fifth scale has a maximum score of 96.

For the German version of the GSCL, a test handbook (Brähler and Scheer 1983), a book of tables listing empirical findings (Brähler et al. 1983), and a discussion of various individual aspects (Brähler and Scheer 1984) have been published. In the present chapter, all the results obtained so far will be summarized and some of them discussed in more depth. The mass of material makes certain restrictions necessary, however, and the quantities of numbers may appear daunting at first. Nevertheless, we are convinced that a comprehensive survey of the data will help individual users to place their own results in better perspective and acquaint the general reader with the entire field in which the nature and degree of bodily complaints has been found to be of significance. Particular emphasis is placed on somatic complaints in the context of partner relationships. Many results from single applications in specialized fields are not included; most of these can be found in the references quoted.

Results of Sample Studies with the GSCL

Tables 1-3 show the means for the 5 scales of the GSCL, obtained from studies carried out by ourselves and others. Numerous further investigations have not been included, either because too little information was available to us or because the samples were too small, taking into account the relative accessibility of the group of patients involved. At the same time, the tables provide a useful survey of the areas in which the GSCL is most commonly applied. It is used most frequently in work with psychosomatic and psychoneurotic patients, for investigating various

Table 1. Profile of GSCL scale means for women

	Source	Scale					
		n	E	G	L	C	D
Peptic ulcer (Frankfurt) (M)	[68]	14	10.7	10.6	12.9	8.3	42.6
Psychosom. clinic Heidelberg (in-patients) I (M)	[24]	22	13.0	9.8	10.1	9.1	42.0
Mixed psychosom./psychoneur. (Frankfurt) (M)	[67]	62	12.5	6.9	10.7	9.3	39.4
Depression (Bad Berleburg) (M)	[35]	59	12.4	5.8	9.0	9.4	36.7
Psychosom. clinic Heidelberg (catamnesis) II (M)	[24]	22	11.0	8.5	8.2	7.6	35.4
Psychosom. disorders (Frankfurt) (M)	[67]	60	10.8	6.2	9.4	7.1	33.5
Headache patients (Heidelberg) (M)	[32]	36	8.8	6.2	13.7	4.8	33.5
Turkish gynaecol. patients (Hamburg)	[73]	76	9.8	5.3	10.4	7.4	32.9
Psychosom./psychother. out-patients (Ulm) (M)	[39]	494	10.9	5.5	8.6	7.6	32.6
Sanatorium Bad Nauheim (admission) I (M)	[12]	73	11.3	4.4	9.2	6.9	31.9
Headache patients (Giessen) (M)	[80]	25	8.4	6.3	13.4	3.6	31.8
Lipometabolic disorders (without infarction)	[48]	44	8.6	5.6	11.3	6.1	31.5
Psychosom./psychother. out-patients Giessen (M)	[15]	2011	10.7	8.0	5.4	7.0	31.2
Psychosom. clinic Giessen (in-patients) (M)	[41]	20	10.4	4.6	7.7	8.4	31.0
Cardiovalvular surgery (catamnesis) (M)	[44]	85	9.3	4.2	9.2	7.6	30.2
Cardiosurgery (pre-operative) I (M)	[23]	21	8.2	5.8	7.1	9.1	30.2
Pituitary adenoma surgery (M)	[74]	23	10.5	4.8	9.8	4.7	29.8
Cardiosurgery (6 years catamnesis) III (M)	[54]	18	8.5	4.8	8.4	8.1	29.8
Cardiac catheter (M)	[76]	21	9.5	3.0	8.3	8.7	29.5
Wives of coronary patients with operation	[7]	10	7.7	6.1	10.6	5.0	29.4
Women after hysterectomy (Vienna)	[63]	33	7.4	6.3	9.7	5.3	28.6
Women after curretage or gall bladder op. (Vienna)	[63]	118	7.8	4.6	9.7	5.8	27.8
Genital carcenoma (5-10 years survival) (P)	[61]	46	8.0	4.1	10.0	5.3	27.4
Wives of coronary patients without operation	[7]	15	6.5	4.3	11.0	5.1	26.9
Rectectomy (Marburg) (P)	[55]	40	7.6	3.5	9.1	6.7	26.8
Psychother. student counselling Giessen (M)	[12]	498	10.4	4.9	5.9	5.5	26.2
Cardiac infarction (discharge from intensive care) (M)	[49]	11	9.6	3.6	6.8	5.9	25.9
Vascular disease (M)	[9]	18	7.4	3.6	8.8	4.7	24.5
Genital carcinoma (10 years survival) (P)	[62]	60	6.6	4.2	9.1	4.5	24.4
Arthritis (M)	[5]	61	7.4	2.9	10.9	3.2	24.3
Hysterectomy, post-operative (Marburg)	[83]	41	5.2	3.6	9.6	5.1	23.5
Partners of peptic ulcer patients (Frankfurt)	[68]	45	7.3	4.1	6.9	5.1	23.4
Wives of men with cardiac infarction	[7]	25	6.1	3.4	9.2	4.4	23.1
Couples psychotherapy Vienna (P)	[70]	60	7.8	3.0	6.4	5.2	22.3
Cardiosurgery (post-operative) II (M)	[23]	21	8.5	3.5	6.0	4.2	22.1
Couples group, waiting list (P)	[57]	38	8.3	3.4	5.8	4.4	21.9
Secondary amenorrhoea	[8]	26	7.5	3.1	6.4	4.9	21.9
Sanatorium Bad Nauheim (discharge) II (M)	[12]	73	7.9	3.1	6.3	4.3	21.5
Couples psychotherapy Giessen (P)	[12]	170	7.3	3.4	5.6	4.6	21.0
Women before brief couples psychotherapy I (P)	[82]	38	7.3	3.1	6.3	3.8	20.6
Gynaecological practice	[50]	48	5.4	3.9	7.3	4.0	20.5
General practice (M)	[16]	53	5.7	2.9	7.6	3.9	20.1
Schoolgirls 12-14 years (M)	[85]	61	5.9	3.4	5.4	4.9	19.7
Partners of patients with testicular carcinoma	[61]	57	5,5	3.3	7.1	3.8	19.7
Expectant mothers	[83]	50	6.8	3.0	6.5	3.0	18.5
Standard sample (M)	[9]	834	5.6	2.7	6.5	3.4	18.2
Gynaecol. out-patients dept. (Marburg)	[83]	62	4.2	2.9	7.5	3.5	18.1
Partners of psychosom. in-patients (Giessen)	[41]	23	5.6	2.7	6.0	3.8	18.1
Married couples, representative sample (P)	[9]	201	5.2	2.7	6.3	3.0	17.2
Women after brief couples psychotherapy II (M)	[82]	38	6.8	2.2	5.9	2.4	17.2
Menstrual disorders (Marburg)	[83]	31	4.5	3.6	5.7	3.2	17.0
Mothers of disturbed children (family ther. out-pats.) (M)	[64]	152	4.6	2.0	5.9	3.2	15.7
Hormone therapy out-pats. (Marburg)	[83]	23	5.4	2.4	5.3	2.4	15.5
Infertile couples (P)	[11]	25	4.6	2.4	5.6	2.8	15.4
Ante-natal clinic (Marburg)	[83]	32	4.2	3.3	4.0	2.0	13.6
Birth control clinic (Marburg)	[83]	20	2.6	2.4	6.1	2.5	13.5
Swiss women (Zürich) (P)	[33]	220	3.1	1.1	4.0	1.4	9.7
Women seeking refertilization (P)	[56]	37	2.9	1.2	2.7	1.3	8.1
Couples seeking artificial insemination (P)	[11]	25	2.5	1.0	2.6	1.4	7.5

Table 2. Profile of GSCL scale means for men

	Source	Scale					
		n	E	G	L	C	D
Psychosom. clinic Giessen (in-patient) (F)	[41]	23	12.2	8.0	10.4	10.4	41.0
Coronary patients without operation (P)	[7]	15	11.1	4.1	10.7	13.5	39.3
Depression (Bad Berleburg) (F)	[35]	63	12.0	6.5	9.5	8.8	36.9
Sanatorium Bad Nauheim (admission) I (F)	[12]	27	12.4	5.1	10.2	6.9	34.6
Mixed psychosom./psychoneur. (Frankfurt) (F)	[67]	39	10.4	7.2	9.2	7.6	34.5
Headache patients (Heidelberg) (F)	[32]	13	9.8	4.6	14.8	4.6	33.8
Lipometabolic disorders (with infarction)	[48]	22	9.3	4.1	9.2	10.8	33.3
Psychosomatic disorders (Frankfurt) (F)	[67]	46	9.9	6.3	7.3	8.7	32.2
Psychosom. clinic Heidelberg (in-patients) I (F)	[24]	24	9.6	6.5	8.7	6.9	31.7
Cardiac pacemakers (8 months catamnesis) II	[34]	22	8.9	4.9	8.8	7.3	29.8
Peptic ulcer (Frankfurt) (P)	[68]	45	6.3	9.4	8.1	5.3	29.9
Cardiovalvular surgery (catamnesis) (F)	[44]	111	9.2	4.1	7.1	8.2	28.6
Cardiac catheter (F)	[76]	48	7.4	4.8	7.6	8.6	28.3
Multiple sclerosis	[53]	23	11.7	3.7	9.4	3.5	28.1
Psychosom./psychother. out-patients (Ulm) (F)	[39]	411	9.2	5.1	7.1	6.4	27.7
Headache patients (Giessen) (F)	[80]	14	7.8	4.6	11.6	3.3	27.2
Bechterew's disease	[5]	27	7.4	2.6	11.3	5.1	26.5
Psychosom./psychother. out-patients Giessen (F)	[15]	2045	8.7	6.3	5.4	6.2	26.5
Cardiac infarction (9 months catamnesis) III	[49]	20	6.7	2.0	9.4	7.5	25.6
Cardiosurgery (6 years catamnesis) III (F)	[54]	33	8.5	2.8	6.6	7.3	25.2
Duodenal ulcer (pre-operative) I	[26]	76	6.0	9.5	5.3	4.0	24.8
Cardiac pacemakers (2 months catamnesis) I	[34]	22	7.7	4.4	6.5	5.4	24.0
Psychosom. clinic Heidelberg (catamnesis) II (F)	[24]	24	7.7	4.0	5.8	4.8	22.3
Sanatorium Bad Nauheim (discharge) II (F)	[12]	27	8.3	3.4	5.9	4.4	22.1
Psychother. student counselling Giessen (F)	[12]	591	8.4	4.0	4.4	4.5	21.3
Duodenal ulcer (4 years post-operative) II	[60]	33	5.0	5.8	6.1	4.5	21.3
Partners of genital carcinoma survivors (10 years)	[62]	60	5.3	3.7	7.3	5.0	21.3
Vascular diseases (F)	[9]	56	5.8	3.4	7.7	4.0	20.8
Coronary patients with operation (P)	[7]	10	5.6	2.5	6.0	6.6	20.7
Lipometabolic disorders (without infarction)	[48]	32	6.3	3.1	6.7	4.4	20.4
Cardiac infarction (P)	[7]	25	6.5	2.1	6.4	5.5	20.4
Cardiosurgery (pre-operative) I (F)	[23]	29	5.5	2.3	4.2	7.4	19.5
Partners of genital carcinoma survivors (5 years)	[61]	46	4.6	3.2	7.9	3.6	19.3
Arthritis (F)	[5]	26	5.8	1.7	8.8	2.9	19.2
Partners of rectectomy patients (Marburg)	[55]	40	4.3	3.4	7.2	4.0	18.9
General practice (F)	[16]	56	4.4	3.9	6.5	3.3	18.1
Cardiosurgery (post-operative) II (F)	[23]	29	6.5	1.8	5.4	4.1	17.8
Testicular carcinoma (5-year survival) (P)	[61]	57	5.7	3.4	5.7	2.9	17.6
Kidney stones	[69]	27	4.2	3.5	6.1	3.7	17.4
Prostatitis	[14]	101	4.7	3.1	6.5	2.8	17.1
Cardiac infarction (discharge intensive care) I (F)	[24]	29	7.8	1.8	3.9	3.4	16.9
Pituitary adenoma surgery (F)	[74]	20	6.5	2.5	5.5	2.2	16.6
Couples psychotherapy Vienna (P)	[70]	60	5.7	3.5	4.4	2.5	16.2
Couples group (waiting list) (P)	[57]	38	4.9	3.1	4.7	2.8	15.5
Infertile couples (Giessen) (P)	[11]	25	3.6	4.3	4.6	3.0	15.5
Couples psychotherapy Giessen (P)	[12]	170	4.4	3.0	3.5	2.6	13.5
Men after brief couples psychotherapy II (P)	[82]	38	3.8	2.9	4.1	2.6	13.4
Schoolboys (Ulm) (12-14 years) (F)	[85]	61	4.1	2.9	3.3	2.7	13.3
Married couples, representative sample (P)	[9]	201	3.6	2.5	4.6	2.2	13.0
Partners of psychosom. in-patients	[41]	20	3.3	2.6	4.2	2.8	12.9
Standard sample (F)	[9]	723	3.5	2.7	4.1	2.5	12.8
Men before brief couples therapy I (P)	[82]	38	3.9	2.2	3.6	2.3	12.0
Cardiac infarction (discharge) II (F)	[24]	19	5.7	0.9	2.9	1.9	11.5
Fathers of disturbed children (family therapy, out-pats.) (P)	[64]	152	2.7	2.2	3.6	2.0	10.4
Couples seeking artificial insemination (P)	[11]	25	2.3	2.1	3.9	1.6	10.0
Swiss men (Zürich) (P)	[33]	220	2.3	1.9	2.7	1.3	8.2

Table 3. Profile of GSCL Scale Means for Mixed Samples

	Source	Scale					
		n	E	G	L	C	D
Cardiac neurosis (various clinics)	[20]	30	12.1	6.6	10.0	13.3	42.0
Cardiac neurosis (Giessen)	[72]	79	10.9	6.0	8.7	12.5	38.0
Cardiac phobia	[52]	56	10.6	6.1	7.6	13.2	37.5
Anxiety neurosis	[52]	61	11.2	6.1	8.6	9.2	35.1
'Psychoneurotic disorders'	[28]	103	11.9	5.8	8.9	8.6	35.1
'Psychosomatic disorders' (Giessen)	[66]	62	10.6	6.8	8.3	8.6	34.2
Mixed psychosom./psychoneur. (Giessen)	[66]	42	11.2	6.4	8.3	8.0	33.9
Psychosomatic clinic (Umkirch)	[51]	440	10.5	6.8	8.4	7.8	33.5
Phobia	[52]	52	10.8	6.0	7.9	8.9	32.9
Depression	[52]	114	12.4	6.3	7.6	6.5	32.7
'Psycho-autonomic disorders'	[28]	104	9.9	5.0	9.0	6.7	30.7
Peptic ulcer (internal medicine)	[3]	35	7.3	10.6	6.4	5.7	30.0
Asthma	[25]	74	8.7	4.3	7.8	9.0	29.8
Psychosom. in-pats. Giessen (admission) I	[59]	23	9.3	5.0	7.0	6.8	28.1
Homeless people (Giessen)	[79]	55	7.1	4.7	7.5	5.1	24.4
Engineering students	[46]	403	7.1	4.7	7.5	5.1	24.4
Anorexia	[52]	28	8.8	7.2	4.2	3.9	24.1
Psychother. student counselling Giessen 1968/9	[58]	301	9.6	4.1	4.9	4.6	23.1
Psychosom. in-pats. Giessen (1 months after admission) II	[59]	23	7.1	4.1	5.8	6.1	23.1
Psychoneurotics (Giessen)	[66]	59	8.4	4.2	5.1	5.3	23.0
Cardiosurgery I	[77]	86	6.2	2.7	5.5	7.8	22.1
Psychother. student counselling Kassel	[45]	72	7.4	4.3	5.7	4.6	21.9
Civil service (Vienna)	[6]	167	5.4	2.9	6.3	3.1	17.7
Cardiosurgery II	[77]	65	5.6	1.4	5.0	3.8	15.8
Psoriasis	[37]	28	5.2	2.4	4.1	3.9	15.6

acute and chronic physical conditions, in general practice and gynaecology, in sanatoria and other hospitals and for gathering information from various social groups – not only in the Federal Republic of Germany. This enormous range of fields and topics of investigation is responsible for the heterogeneous mixture of samples. The diagnostical criteria underlying sample selection are likewise very varied, since the definitions used by different researchers stem from their differing objectives. For this reason, only abbreviated sample descriptions are given here; more detailed information can be found in the references. All these things must be taken into account in interpreting the data, with the result that only generalized conclusions that are not dependent on a detailed knowledge of the selection criteria involved in each study will be drawn.

Data on variability are also not included, partly because this would overcomplicate the presentation and partly because, in the standard sample at least, the frequency curves have a negative logarithmic distribution, so that the mean values given actually supply all the information needed, even for testing whether a certain sample deviates from the standard sample. The samples in each table are listed in descending order according to their scores on scale 5, 'Overall distress'. Sex differences are taken into account by the division of the data into three separate tables (men, women and mixed), but age differences must be considered separately. For all samples, including the standard sample, no information is offered here on age distributions as we decided that this, too, would detract from the clarity of the tables. Information on the scores for the various age groups in the standard sample can be found in Brähler and Scheer (1983). Where samples are defined in the same way, the place of the inquiry is also given for purposes of differentiation. Where the same sample was tested at more than one point in time, this is indicated by Roman numerals. In Tables 1 and 2, samples are marked with a (P) where the partners' equivalent data are listed on the other table. Where men and women were included in the same inquiry but presented separately in the tables, these are marked with an (M) in Table 1 and an (F) in Table 2. The mass of information presented here precludes a comprehensive review of all the results. The discussion below is limited to a few selected aspects.

Groups with High Complaint Frequency

We shall begin our discussion of the results in the tables by taking a look at the groups with the highest number of subjective complaints. These we have defined somewhat arbitrarily as the first 10 samples in each list, i. e. those with the highest scores in the last scale, 'Overall distress'.

Among these we find a marked accumulation of groups with psychosomatic and psychoneurotic diagnoses or mixed forms of these. The only exceptions to this rule are the men with coronary conditions and the Turkish gynaecological patients. This we see as further evidence of the fact that frequent somatic complaints do not automatically indicate an organic disorder. Patients with clearly defined organic diseases are to be found more in the regions of medium complaint frequency, along with some, albeit few, groups in psychotherapy. From this we draw the following conclusions: there is clearly a tendency in psychosomatic and psychoneurotically ill people to complain more of physical ailments than other groups of patients, making bodily complaints of a high intensity, particularly without a definable organic diagnosis, a typical characteristic of this group of patients. This finding supports Bastiaans' hypothesis (1974), which interprets patients' complaints in general as expressions of their psychosocial state, and exaggerated distress signals in particular as a form of neurotic behaviour. The further explanation of psychosomatic diseases as suppressed distress signals (Bastiaans 1974) is not confirmed by the present data on the degree to which psychosomatic patients give expression to their body complaints. According to this last hypothesis the psychosomatic patients should be at the bottom of the list, whereas in fact they are so very mixed up with the psychoneurotic patients that, according to our findings, it is impossible to separate psychosomatic from psychoneurotic on the basis of complaint frequency. From this it follows that it would also be extremely difficult to separate various different psychosomatic diseases from one another on the grounds of general complaint frequency, although it may be possible to do this using individual scales, such as the scale 'Gastric complaints' for peptic ulcers, or by means of a typological approach, whereby typical patterns of complaints are identified as typical of certain diagnostic or other, e. g. social, groups.

A further significant observation is that in the high-complaints group there are many groups of psychosomatic and psychotherapeutic in-patients. These can best be defined in terms of a group with a common social characteristic, namely that their suffering has reached such a pitch that the ambulatory setting of the out-patient departments cannot treat them adequately. Their score on scale 5 ('Overall distress') is a reflection of the intensity of their distress. Here again we can see the expression of complaints as a measure of suffering in the broadest sense of the word.

Groups with Low Complaint Frequency

Particularly few complaints were registered by women attending the out-patient departments of gynaecological clinics: women seeking refertilization, women with fertility problems, women with menstrual problems, women attending the antenatal clinic with high-risk pregnancies, women with special difficulties connected with birth control and above all women seeking artificial insemination. The striking common feature here is that all of these women are attending clinics because of problems related with reproduction. It seems quite feasible that these could be response sets, in the sense that women who come to an institution on account of an intimate problem tend on the whole to present themselves as especially healthy. But even more probable is the explanation that many of these women have a rather removed attitude towards their bodies – that they fail to perceive body signals and tend rather to experience themselves as basically healthy but with a technical problem in their bodies. Men with infertility problems likewise have a low complaint frequency.

Interpreting a striking lack of complaints as hypoaesthesia would imply that this phenomenon, like the complaints themselves, is another expression of a disturbed relationship with one's body. The parents of emotionally disturbed children also report very few complaints. For these couples, the child is the symptom-bearer; they frequently refuse to understand that they may have something to do with their children's problems and tend instead to present themselves as very normal (Neraal et al. 1983). The hypothesis that this attitude leads to the children's taking on the family's symptoms has, with respect to somatic omplaints, never been more closely investigated. Preliminary investigations on children's complaints indicate that ill children tend on the whole to record fewer complaints than healthy ones (Brähler et al. 1984).

The Complaints List as an Instrument for Screening or Differential Diagnosis

The symptom checklist by Höck and Hess (1975) was constructed as a screening instrument for identifying 'neurotics': depending on their score, subjects are classified as 'neurotic', 'questionable' or 'not neurotic'. The method is reputed to be highly sensitive and accurate; for example, with a certain threshold score only 13,4% of male neurotics and 18,3% of normal subjects were wrongly classified. A major problem here is the definition of 'neurotic' and 'healthy' or 'not neurotic'. For the test described, neurosis is defined as 'disturbances in cerebral stimulus processing, arising from experience and with illness value'. The underlying principle here is that every complaint is automatically attributed illness value and that those with few complaints are assumed to be mentally healthy. This assumption is sometimes also to be found in studies on the success of therapy, where every reduction in the number of symptoms is interpreted as a sign of 'recovery'. However, it should not be ignored that even minor complaints can indicate a disturbance in body experience.

With regard to our questionnaire, we have often been asked whether we could develop just such a 'neurosis scale' for filtering out neurotics.

In our view, such an undertaking is very problematical, as it cannot be the purpose of a questionnaire to replace the consultation between doctor and patient; it should serve rather as a supplementary instrument. On this question we can only say that the groups diagnosed as 'neurotic', 'psychosomatically ill' and 'mixed' forms of these, i.e. the usual clientele of centres for psychosomatics and psychotherapy, regularly have raised scores on the following items: all items in the scale (E) 'Exhaustion', i.e. weariness, exhaustability, tiredness, physical weakness, excessive need for sleep and generalized numbness; also on the following items: inclination to cry, lump in the throat, frequent urination, disturbed sleep, loss of appetite, hot flushes, shakiness, blushing, a pressurized feeling in the head and speech disturbances. With a scale consisting of these 16 items, one can obtain very high specificity and sensitivity scores with respect to the diagnosis 'neurotic' v. 'not neurotic'.

In this connection it is interesting to consider lay aetiologies about the psychological origin of physical symptoms. In the representative standard sample (described in Brähler 1978), a number of items are highly correlated with the answers to a question at the end of the form on the psychological (v. purely physical) origins of bodily complaints in general. These items are: physical weakness, heart palpitations, heavy stomach, inclination to cry, headaches, exhaustability, insomnia, tiredness, general numbness, weariness, chest pains, shakiness, blushing, stomach ache, abdominal pains, head-pressure and speech disturbances.

This means that people who view their own complaints in psychological terms tend to report having more of the sorts of complaints which the doctors also see as typical 'neurotic disorders'.

Expert and lay aetiologies agree on this point. The variety of terms adopted by the experts to describe disturbances which are assumed to be of mental origin, e.g. neurasthenia, vegetative lability, neuroticism, nervousness, etc. (see Netter 1981), reflects a good deal of insecurity in this area. The scientific label is a relief to both doctor and patient, in that it defines a 'proper' illness, even though a palpable organic basis is usually lacking. All the same, such a diagnosis still smacks of hypochondria. Applying the GSCL as a screening instrument for filtering out neurotics could easily lead to a labelling approach to diagnostics. In the interests of their employers, personnel psychologists could be tempted to try and separate the potentially mentally instable from those who have no complaints and are thus thought to be best suited to the demands of modern working life – although such an assumption can prove to be a fallacy.

As well as such attempts at using the GSCL as a screening instrument for identifying neurotics, researchers have repeatedly tried to use it for purposes of differential diagnosis, e.g. for identifying 'psychosomatic' v. 'psychoneurotic' clients, 'psychovegetative' v. 'psychoneurotic' disorders, 'real' v. 'vegetative' prostatitis, 'organic' v. 'psychogenic' impotence or 'organic' v. 'neurotic' heart troubles. To this end, highly specific items are selected and combined to form a new scale. The results achieved in this way are not convincing. For example, we discovered to our surprise that patients with 'real' prostatitis differ from those diagnosed as having 'vegetative' prostatitis in that the former group have *more* 'neurotic' complaints than the latter. On the one hand, somatopsychic aspects are surely involved to a certain extent in this case, but on the other it becomes clear that the difficulties arising from such diagnostical divisions into 'organic' v. 'psychogenic' as the above, which is based largely on a process of elimination, cannot be solved by the use of questionnaires. The fact remains that this sort of dichotomizing is highly problematical.

The GSCL in Case-Control Studies

As can be seen in Tables 1-3, the GSCL is frequently used for case-control or follow-up studies; for example, for duodenal ulcer patients before and 4 years after their operation, for cardiac surgery patients, and in sanatoria and psychotherapy departments.

The results of reliability studies have shown that the GSCL, at the same time as being highly reliable for measuring complaints (Brähler and Scheer 1983), is also sensitive to changes. In two-point studies carried out before and after a medical intervention, such as the removal of a peptic ulcer, a heart operation, a stay in a sanatorium or as an in-patient in a psychosomatic clinic, it usually reflects a reduction in complaint level. In such cases, the questionnaire is clearly suitable as an instrument for checking therapeutic success.

This also applies to cases in which therapy aims at improving body perception, such as in forms of brief couples therapy where the mens' attitude of denial to their bodies is a focus of treatment (Wirth and Richter 1980).

Less common are repeated studies of the sort which measure complaint frequency not only immediately before and after medical treatment but also after a certain interval of time, in order to investigate the permanency of the patient's subjective physical improvement. In a follow-up study carried out 5 years after heart surgery it could be demonstrated that, following an initial marked reduction of overall subjective distress shortly after the operation, the women's complaint frequency 6 years later had returned to its original pre-operative level, and the men's was even higher (Landeck and Möhlen 1985).

Similarly, a single follow-up study after cardiovalvular surgery found that the women's complaints had reached the level typical for heart patients prior to an operation and the men's, again, had exceeded it (Ibe 1983).

Patients with cardiac pacemakers also registered an increase in complaints between 2-month and 8-month follow-ups (Friedrich 1981).

The same applies to cardiac infarction patients; after hospital treatment they have few complaints at first but 9 month later they have considerably more, even more than they had on leaving the intensive care unit (Klapp et al. 1985, unpublished data).

With these groups of patients, the medical intervention clearly only leads to a temporary improvement in their subjective condition. For this reason it is imperative that effectivity studies always include longer term catamneses, which can also offer important indications about after-care requirements. A patient-centred approach demands that more attention be paid to the patient's subjective state after operations and other medical interventions.

Cross-Cultural Aspects

From Tables 1 and 2 one can see that married couples in Switzerland have considerably lower scores on all scales than German couples, this applying equally to the men and the women (Brähler 1978). It is further striking that the Swiss couples' complaints are less clearly sex-linked, the women even registering fewer gastric complaints than the men. The German statistics are taken from a representative sample of married couples between the ages of 18 and 75; the Swiss figures are from a sample of married couples who, after the birth of their first child in 1970, were still living together in Zürich in 1975. The age difference between these two samples is not in itself enough to explain the difference in complaint level, as the Swiss couples still have fewer complaints when compared with their own age-group among the Germans. So the discrepancy must go back to cultural differences. One reason could of course be that the Swiss really are healthier. Another more probable explanation is that the calvinistic, mercantile influence on the Swiss national character makes it socially undesirable to have many complaints. The body is expected to function independently and is not perceived intensely. Buddeberg (1985) also reports very low scores for the husbands in the couples studied.

Figures are also available for comparable clinical groups in Austria and the Federal Republic of Germany. Couples attending out-patient couples psychotherapy in Vienna had a similar complaint level to those in Giessen. Hysterectomy patients in Vienna had rather more complaints than those in Marburg (FRG). Particularly striking is the very high level of complaints among Turkish gynaecology patients in Germany as compared with equivalent groups of German women. This may be an expression of the real degree of suffering of these women (usually the families of immigrant workers), living as they do as strangers between two cultures and so subject to very great stress. However, it may also be an indication of their greater body-relatedness: their complaints are expressed less in abstract categories and more in the concrete and immediate language of the body. Cross-cultural differences in the expression of pain have been pointed out by Cohn (1983).

Sex Differences

That bodily complaints are frequently sex-related is well known (see Brähler and Scheer 1984). Many different approaches to the phenomenon have so far produced no conclusive explanation as to why women have more complaints than men. Before going into the question of what the questionnaire data presented here can contribute to this discussion, we would like to point out that in this controversy – which has arisen largely to counter the prejudice against women that can be encouraged by over-hasty and incorrect interpretations – one should not ignore the fact that other factors, such as age and especially the subject's partner, have a greater influence on complaint level than sex alone.

In a representative sample of 201 married couples who filled out the GSCL, the correlation between the scale 'Overall distress' and sex of subject was 0.13, but with age (younger/older) it was 0.21 and with the partner's 'Overall distress' (low/high) it reached 0.41 (Brähler and Scheer 1983).

In attempting to explain the greater complaint frequency prevalent among women, two approaches stand in mutual opposition. A psychological approach, whose protagonists in West Germany are led by names such as Richter (1974) and Beckmann (1976), both from Giessen, interprets this finding as an expression of women's greater capacity for subjective suffering and emotional openness, as opposed to the inner defence against feelings and denial of weakness which is typical of the male mentality. On the other side we find the sociological approach, which claims that women have more physical complaints because their lot is objectively harder than men's (e.g. Rodenstein 1980). This author fears that the psychological explanation could result in women's complaints being taken less seriously and she points out that women suffer more from mental illness and physical symptoms of a less serious nature than men, whilst men's reduced life expectancy is largely because of the fact that they suffer more frequently from serious physical diseases. Since this female advantage is less frequent among women in employment, great emphasis is laid upon employment and the stresses associated with it in explaining the difference in mortality. If differences in subjective experience are explained purely in terms of objective circumstances, this is a form of reductionism which ignores the great variety of psychological responses which can occur in answer to the same conditions. When Beckmann (1976) and Richter (1974) interpret women's more frequent expression of complaints as demonstrating their greater emotional openness and capacity for suffering, no statement is made about objective differences. That women are supposed to suffer from mental illness more frequently than men is no argument against this interpretation; on the contrary, it shows that those with the highest rate of mental disturbance have the highest complaint scores, the complaints being a further expression of their suffering. If men report having fewer complaints than women, this can very well mean that they are less ready to articulate their complaints, because this form of self-expression is not as available to them; again nothing is said here about objective conditions. If all social inequalities were as small as the differences in complaint frequency between the sexes, a high degree of equality would have been achieved already.

If such controversies are overinfluenced by fears of discrimination, the further danger arises that the various explanations, which have their validity in their own spheres, will be played out against each other.

The present data show unequivocally that in all the samples, apart from those defined through depressive states, the women always have higher complaint scores; the heterogeneity of the samples involved is further clear evidence of the fact that this is a general phenomenon. It is hard to understand why the groups suffering from depression form an exception. Depressive states are more frequent among women, but who can say that in men they are worse or more readily expressed through somatic complaints than in women? We must await further research to clear up this question. However, for all other cases it holds true that women have more complaints than men, even when both have the same illness.

In the representative enquiry using the GSCL, the subjects were also asked, among other things, whether they had in the past been troubled by one or more of 28 illnesses listed. These included lumbago, sciatica, slipped disc, angina, stomach ulcers, gastritis, high blood pressure and nervous disorders. 18.9% of the women and 30.4% of the men answered that they had had none of the listed illnesses. Table 4 shows the unweighted three-way analysis of variance that was performed for evaluating this data, with the three independent variables age (18-34, 36-60), illness (yes/no) and sex. The results show that the illness effect is the strongest of the three. In spite of this, scales 1 and 3 still show a strong sex-dependency (age-dependency will be left out of this discussion). In other words, the women suffered more than the men, regardless of whether they had had one of the illnesses listed or not.

This cannot be explained in terms of their complaints being objectively more severe. The sociological argument could claim that additional stresses which were not investigated here are responsible for the higher scores. From the psychological side we assume the discrepancy to be due to a sex-linked difference in the attitude towards illness. Given the same diagnosis, this takes the form of women being more prepared to articulate their complaints and men tending to express themselves in this manner as little as possible. This hypothesis is supported by Gellert (1975), who found that adolescent girls have more developed body images than boys of the same age, and by Secord and Jourard (1953), who showed that women are more body-oriented and have more differentiated ideas about their bodies than men. In this light it seems reasonable to conclude that, if women generally relate more closely to their bodies, they will notice complaints more readily and be more likely to use their bodies as a medium for expression.

Our own investigations have shown that women see psychological factors behind their complaints more frequently than men (Beckmann et al. 1977). Hampel and Fahrenberg (1982) found that women inclined rather to attribute their complaints to problems in personal relationships and men to difficulties at work. According to Horn et al. (1983), women on the whole tend to understand illness in a biographical context, strongly influenced by personal relationships, whereas men as a rule prefer to ascribe any symptoms or states of physical or mental discomfort

Table 4. Three-way analysis of variance (illness/sex/age), representative sample ($n = 1547$)

Scale	Illness	Sex	Age	I × S	I × A	S × A	I × S × A
Exhaustion	83.32***	18.21**	1.01	3.54	1.05	1.34	0.21
Gastric complaints	50.25***	0.03	0.20	0.55	0.59	0.59	0.04
Pains in limbs	105.49***	30.54**	7.80**	0.96	2.70*	0.07	0.84
Cardiac complaints	90.01***	4.98*	3.89**	0.09	2.13	0.24	0.56
Overall distress	127.82***	16.12***	2.81*	0.78	2.10	0.37	0.45

* $p < 0.05$
** $p < 0.01$
*** $p < 0.001$

to external circumstances, especially conditions at work (occupational diseases, stress, wearing out).

In the same vein, Forster (1977) could demonstrate only for women a connection between bodily complaints and marital role-divisions or other partner-related problems. Eger and Pelchen-Baumann (1985) found a strong relationship between women's complaints and partnership structure; this link was less evident among their male partners.

Body Complaints and Partner Relationships

Tables 1 and 2 show that in various samples involving married couples, the 'healthy' partner has a very high complaints score as well: the wives of coronary patients (with and without surgery), of cardiac infarction patients and of men with peptic ulcers are examples. Correspondingly, the husbands of women with genital carcinoma and of rectectomy patients also have raised scores.

In general, the influence of a spouse or partner on the articulation of complaints is far greater than that of age or sex (Brähler and Scheer 1983, 1984).

Table 5 shows the congruence with respect to complaint frequency between married couples in various samples. It shows that a relatively high degree of convergence is the norm in these marriages. This can be explained in terms of the choice of partner, the nature of the marital interaction or through shared living conditions (Brähler and Scheer 1984). In psychopathological terms, it is an effect of mutual identification, a psychological mechanism familiar to developmental psychologists and psychoanalysts (who regard it as a defence mechanism) and which is apparently at work here as well, influencing the partners' complaint scores. The manner in which married couples tend to build up boundaries separating them – including their body experience – from the outside world is described by Willi (1985). On a closer examination of the figures in Table 5, one is struck by the particularly high correlations between the couples in the three samples with genital carcinoma. These groups have in common that they have had to struggle not only with the malignant illness itself but also with the awareness that the life of the ill partner is in imminent danger, so that the high congruence can be understood as a defence against the fear of this threat: the partners draw closer together and observe their bodies carefully.

A further striking feature of Table 5 is that, of the other four groups, the repre-

Table 5. Congruence of bodily complaints between husbands and wives in various samples

	E	G	L	C	D
Married couples	0.31	0.22	0.38	0.27	0.41
Couples therapy	0.14	0.31	0.03	0.11	0.19
Genital carcinoma (10-year survival)	0.41	0.51	0.25	0.51	0.51
Genital carcinoma (5-year survival)	0.31	0.53	0.40	0.59	0.60
Testicular carcinoma survivors	0.21	0.16	0.40	0.44	0.46
Peptic ulcer	0.23	0.00	0.08	0.23	0.18
Family therapy	0.17	0.16	0.09	0.16	0.23

sentative sample of marriages shows the highest degree of congruence. In the case of the peptic ulcer patients, the lower congruence is understandable in view of the differences to be expected on the gastric complaints scale, but with the other samples this deviation from the general tendency can hardly be connected directly with their symptoms. A possible explanation is that the lack of congruence found in these marriages is an indication of greater dissonance in the relationship: conflicts in the interaction may have disturbed the normal process of mutual assimilation. In the couples therapy sample this would seem to be a likely explanation and, assuming that family dynamics and psychosomatic factors are involved in the growth of peptic ulcers, may also be the reason for the relatively low correlations in the other groups as well.

The discussion so far – including the consideration of sex-linked differences – has been based entirely on the data from whole samples i.e. on an assumption of homogeneity. In addition, this approach also involves implicit assumptions about specificity when talking about a certain sample. In our view, it is therefore useful to take a typological approach as well, as we shall demonstrate. For the samples considered above, the different selection criteria reduce the validity of the homogeneity assumption and point rather in the direction of a certain inhomogeneity within the groups so defined.

The typological approach we have chosen to apply to a representative sample of married couples. With the help of the self-image and other-image forms of the Giessen Test, we have identified 12 typical marital relationship patterns (Brähler et al. 1985). These 12 patterns also differ considerably with respect to the complaint scores reached by the husbands and wives.

In Table 6, the scores for three of the 12 marriage types are shown. Type A is characterized by very low complaint scores for husband and wife. In Type B, the wives have very many complaints and the husbands very few. In Type C, both partners have a lot of complaints.

Figure 1 shows the Giessen Test profiles (Brähler and Beckmann 1984) characteristic of Type A couples. In this test, six items each from the four self- and other-image forms are grouped into the following 5 scales: social response (negative/NR v. positive/PR); dominance (dominant/DO v. submissive/SU); self-control (uncontrolled/UC v. compulsive/CO); underlying mood (hypomanic/HM v. depressive/DE) and permeability (permeable/PE v. retentive/RE). Type A includes couples where both partners have very few complaints, which are seen particularly by the wives as not being of psychological origin.

The Giessen Test profiles of these couples show them to be unexceptional, conventional, but also socially rather disregarded people. They have no particuar

Table 6. Complaint scores for 3 typical partnership patterns

	Husbands					Wives				
	E	G	L	C	D	E	G	L	C	D
Type A	3.5	2.2	3.7	1.4	10.8	2.7	1.1	2.4	1.5	7.7
Type B	3.1	1.3	3.8	2.2	10.4	7.1	4.6	7.6	4.4	23.9
Type C	10.3	3.9	8.0	4.6	26.8	6.8	3.5	7.1	4.5	21.9

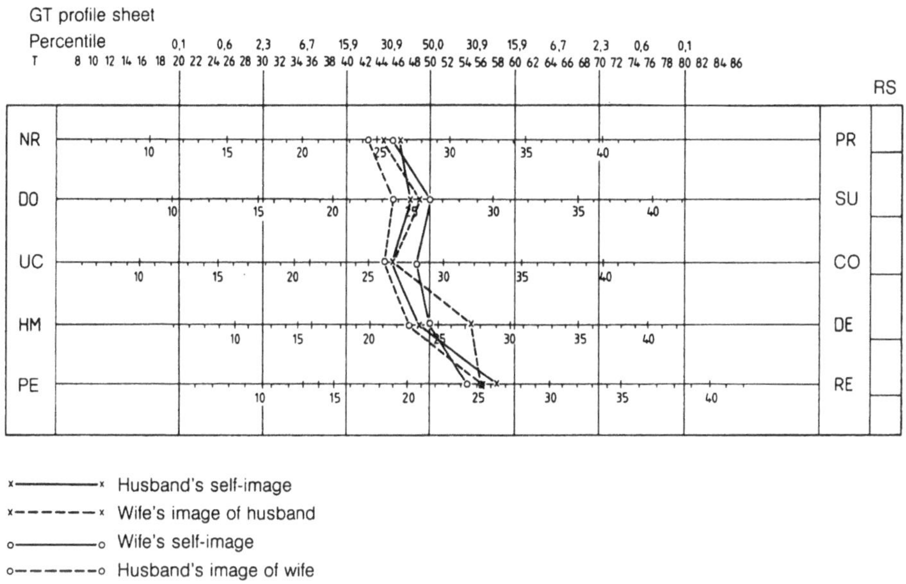

Fig. 1. Giessen Test profile for Type A couples

distinguishing characteristics and there are very few points of difference between the partners. The men describe their wives as they describe themselves, but with the common characteristics slightly more accentuated. The wives see a difference only with respect to underlying mood: they describe their husbands as rather depressed, but the husbands do not confirm this. The relationship is very symmetrical.

The striking quality of these couples is their social adjustment. They are very concerned to fit in with the norm, but attain no great social recognition, have rather poor self-control and are emotionally rather unresponsive; they conform without success or gratification. These couples may be seen as representatives of dreary everyday married life.

Type A partnerships are frequently to be found among neurotics and the parents of ill or disturbed children. In the clinical samples, similar patterns often occur among couples seeking sterilization, the parents of schizophrenics, in marriages where breast cancer has been suspected in the past and after cardiovalvular surgery. In such cases, this sort of relationship would appear to occur as a way of coping with a serious problem (see Brähler et al. 1985).

Figure 2 shows the Giessen Test profiles of Type B couples. In these marriages, the men report few complaints, in contrast to the obvious suffering of their wives.

Judging from the profiles they present, it would appear that the men 'camouflage' themselves. They describe themselves as completely normal, without any special personal characteristics. Their wives however – lacking self-confidence, dominant, withdrawn and depressive – experience their husbands as successful, emotionally open (permeable) and submissive. The wives carry the burdens and worries whilst their husbands apparently have no problems, preferring to take the

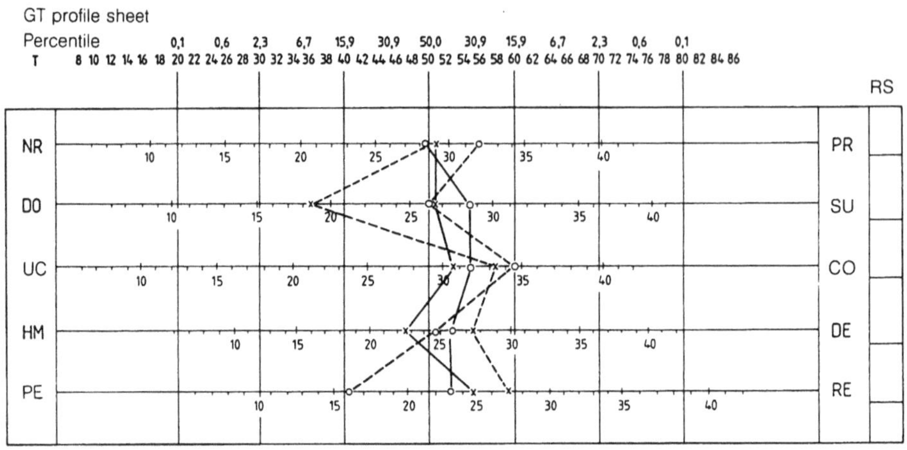

x———x Husband's self-image
x- - - - - -x Wife's image of husband
o———o Wife's self-image
o- - - - - -o Husband's image of wife

Fig. 2. Giessen Test profile for Type B couples

line of least resistance. In spite of this conventionality and tendency to subordination in the men, the wives see their husbands as especially attractive and emotionally responsive. This constellation points in the direction of a phallic, narcissistic injury to the wife's self-esteem, which she overcomes by dominating her envied husband.

Type B occurs frequently among couples with sexual problems and in the clinical groups defined through the wife's sexual difficulties. This type of marriage seems to be particularly conflict-ridden (see Brähler et al. 1985).

Figure 3 shows the Giessen Test profiles typical of Type C couples. Here, the husbands complain of a great many physical symptoms, especially exhaustion, and emphasize the somatic nature of their troubles. The wives suffer particularly frequently from heart trouble and see their complaints in a more psychological light. From the profiles, these are conventional, unexceptional marriages, with discontented wives experiencing their husbands as extremely dominant. The men deny this conflict and describe their marriages as harmonious. The only differences they see lie in their wives' greater popularity and emotional openness which, however, is not confirmed by the wives themselves. On the whole, the similarities outweigh the differences, although the wives complain of their husbands' inability to co-operate. The differences perceived by the men, on the other hand, take the form of a tribute to their wives' attractiveness and capacity for love. Their obvious striving for harmony and normality and the difficulties they have in coping with deviations or disharmony is reminiscent of symbiotic partnership structures in which, however great the agreement may be, both partners ultimately avoid opening themselves to each other in trust, for fear of being swallowed up or exploited by the other (Scale 5, permeability, of the Giessen Test).

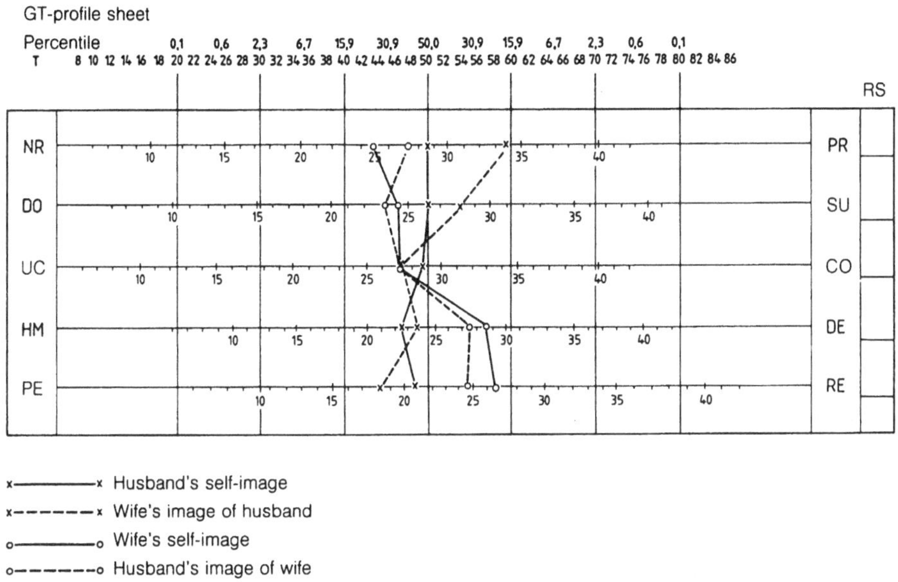

Fig. 3. Giessen Test profile for Type C couples

This sort of partnership is relatively rare among neurotics and did not prevail in any of the clinical samples. But whether such marriages can be considered 'healthy' is to be doubted.

Résumé

The influence of marriage and partnership on body complaints – compared with that of age, sex or social class – has so far been neglected in the research. If the partner has a greater influence on a person's complaints than all these other factors, then both diagnostic and therapeutic measures should take this into account, since the individual style of each family clearly leads to very considerable differences in their articulation of complaints. The inclusion of a partner in therapy, an extension of the therapeutic setting, is a new challenge which requires interactional thinking and at the same time offers the possibility of improving both diagnostic precision and the effectiveness of therapeutic interventions, for example, through couples therapy. What is more, findings such as these make the necessity of taking the whole family environment into account and working towards a family-oriented medicine clearer than ever. The GSCL is a useful instrument for observing therapeutic processes.

In a number of samples, the sensitivity of the instrument for registering changes in the patient's subjective condition as a result of medical treatment, usually in the direction of an initial improvement, has been demonstrated. Studies over longer periods of time, on the other hand, have shown that after this temporary improvement complaints can increase again, as in the case of the heart surgery patients whose subjective condition got progressively worse. Thus, the GSCL can be of help in recording the more long-term consequences of treatment and pointing out where further rehabilitation measures are necessary at a later date.

The frequent attempts made by many researchers to divide psychosomatic from psychoneurotic patients will be unlikely to succeed with the GSCL either. The frequency and intensity of somatic complaints is very high for both groups and it is hardly to be expected that this picture will be so different at item level as to make such a separation possible. On the contrary, the results already obtained could help to put into perspective the conception of illness which persists in trying to draw such clear distinctions.

Experience with the GSCL so far indicates that in general it would probably be more productive, along with data on central tendencies in defined samples, to make far more use of the typological approach, which allows for more differentiated findings on complaints and their significance. From the figures, it is clear that suffering from physical complaints is a very human phenomenon. Freedom from complaints appears not even to be a desirable utopian objective, for this turns out more often than not to be a form of hypo-aesthesia, a lack of relatedness with the body. 'Give the body its due' would seem to be the consequence of all this: a certain amount of physical discomfort belongs to every life, whether it is in Switzerland, Germany or Austria, whether one is homeless, a patient in treatment or a civil servant; also; those at the lower end of the frequency tables may be assumed rather to have a disturbed relationship with their bodies than to be exceptionally healthy people.

Cultural differences in the expression of complaints are a factor which have to be considered when applying an instrument like the GSCL. For research, this means that each ethnic group must be seen in relation to its own norms, taken from suitable standard samples. At the same time, the results so far have shown that the GSCL can well be used for transcultural research, demonstrating once more the subjective nature of the answers, i.e. the expression of complaints in their psychological dimension.

The GSCL was developed and applied on the basis of a patient-centred conception of illness which aims to raise the patient's subjective condition to a more important status, since this is an aspect which has been increasingly pushed into the background by the doctor-centred approach to illness in recent years.

References

1. Bastiaans J (1974) Neue psychosomatische und psychobiologische Aspekte der Hysterie. Prax Psychother 19: 159-166
2. Bayer E (1971) Validierung des Giessener Persönlichkeitsinventars an Ulcuspatienten. Dissertation, University of Giessen
3. Beckmann D (1976) Paardynamik und Gesundheitsverhalten. Einige Ergebnisse einer repräsentativen Erhebung. In: Richter H-E, Strotzka H, Willi J (eds) Familie und seelische Krankheit. Rowohlt, Reinbek
4. Beckmann D, Brähler E, Braun P (1977) Zur Scheinkorrelation zwischen neurotischen Körperbeschwerden und sozialer Schichtzugehörigkeit. Z Psychosom Med Psychoanal 23: 251-261
5. Biefang S (1981) Auswertung und Analyse des 'Fragebogens für Rheuma-Patienten', Teil 1: Skalen. (unpublished documentation, Schloß Reisensburg)

6. Biehal-Heimburger E (1982) Ein Beitrag zum Zusammenhang zwischen Arbeitszufriedenheit und psychosomatischen Beschwerden im Bereich der öffentlichen Verwaltung. Dissertation, University of Vienna
7. Biskup J (1982) Die psychosoziale Situation von Koronarpatienten. Lang, Frankfurt
8. Boecker HH (1980) Sekundäre Amenorrhoe und Psychosomatisches Phänomen - Empirische Untersuchungen zu Persönlichkeitsstrukturen und Objektbeziehungen von Amenorrhoe-Patientinnen. Dissertation, University of Giessen
9. Brähler E (1978) Der Giessener Beschwerdebogen (GBB). Thesis, University of Giessen
10. Brähler E, Beckmann D (1984) Die Erfassung von Partnerbeurteilungen mit dem Gießen-Test. Diagnostica 30: 184-197
11. Brähler C, Meyhöfer W (1985) Psychologische Aspekte der Fertilitätsstörungen. Med Welt 36: 230-241
12. Brähler E, Scheer JW (1983) Der Giessener Beschwerdebogen (GBB) - Testhandbuch. Huber, Bern
13. Brähler E, Scheer JW (1984) Subjektive Beschwerden und objektiver Befund. In: Scheer JW, Brähler E (eds) Ärztliche Massnahmen aus psychologischer Sicht. Springer, Berlin Heidelberg New York
14. Brähler E, Weidner W (1982) Psychodiagnostische Aspekte der Prostatitis. Symposium on the occasion of the 10th anniversary of the Departmnt of Medical Psychology, University of Giessen
15. Brähler E, Beckmann D, Müller S (1977) Psychosomatische Beschwerden und Schichtzugehörigkeit. Med Psychol 3: 214-223
16. Brähler E, Scheer JW, Meyer A (1978) Psychosomatische Beschwerdemuster in der Allgemeinpraxis. Med Psychol 4: 217-218
17. Brähler E, Surrey HW, Scheer JW (1983) Der Giessener Beschwerdebogen (GBB) - Tabellenband. Institut für Medizinische Psychologie. Giessen
18. Brähler E, Klein H, Ernst R (1984) Körperbeschwerden bei Kindern und Jugendlichen. Paper presented at the 5th congress on psychology in medicine, Munich
19. Brähler E, Ernst R, Brähler C (1985) Typische Paarbeziehungsstrukturen im Giessen-Test. Psychother Psychosom Med Psychol (im Druck)
20. Bruns M, Wöbbe E (1977) Untersuchungen zur Struktur der Partnerbeziehungen neurotischer und neurotisch-depressiver Patienten mit dem 'Giessen-Test'. Dissertation, University of Göttingen
21. Buddeberg C (1985) Ehen krebskranker Frauen. Urban und Schwarzenberg, Munich
22. Cohn N (1983) Psychologische Faktoren und Prozesse bei der Entstehung und dem Verlauf von psychogenem Schmerz. Psychother Psychosom Med Psychol 33: 13-19
23. Davies-Osterkamp S, Möhlen K (1978) Postoperative Genesungsverläufe bei Patienten der Herzchirurgie in Abhängigkeit von präoperativer Angst und Angstbewältigung. Med Psychol 4: 247-260
24. Deter H-C (1984) Körperbeschwerden von Patienten vor und nach stationärem Aufenthalt in einer psychosomatischen Klinik. (unpublished work, Heidelberg)
25. Deter H-C (1984) Körperbeschwerden von Asthmapatienten aus der Medizinischen Klinik, der Hautklinik, Allgemein- und Pulmologenpraxis in Heidelberg (Unpublished work, Heidelberg)
26. Eckensberger D, Overbeck G, Biebl W (1976) Subgroups of peptic ulcer patients. J Psychosom Res 20: 489-499
27. Eger P, Pelchen-Baumann M (1985) Validierung von typischen Beziehungsmustern bei neurotischen Paaren. (Unpublished work, Giessen)
28. Ermann M (1978) Psychovegetative Störungen aus analytisch-psychosomatischer Sicht. Thesis, University of Mannheim
29. Fahrenberg J (1975) Die Freiburger Beschwerdeliste FBL. Z Klin Psychol 4: 79-100
30. Fahrenberg J (1983) Psychophysiologische Methodik. In: Groffmann KJ, Michel L (eds) Enzyklopädie der Psychologie. Psychologische Diagnostik, vol 4. Verhaltensdiagnostik. Hogrefe, Göttingen
31. Fisher G (1983) Untersuchungen zum Körperbild der Frau. Dissertation, University of Giessen
32. Fischer MV (1985) Körperbeschwerden von Kopfschmerzpatienten. (Unpublished work, Heidelberg)

33. Forster J (1977) Körperliche Beschwerden bei Ehepaaren. Thesis, Zürich
34. Friedrich R (1981) Aspekte der psychischen Adaptation an einem implantierten Herzschrittmacher - unter besonderer Berücksichtigung der Bewältigungs- und Abwehrmechanismen. Haag und Herchen, Frankfurt
35. Gellermann G (1976) Zusammenhänge zwischen physiologischen Variablen und Fragebögen bei psychiatrischen Patienten. Dissertation, University of Marburg
36. Gellert E (1975) Children's constructions of their self-images. Percept Mot Skills 40: 307-324
37. Gieler U, Ernst R, Fritz J, Rohjahn J (1984) Mein Schuppenpanzer schützt mich! Persönlichkeitsbild und Körperbeschwerden bei Psoriasis-Patienten. Paper 60, congress of North-west German Dermatologists, Hanover, September 1984
38. Gieler U, Ernst R, Neraal T, Welp (1985) Psychosomatische Aspekte bei der Akne vulgaris. Paper 113, Dermatological Society Conference, Zürich 1985
39. Grünzig H-J, Kächele H (1978) Körperbeschwerden in der psychosomatisch-psychotherapeutischen Ambulanz Ulm. (Unpublished work, Ulm)
40. Hampel R, Fahrenberg J (1982) Freiburger Beschwerdenliste FBL. Gruppenvergleiche und andere Studien zur Validität. Research report, Institute of Psychology, University of Freiburg
41. Hartmann HP (1985) Therapieergebnisse nach stationärer Psychotherapie. Dissertation, University of Giessen
42. Höck K, Hess H (1975) Der Beschwerdebogen (BFB) - Ein Siebtestverfahren der Neurosendiagnostik für Ärzte und Psychologen. VEB Deutscher Verlag der Wissenschaften, Berlin
43. Horn K, Beier C, Wolf M (1983) Krankheit, Konflikt und soziale Kontrolle. Westdeutscher Verlag, Opladen
44. Ibe B (1983) Berufliche und psychosoziale Entwicklung nach einem Herzklappenersatz. Dissertation, University of Giessen
45. Junker H (1981) Zur psychischen Situation ratsuchender Studenten - in Selbsteinschätzungen, Psychodiagnostik und Therapeutenurteilen. Second report of the psychotherapeutic research and advice centre, Gesamthochschule, Kassel
46. Kächele H (1977) Körperbeschwerden von Ingenieurschulstudenten. (Unpublished work, Ulm)
47. Kerekjarto M, Meyer AE, Zerssen D von (1972) Die HHM-Beschwerdenliste bei Patienten einer internistischen Ambulanz. Psychosom Med Psychoanal. 18: 1-16
48. Klapp C (1982) Genetisch bedingte, isolierte Hypercholesterinämie - Inadäquate Krankheitseinsicht und mangelnde Therapieadhärenz als Wegbereiter eines schicksalhaften Krankheitsverlaufs. Dissertation, University of Giessen
49. Klapp B, Laubach W, Scheer JW (1985) Körperbeschwerden von Infarktpatienten. (Unpublished work, Giessen)
50. Klein H (1985) Die Gynäkologen aus Sicht der Patientinnen. Dissertation, University of Giessen
51. Kokott HOJ (1980) Aufarbeitung des Umkircher Dokumentationssystems mit einer Beispielauswertung zu einer körperlichen Beschwerdeliste - unter weiterer Berücksichtigung der Beziehungen zwischen einigen Fragebögen und Tests. Dissertation, University of Freiburg
52. Kordy H (1985) Körperbeschwerden von Patienten der Ambulanz der Psychosomatischen Klinik Heidelberg. Unpublished work, Heidelberg
53. Kronsbein H, Boppel C (1982) Paarbeziehungsstrukturen bei MS-Patienten. Paper presented at the congress of clinical psychology, Berlin
54. Landeck, Möhlen K (1985) Katamnestische Untersuchung an Herzoperierten. (Unpublished work, Giessen)
55. Liffler W (1982) Verarbeitungsmuster bei Mastektomiepatientinnen und ihren Partnern. (Unpublished work, Marburg)
56. Meyer A, Davies-Osterkamp S (1984) Zur Paardynamik bei Refertilisierungspatientinnen und ihrer Partner. In: Tewes U (ed) Angewandte Medizinpsychologie. Fachbuchhandlung für Psychologie, Frankfurt
57. Moeller ML (1978) Psychodiagnostische Befunde von Paargruppenanwärtern. (Unpublished work, Giessen)
58. Moeller ML, Scheer JW (1974) Psychotherapeutische Studentenberatung. Probleme der Klientel - Probleme der Institution. Thieme, Stuttgart
59. Möhlen K (1982) Körperbeschwerden von Patienten einer psychosomatischen Station. (Unpublished work, Giessen)

60. Möhlen K, Brähler E (1984) Beschwerdebild und Selbstkonzept von Patienten mit Ulcus duodeni vor und 4 Jahre nach einer Operation. Psychosom Med Psychoanal 30: 150-163
61. Möhring P, Brähler E this volume
62. Möhring P, Wittmeyer H, Brähler E (1985) Paarbeziehungsstrukturen und Körpererleben bei ehemaligen Krebspatientinnen und ihren Partnern. Geburtshilfe Frauenheilkd 45: 784-788
63. Morgenthaler A (1981) Die Bedeutung der Hysterektomie im weiblichen Lebenszusammenhang. Dissertation, University of Vienna
64. Neraal T, Meyer A, Brähler E (1983) Zur Anwendung des GT-Paartests in der Familiendiagnostik. Prax Kinderpsychol Kinderpsychiatr 32: 278-285
65. Netter P (1981) KFA von funktionellen Beschwerden bei Spontanangabe und standardisierter Befragung. In: Janke W (ed) Beiträge zur Methodik in der differentiellen diagnostischen und klinischen Psychologie. Hain, Königstein im Taunus, pp 393-420
66. Overbeck G (1975) Objektivierende und relativierende Beiträge zur Pensée operatoire der französischen Psychosomatik. Thesis, University of Giessen
67. Overbeck G (1979) Körperbeschwerden bei Patienten der psychosomatischen Ambulanz. (Unpublished work, Frankfurt)
68. Overbeck G (1979) Beziehungsmuster von Ulcus-Kranken und ihren Partnern. (Unpublished work, Frankfurt)
69. Paar G (1982) Körperbeschwerden von Nierensteinerstträgern. (Unpublished work)
70. Reiter L (1983) Gestörte Paarbeziehungen. Theoretische und empirische Untersuchungen zur Ehepaardiagnostik. Vandenhoeck und Ruprecht, Göttingen
71. Richter H-E (1974) Lernziel Solidarität. Rowohlt, Reinbek
72. Richter H-E, Beckmann D (1973) Herzneurose. Thieme, Stuttgart
73. Richter R (1982) Körperbeschwerden von türkischen Frauen, die den Gynäkologen aufsuchen. (Unpublished work, Hamburg)
74. Richter R, Trittmacher (1983) Körperbeschwerden von Patienten mit operierten Hypophyseadenom und Hormonsubstitution. (Unpublished word, Hamburg)
75. Rodenstein M (1980) Fraueninteressen in Gesundheitspolitik und -forschung. Soziale Welt 2: 176-190
76. Salm A (1980) Psychologische Aspekte der Herzkatheterisierung. University of Giessen
77. Salm A (1983) Katamnestische Untersuchungen von Herzklappenoperierten. (Unpublished work, Giessen)
78. Secord PF, Jourard SL (1953) The appraisal of body cathexis: Body cathexis and the self. J Consult Psychol 17: 343-347
79. Strupowski R, Dierking W (1979) Einige Aspekte des Gesundheitsverhaltens bei Giessener Obdachlosen. Dissertation, University of Giessen
80. Weihrauch E (1979) Migräne- und Akupunkturtherapie. Lecture, University of Giessen
81. Willi J (1985) Koevolution. Rowohlt, Reinbek
82. Wirth H-J, Richter H-E (1980) Veränderungen der Paarbeziehung und der Körperbeschwerden durch Zwei-Wochen-Paarkurztherapie. Lecture, University of Giessen
83. Woynar W (1979) Körperbeschwerden von verschiedenen Gruppen von Patientinnen in der Gynäkologie. (Unpublished work, Marburg)
84. Zenz H (1971) Empirische Befunde über die Giessener Fassung einer Beschwerdeliste. Psychother Med Psychol 21: 7-13
85. Zenz H, Marschall P, Balzer-Böken B (1983) Untersuchungen über Leistungsverhalten und körperliches Wohlbefinden von Schülern. Research report, Department of Medical Psychology, University of Ulm
86. Zerssen D von (1971) Die Beschwerdenliste als Test. Therapiewoche 21: 1908
87. Zerssen D von (1976) Beschwerdenliste. Beltz, Weinheim

Body Complaints in Children from 8 to 15 Years of Age

E. Brähler, R. Ernst, W. Hettich, H. Felder and A. Otten

During their years at school, children are subjected to a great many tests of achievement, be these in the form of school tests, examinations, intelligence tests or other methods developed by psychologists and educationalists. The latter are especially concerned to find out how school subjects can be made more attractive, how the children's motivation can be increased, and endless discussions are in progress about what belongs in the curriculum and what not. Although it is surely fair to say that many teachers and educators have taken it into their heads to do something educationally useful for their pupils' bodies as well, it is equally true that 'the sort of education which took the body seriously missed its target, because in striving for perfection it lost sight of its object' (Wünsche 1982). The overemphasis on teaching cultural skills in schools these days – this applies especially, but by no means only, to schools in the Federal Republic of Germany – has often been criticized and there has been no lack of calls for giving more room to social and emotional aspects in education. Nevertheless, the school situation today is largely hostile to the body. Subjects like music have been pushed into the background: they are the first hit when timetables are reduced, as in West Germany in recent years, to save employing more teachers. At school, the children's bodies play only a marginal role; they are expected to sit still, behave in a disciplined manner and not to disturb the brain at its work. Admittedly, there are subjects known as physical education and sports, which are intended to keep the body fit. But these, too, are taught as school subjects, demanding discipline and, once again, achievement. The children's experience of their own bodies is their private affair and not the school's responsibility.

Should disturbances occur in the schoolchild's body experience an expert is consulted, the doctor, who attempts to trace the disturbance back to an organic cause and so, through suitable treatment, to eradicate it – not always with success.

The result is that not a small percentage of schoolchildren are even supplied with psychoactive drugs (Hildebrandt and Schultz 1984).

Through immunization programmes, medical examinations in infancy and mass health checks for preschool and schoolchildren, including dental checks, everything is done to reach a high standard of health among the population. However, this is necessarily limited to organic disorders which are easily identified in mass screenings.

In the field of medicine, the specific situation of children does have its special place in the area of paediatrics, which deals with infants, children and adolescents alike, regardless of the nature of their disorders. Thus the developmental aspect of the body at least is given its due. The books on paediatrics give a great deal of detailed information on aspects of physical development as well as on illnesses which can occur in infants and children. The situation of adolescents is usually dealt with in short chapters on puberty and the physical changes taking place during it (see Wiscott et al. 1977; von Harnack 1971). The subjective feelings of children and adolescents are paid no attention whatever.

Developmental psychology, for its part, has been quicker to point out the close links between somatic and psychic development (Nickel 1974), although the greatest emphasis here is still laid on cognitive aspects (Oerter 1974). Of the psychoanalytical theories, the works of Mahler et al. (1984) and Kestenberg (1968) especially have stressed the importance of bodily processes in children's psychic development, but here again, the child's own experience of its body is always seen as being of only secondary importance.

In adults, the discrepancy between subjective body experience and objective organic findings has been observed so often that a whole variety of terms have been invented for the illness or disturbance attributed to patients who have many complaints but no equivalent organic disorder: nervousness, neuroticism, vegetative lability, and dozens more (Netter 1981).

Paediatricians in particular are very often confronted with the fact that children and adolescents experience their bodies in a very special way; especially for children, the body has the function of a medium of communication for expressing emotions, so that here subjective feelings and objective findings frequently diverge even more than with adults. Recent discussions on anorexia nervosa demonstrate just this fact very clearly (Bruch 1980).

All the same, children are taken less seriously than adults and are often accused of imagining things, malingering or hypochondria. Children's symptoms are frequently played down as 'children's' illnesses', 'growing pains', etc. Children are often denied any right to have complaints, these being explained away as passing, imagined or natural. A myth of the immaculate child's body prevails (see also Scherer 1982). Whilst all the books agree (see Bräutigam and Christian 1981) that somatic complaints are strongly linked with sex (women complain more than men) and age (older people complain more than younger), very little is known about the complaints of children and adolescents under 18 years of age. The age-dependency of complaints found to apply to adults is implicitly extrapolated into childhood and adolescence, with the result that the latter are assumed to have correspondingly few such troubles.

For 'problem children' a whole series of questionnaires on physical symptoms has been developed, but these are all constructed to be answered by the parents and so are more likely to reflect the parent's distorted attributions than the child's true subjective state. Investigating a sample of behaviourally and emotionally disturbed children, we could show that the children themselves register considerably more and different complaints than are ascribed to them by their parents (Brähler et al. 1983).

We would like to report here on how we have developed a children's complaints list and tested it empirically on a sample of 303 schoolchildren between

8 and 15 years of age. The aim of the undertaking was to develop a questionnaire for use by paediatricians and general practitioners for gathering systematic information on children's bodily complaints, since the usual spontaneous description given to the doctor by an accompanying parent includes only a few aspects, mainly those which are closely related to the reason for coming to the doctor in the first place. The list is intended to provide a comprehensive picture of the child's subjective complaints and identify the key symptoms. For psychologists and doctors confronted with behavioural disturbances and other psychological problems in children, it offers an indication of the degree of subjective distress experienced by the child.

The Construction of the Children's Complaints List

The children's complaints list was originally developed as a special form of the *Giessener Beschwerdebogen* (English version: Giessen Subjective Complaints List, GSCL), which is by now a standard instrument for use with adults in the Federal Republic of Germany and has proved its worth in many studies (see Brähler and Möhring, this volume, and Brähler and Scheer 1983). Certain items from this questionnaire were excluded as not applying to children at all and others were worded differently to make them easier for children to understand. A number of other complaints were added, which are irrelevant for adults but in the opinion of experts (paediatricians, psychologists and family therapists) important for children. There is also space for the children to add complaints not included in the list. After a trial application with 40 emotionally disturbed children, the list was extended to include some of these supplementary complaints. The children are asked to show how often they suffer from each complaint.

The three-point scale originally planned ('never', 'sometimes' and 'often'), on the assumption that children are unable to differentiate further in their replies, was subsequently extended because many children in the trial run chose to answer more precisely by putting their crosses in the spaces between the answers provided. The answer alternatives now offered are: 'never - rarely - sometimes - often - always'.

The 80 items in the final form cover the areas of general wellbeing, vegetative disturbances, pains and emotionality, as well as special 'children's complaints' like 'stitches', etc. Figure 1 shows the localization of the complaints in the body.

The questionnaire was offered to a total of 12 classes from one primary school and two comprehensives, containing altogether 303 schoolchildren between the

Table 1. Age and sex distribution of sample

Sex	8-10 years	11-12 years	13-15 years	Total
M	31	81	44	156
F	25	80	39	144
	56	161	83	300

Three children forgot to state their sex

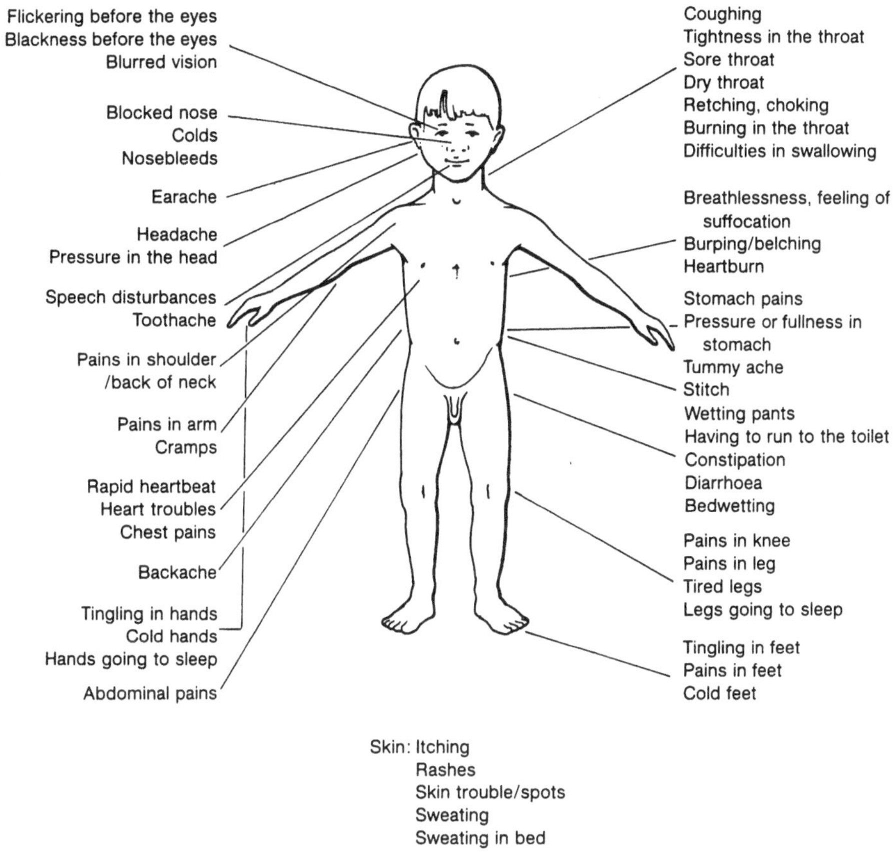

Fig. 1. Localization of complaints in children

ages of 8 and 15; the forms were usually distributed by the biology teacher. The children filled them out with great enthusiasm, clearly seeing this as a welcome change from the usual achievement-orientated tests and moreover as a chance to vent their feelings about their physical complaints. Table 1 shows the distribution of the children in the sample according to age and sex.

On the whole the items were all well understood; 98.9% were answered. The items most frequently not answered were:

73	Pressure or fullness in the stomach	5.0%
30	Heartburn or burping	3.6%
21	Getting fat	3.3%
43	Hunger	3.0%

These items were presumably left out not so much because they were not understood as out of embarassment or awkwardness. This explanation was suggested partly by the fact that it was mostly girls who refused to answer them.

Figure 2 shows which complaints occur at least 'rarely' in more than 70% of the children, ordered according to the sum of the affirmative answers ('rarely', 'sometimes', 'often' and 'all the time').

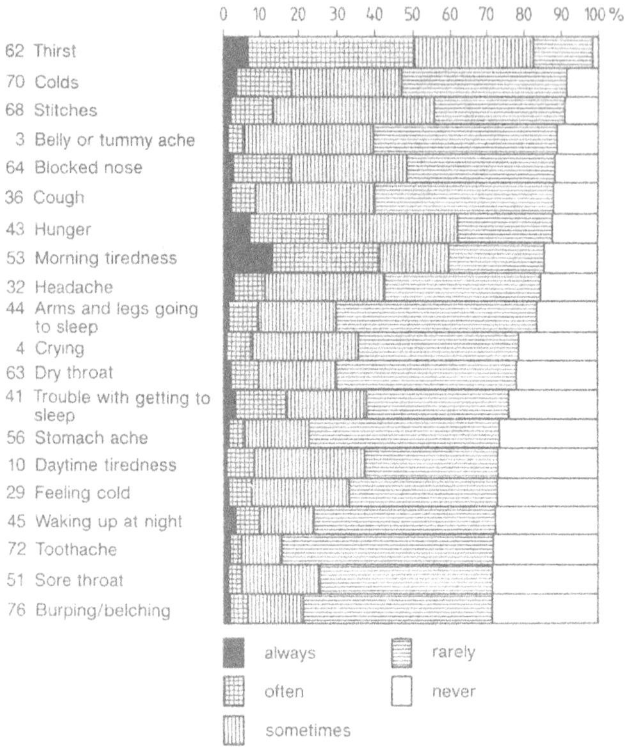

Fig. 2. Children's most frequent complaints

It is surprising that more than 20 of the 80 complaints on the list occur in over 70% of the children at least 'rarely', whereas this is not true of any of the items on the adult form. Altogether, over 50% of the children report that they have had 47 of the 80 complaints at least 'rarely', whilst this applies to only 5 of the 57 items in the adult form. Even if one sees the key complaints – thirst, morning tiredness, hunger, stitches, colds and blocked nose – as relatively minor, there are a number of more serious complaints which occur quite frequently.

Table 2 shows a comparison between the physical complaints of adults (18–60 years, standard sample; Brähler and Scheer 1983) and children. Comparison is only possible for these items, which are identically worded. Of the 22 items in question, 19 are reported more frequently by the children than the adults and only three less frequently.

Our results show that children between the ages of 8 and 15 have more complaints than any of the adult age-groups, even more than the old people. This raises many questions, since a high frequency of complaints among adults is usually interpreted as an indication of nervousness, depression or neuroticism. Are the children's many complaints to be interpreted as developmental phenomena, a sign of permanent stress induced by school pressures, or is it that children feel they can admit to having complaints more easily than adults? It is well-known that women complain more than men, who may not be and do not wish to be seen as

Table 2. Comparison between children (8-15 years) and adults (18-60 years) for selected complaints ('slightly' to 'very much' and 'rarely' to 'always' combined and expressed as a percentage)

Complaint	Children ($n=303$)	Adults ($n=1557$)
General physical weakness	46.2	38.6
Excessive sweating	67.7	50.7
Vomiting	58.4	10.5
Nausea	69.3	18.8
Heartburn or belching	43.6	22.2
Headaches	84.5	59.3
General numbness	36.3	23.3
Constipation	25.1	28.9
Weariness	60.7	43.4
Diarrhoea	67.3	12.8
Shakiness	45.5	19.3
Sore throats	71.0	26.3
Cold feet	61.4	40.4
Stomach pains	74.3	32.8
Pressure in the head	39.9	33.5
Speech disturbances	32.7	5.7
Heavy stomach	88.4	39.9
Excessive need for sleep	39.9	50.0
Lump, tightness or choking in throat	18.5	17.1
Belching	71.0	32.2
Dragging or tired legs	51.2	39.5
Bouts of heart trouble	14.9	26.7

complainers. Could it be that children have a better perception of their bodies, so that their greater awareness of complaints is a good sign? Studies have been carried out with children in which complaint frequency is used as an indicator for health v. illness (Schrör 1984). In a parallel study which we carried out in the outpatient department of the Children's Hospital in Giessen, however, we found that ill children on the whole reported considerably fewer complaints than the schoolchildren. A possible explanation for this could be that children undergoing hospital treatment avoid admitting to too many complaints for fear of further medical interventions, or it is possible that their particular illness, with all its own special symptoms, pushes all other complaints into the background.

If one takes the WHO definition of health seriously, one cannot necessarily assume that our children all feel thoroughly well and are always the picture of health, but on the other hand it is perhaps a healthy sign if they can react so directly to external stresses with their bodies.

Complaint Complexes

By means of factor and item analysis the complaints were grouped into complexes of items which generally occur together. The first finding was that a strongly dominant factor reflecting a general tendency to complain, or 'overall distress', was just as clearly present in the childrend as in adults. Almost all correlations between the items are positive. For the 11 – 15 year-olds, five relatively independent complaint complexes, applying to boys and girls alike, could be identified. The sex-linked complexes that were also found will be left out of the present discussion. The following complaint configurations did not hold true for the 8 – 10 year-olds; their complaints were grouped differently.

Complex 1 contains the following complaints:

3 Tummy ache
17 Being sick (vomiting)
20 Feeling sick (nausea)
48 Diarrhoea
56 Stomach pains
73 Pressure and fullness in the stomach
76 Burping
79 Heartburn

This complex is very similar to the scale 'Gastric complaints' for adults; for the children it is extended by the items 'Tummy ache' and 'Diarrhoea', but we shall still call it *Gastric complaints.*

Complex 2 includes:

36 Coughing
42 Cold hands
51 Sore throat
54 Cold feet
64 Blocked nose
70 Colds

This complex does not occur in adults and could be described as *Cold symptoms,* although the items 'Cold hands' and 'Cold feet' seem a little out of place.

Complex 3 is made up of:

8 Pains in arm
11 Pains in knee
24 Pains in leg
35 Difficulty in swallowing
40 Pains in feet
77 Dragging or tired legs

This complex consists of *Motility complaints.* It is not comparable to the scale 'Pains in Limbs' from the adult version, since neck, shoulder and back aches are not included and only pains in the extremities appear. The item 'Difficulty in swallowing' seems to be the odd one out here. The complaints in this complex are altogether not very common among children.

Complex 4 includes:

10 Daytime tiredness
14 Excessive sweating
33 Getting tired quickly
47 Weariness

53 Morning tiredness
68 Stitches
74 Excessive need for sleep

This group of complaints is similar to the scale *Exhaustion* in the adult form and has the same name.

Complex 5 consists of:

9 Going black before the eyes
12 Feeling dizzy
18 Blurred vision
27 Flickering before the eyes
34 Staggering and reeling
37 Feeling numb all over

This complex does not occur with adults. It may be described as *Circulatory problems*. These complaints, too, are relatively rare among children.

The adult scale 'Cardiac complaints' is not relevant for children. Of the four scales belonging to the adult version, only 'Exhaustion' and 'Gastric complaints' have equivalents in the children, whereas three of the children's complexes – 'Cold symptoms', 'Motility complaints' and 'Circulatory problems' – have no adult equivalent. This indicates that in certain respects children's body perception differs very considerably from that of adults.

Influence of Sex and Age on Children's Complaints

In order to investigate the dependency of the complaints on sex and age, a two-way analysis of variance was carried out with the factors sex (girls/boys) and age (8-10, 11-12, 13-15 years). Thirty items proved to be sex-linked. The greatest differences were found in the following items ($p < 0.001$), all of which were registered more often by the girls than the boys:

3 Tummy ache
4 Crying
6 Pains in the abdomen
13 Backache
38 Burning or tingling in hands and feet
42 Cold hands
50 Shakiness
51 Sore throat
52 Blushing easily
54 Cold feet
55 Stomach pains

Of the 80 items, 17 proved to be age-dependent, particularly the following ($p < 0.001$):

4 Crying
10 Daytime tiredness
16 Stumbling and falling over

26 Sweating in bed
48 Diarrhoea
67 Unclear skin

Stumbling and falling over, sweating in bed and diarrhoea decrease continuously as the children grow older, whilst daytime tiredness and unclear skin increase. The 13-15 year-olds report crying less than the younger age-groups.

Sixteen items showed interaction effects between age and sex, which were strongest for the following complaints ($p < 0.01$):

1 Feeling weak
15 Pains in shoulder and back of neck
17 Being sick (vomiting)
19 Earache
20 Feeling sick (nausea)
75 Lump in throat

The girls complained more frequently of all of these than the boys in the age-group 11-12 years, whereas this tendency was either lacking or reversed for the other age-groups. All these complaints become less frequent among the boys aged 11-12 and more frequent with the girls. To demonstrate this, the scores for boys and girls in the three age-groups on items 1, 20 and 75 are shown in Fig. 3.

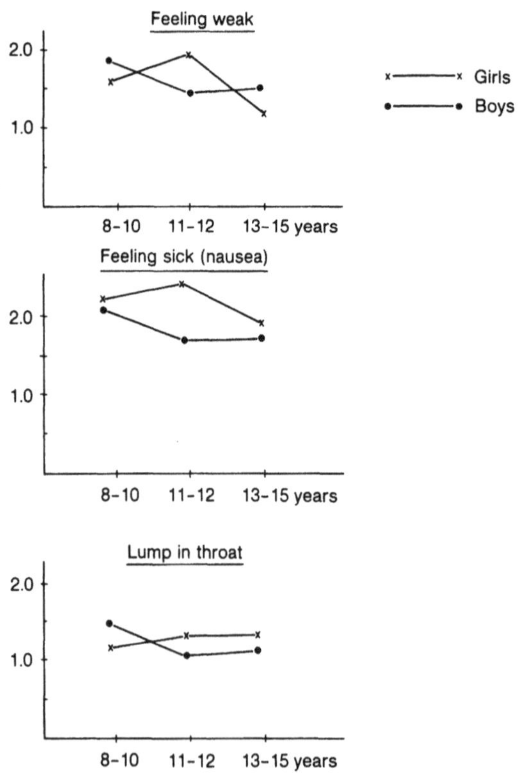

Fig. 3. Age and sex dependency of selected items

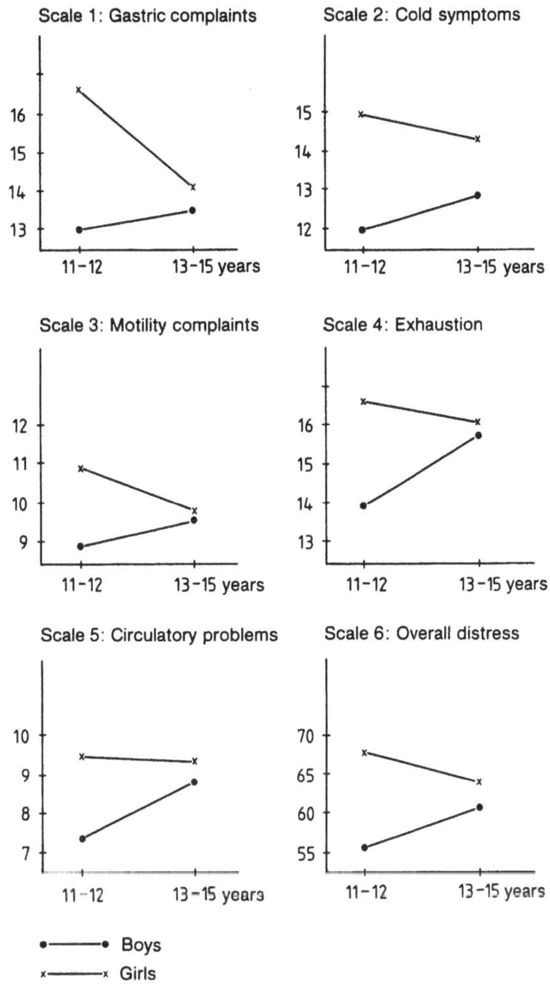

Fig. 4. Scale values for boys and girls in age-groups 11-12 and 13-15 years

Figure 4 shows the boys' and girls' scores on the six scales (complexes), for the age-groups 11-12 and 13-15 years. On all scales the girls have higher scores. Age-dependency can only be identified on scale 1, 'Gastric complaints', where the scores decrease as age increases.

On scales 1, 4, 5 and 6, there is a significant interaction between age and sex; interaction is visible on scales 2 and 3 as well, but is not significant.

Discussion of Results

Reviewing the results obtained so far, the degree to which children and adolescents feel hampered by physical complaints is very striking. As we know from the research on old people's visits to the doctor, physical changes at certain times in life are in danger of being attributed to ageing processes, with the result that serious conditions are often overlooked (Haug 1981). With children and adolescents something similar often happens: their complaints are explained away as growing processes and true distress may remain unnoticed, or they are comforted with reassurances that they will grow out of it. Body complaints are reduced to passing phenomena. At the same time, the experts point out how troubling it is for most children and adolescents to perceive changes in their bodies (Zenz et al. 1983). If one considers how much closer children often are to their bodies than adults (Hildebrandt and Schultz 1984), then one can begin to imagine with what anxiety children react to the perceived loss of their bodily integrity, being as it is the vital foundation for the development of their autonomy in other directions as well. Being ill and feeling physically impaired or unwell amounts to reverting to dependency on their parents.

Furthermore, the ideas children and young people associate with illness are to be considered: being ill means being vulnerable; illness and physical complaints are often interpreted as a punishment for some misdemeanour (Cohn 1983). The threats of many parents that if the child does not behave it will be sent to the doctor or to hospital fit in with these phantasies (Robertson 1974). At the same time, children's knowledge about the ways in which the individual parts of their body function and about its inner processes is always on a level with their general cognitive development, so that a rational interpretation of their complaints is often not possible (Gutezeit and Marake 1984).

Observing children and adolescents at play, one is struck by the pleasure they take in exhibiting themselves, in feeling and experiencing their bodies, in looking and being looked at. The importance of the body for social acceptance and approval is evident (Stutte 1971). To be able to rely on one's own body to look and function to one's satisfaction is very important to children and adolescents (Clifford 1971).

Between the ages of 10 and 16, the permanent irritation caused to children and adolescents by physical growing processes is coupled with increased demands being made on them by others (Baake 1976). The standards set at school rise, the children become more aware of the importance of doing well at school for their later life; at the same time, being forced to sit still on school furniture which is not necessarily beneficial to the muscles and bones of children stands in hopeless contradiction to their natural urge for movement and activity (Zenz et al. 1983).

Whilst the psychosomatic viewpoint has become practically ubiquitous in the field of adults' complaints, children's somatic reactions to emotional stresses have been only partially discussed (Wallis 1971). This may in part be justified as reflecting a reaction against the danger of developing an unhealthy fixation on the doctor and of the children being stigmatized at an early age. However, this consideration is balanced by the danger of unheeded complaints becoming chronic in the course of time.

Some of the complaint complexes that we found may well be due to problems associated with growing up and the physical changes occurring in adolescence. The motility complaints, for example, may point to an uncertainty in relation to the arms and legs. The disproportionate growth of the body and the extremities during adolescence is well-known. At the same time, the arms and legs are important for establishing boundaries and for personal autonomy. Being able to get away, being able to walk and run in safety, to grasp and to hold – these are all relevant functions at this age; they constitute a reactivation of the processes so vital in earlier separation phases (Mahler et al. 1984; Joraschky 1983).

The circulatory problems may be an expression of a generally labile state of the circulation caused by hormonal changes. However, the complaint complexes 'Gastric complaints' and 'Exhaustion' are a clear indication of the degree of stress experienced by the children in everyday life, to which they respond with physical symptoms. The circulatory complaints could well be discussed in relation to stress too (Reissig 1980).

The cold symptoms suggest infection at school. One often reads in the papers about the rapid spread of colds and 'flu in schools and indeed every institution where many people come together. On the other hand, every individual must first have a weakened resistence in order to succumb to the infection, which again points in the direction of stress in the case of our children.

The sex-linked differences in the frequency of certain complaints reflect the girls' poor subjective condition. They are more bothered by their complaints than the boys are; there are hardly any complaints from which the boys suffer more. In connection with the discussion on anorexia nervosa, which is more frequent in girls, the greater conflicts of growing girls have been pointed out. Girls find themselves confronted with more models for their future life (housewife, mother, going out to work, training for a profession or career). The straight-line development prescribed for the boys, in which whether to work and provide for themselves hardly arises as a serious question, protects them from inner conflicts in reaching decisions. Problems manifestly arise for them when these expectations are not fulfilled. Regardless of achievement, girls, however, can always reflect on these more basic questions concerning their future during all their years at school. Success and failure thus have a different meaning for them.

On the other hand, the sex-linked differences in complaints may already be an expression of basically different attitudes towards complaints and illness. Complaints and complaining are socially more accepted in girls. The influence of socialization on the question of complaining comes out clearly in the item 'crying', which occurs far less among the older boys than the girls. When followed through all age-groups, the complaint complexes show a different pattern of development for girls and boys. On the whole, girls report having more complaints. The gap narrows in later years, however, because there is a tendency for the number of girls' complaints to decrease as they get older, whilst the boys' show a parallel increase in all complexes, bringing them closer to the girls' complaint level. This development contradicts a role-related interpretation and suggests instead a dephasing of complaint frequency. We have no figures showing the position of the youngest group with respect to the complexes, as the complaints of the 8–10 year-olds were organized differently. The data so far available would appear to suggest that girls are confronted with general complaints at an earlier age and as they grow older learn to reduce their complaints slightly as a sign of increasing social adjustment, whilst the boys come into the phase of greater physical problems a little later. How far bodily processes associated with puberty are involved here remains to be investigated. All in all, however, the general extent of the complaints cannot be ignored. Complaints are always an expression of stresses and pressures, whether of a physical or social nature. Quite apart from sex and age differences, the greater complaint frequency among all subgroups of the children's sample as compared with adults is striking. Further research on the subject of children's somatic complaints and their relationships with their bodies is clearly called for.

References

Baake D (1976) Die 13- bis 16-jährigen. Urban und Schwarzenberg, Munich

Brähler E, Scheer JW (1983) Der Giessener Beschwerdebogen (GBB) - Testhandbuch. Huber. Bern

Brähler E, Ernst R, Klein H, Overbeck A (1983) Arbeitsbericht zum DFG-Projekt 'Interaktion in familientherapeutischen Sitzungen'. Research report, University of Giessen

Bräutigam W, Christian P (1981) Psychosomatische Medizin. Thieme, Stuttgart

Bruch H (1980) Der goldene Käfig. Das Rätsel der Magersucht. Fischer, Frankfurt

Clifford E (1971) Body satisfaction in adolescence. Percept Mot Skills 33: 71-72

Cohn N (1983) Psychologische Faktoren und Prozesse bei der Entstehung und dem Verlauf von psychogenem Schmerz. Psychother Psychosom Med Psychol 33: 13-19

Gutezeit G, Marake J (1984) Untersuchungen zur Wirksamkeit verschiedener Einflussgrössen auf die Selbstwahrnehmung bei Kindern und Jugendlichen. Prax Kinderpsychol 33: 133-141

Harnack GA von (ed) (1971) Kinderheilkunde. Springer, Berlin Heidelberg New York

Haug MR (1981) Age and medical care utilization patterns. J Gerontol 33: 103-111

Hildebrandt H, Schultz ML (1984) 'Wenn ich traurig bin, bin ich auch krank'. Kinder - Körper - Gesundheit. Jugend und Politik. Reinheim

Joraschky P (1983) Das Körperschema und das Körper-Selbst als Regulationsprinzipien der Organismus-Umwelt-Interaktion. Minerva. Munich

Kestenberg JS (1968) Outside and inside, male and female. J Am Psychoanal Assoc 16: 457-520

Mahler MS, Pine F, Bergmann A (1984) Die psychische Geburt des Menschen. Fischer. Frankfurt

Netter P (1981) KFA von funktionellen Beschwerden bei Spontanangabe und standardisierter Befragung. In: Janke W (ed) Beiträge zur Methodik in der differentiellen, diagnostischen und klinischen Psychologie. Hain, Königstein, p 393

Nickel H (1974) Entwicklungspsychologie des Kindes- und Jugendalters, vol 1. Huber, Bern

Oerter R (1974) Moderne Entwicklungspsychologie. Auer, Donauwörth

Reissig M (1980) Zur körperlichen Entwicklung von Schülern vom 12. bis 16. Lebensjahr. In: Friedrich U, Müller H (eds) Zur Psychologie der 12-22-jährigen. Deutscher Verlag der Wissenschaften, Berlin, pp 64-83

Robertson J (1974) Kinder in Krankenhäusern. Reinhard, Munich

Scherer R (1982) Der Körper des Kindes. In: Kamper D, Wulf C (eds) Die Wiederkehr des Körpers. Suhrkamp, Frankfurt

Schrör E (1984) Psychosomatische Belastungen in der Pubertät. Paper presented at the Sonderforschungsbereich 129 workshop, University of Ulm: Adoleszenz - Weichenstellung zur Gesundheit und Krankheit?

Stutte H (1971) Thersites-Komplex bei Jugendlichen. Dtsch Ärztebl 68: 119-125

Wallis H (1971) Psychosomatische Störungen. In: Harnack GA von (ed) Kinderheilkunde. Springer, Berlin Heidelberg New York, pp 411ff

Wiscott A, Betke K, Kunzer W (1977) Lehrbuch der Kinderheilkunde. Thieme, Stuttgart

Wünsche K (1982) Die Muskeln, die Sinne, die Reden: Medien im pädagogischen Bezug. In: Kamper D, Wulf C (eds) Die Wiederkehr des Körpers. Suhrkamp, Frankfurt

Zenz H, Marschall P, Balzer-Böken B (1983) Untersuchungen über Leistungsverhalten und körperliches Wohlbefinden von Schülern. Research report, Department of Medical Psychology, University of Ulm

Subject Index

Acne vulgaris 69
acting out 81
adolescents 242
age differences 239
aggression 58, 127, 163
Alexithymia 79
Alienation 77
Anorexia nervosa 79, 175, 207
approach
- therapeutic 20, 30, 81, 93
armour, character/muscular 25, 93
asthma, bronchial 91
atopic dermatitis 68

Backache 112
bioenergetics 88
birth 161
body
- biographies 193
- boundaries 46
- complaints 177, 211, 232
-, concept of 3, 23, 36, 77, 133
- episodes 193
- image 28, 37, 65, 92, 125, 131, 201
- language 20
- perception 38, 65, 95, 104
  -, concentrative 104
- posture 24
- scenes 194
- schema 35, 54, 92, 200
- self 28, 45, 83
- therapies 29, 77, 88, 91
Body Focus Questionnaire (BFQ) 48, 196
breast feeding 27, 166

cancer patients 177, 192
children 92, 232
-, complaints list 234
-, desire for 153, 173
conflict 20, 52, 127, 158, 185
contraceptives 154, 204
conversion 20, 26, 52
couples, married 171, 177, 220, 223
culture 220

Depressive states 163
desomatization 20, 82
development
-, psychosexual 19, 82
-, of body perception 42
-, and skin 63
doctor 12, 140, 232

Eczema 69, 92
ego 22, 45, 62, 92, 124

Factitious disorders 65, 69
fear 58, 157
field dependence 44
fluor albus 140

gait disturbances,
-, spinal-ataxic 108
Gießen Symptom Complaints List 180, 211, 234
Gießen Test 224
group therapy 91

Heart patients 55, 219
hirsutism 206
hypochondria 124

Infertility 171
injury 171
Insult 126
interaction
-, mother-infant 28, 64, 94, 166, 174

Lay aetiologies 218
libido 21, 45
love, maternal 166
lying-in 163

Medicine, history of 3, 145
men 119, 131, 180, 221

movement therapy,
-, concentrative 29, 77
multiple sclerosis 111

Neurosis, theory of 19
neurotic 25, 56, 217
NLP technique 194

Orientation, spatial 40

pain 51, 106, 119, 161, 181
partner relationship 177, 223
perception 177, 223
- body- 38, 65, 95, 104
-, exercises 104
- object- 83
- pain- 51
- self- 65
personality 44, 55
phantom limb 38
pregnancy 158
prostatosis 119
psoriasis vulgaris 67
psychoanalysis 10, 19, 45, 52, 77, 92, 124, 155
psychosomatic
- illness 66, 92, 112, 119, 146
- medicine 10, 26
- patients 79, 216

Questionnaire
- BEQ (body experience) 200
- BFQ (body focus) 48, 196
- GSCL (complaints list) 180, 211, 234
- GT (partnership patterns) 224
- childrens' complaints list 234
- MAQ (menstrual attitude) 204

Relaxation
-, functional 30, 96
relevance structures 191
Rorschach test 47

schema
-, body 37
-, postural 37
school 232
screening 217
sex differences 220, 239
sexual
- dysfunctions 119, 147, 207
- ethics 171
sexuality 137, 156, 184
skin 62
- diseases 67

Tension, muscular 25, 93, 105
transference, therapeutic 81, 91

Urethral drive 123
urination 119, 165

Women 149, 153, 184, 206, 221
-, alcoholic 207

Zones, body 19, 45, 82

www.ingramcontent.com/pod-product-compliance
Lightning Source LLC
Chambersburg PA
CBHW061205240926
51846CB00006B/1118
* 9 7 8 3 6 4 2 7 3 4 1 4 4 *